# APHASIOLOGY

*APHASIOLOGY* is covered by the following abstracting and indexing services: *BLLDB (Bibliography of Linguistic Literature), CINAHL, Current Contents, Elsevier Science BV, EMBASE/Excerpta Medica, Linguistic Abstracts, Linguistic and Language Behavior Abstracts, Medical Documentation Service, PsycINFO, PsycBITE, Research Alert, Science Citation Index, SciSearch, SCOPUS, UnCover.*

(Continued from back cover)

# APHASIOLOGY

Volume 24    Numbers 6–8    June–August 2010

CONTENTS

# 39th Clinical Aphasiology Conference
Keystone, Colorado, USA, May 26th to 30th, 2009

**Editor**

Beth Armstrong, School of Psychology and Social Science, Edith Cowan University, Perth, WA, Australia

**Reviewers**

| | | |
|---|---|---|
| Kirri Ballard | Tepanta Fossett | Mary Purdy |
| Pelagie Beeson | Robert Fucetola | Barbara Purves |
| Larry Boles | Jean Gordon | Gail Ramsburger |
| Susan Booth | Brooke Hallowell | Steven Rapcsac |
| Arpita Bose | Julie Hengst | Stacie Raymer |
| Mary Boyle | Anne Hesketh | Don Robin |
| Heather Clark | Ellen Hickey | Margaret Rogers |
| Carl Coehlo | Jackie Hinkley | Katherine Ross |
| Paul Conroy | Audrey Holland | Christos Salis |
| David Copland | Monica Hough | Barbara Shadden |
| Karen Croot | William Hula | Lou Shapiro |
| Madeline Cruice | Jacquie Kurland | Nina Simmons Mackie |
| Bronwyn Davidson | Jiyeon Lee | Jackie Stark |
| Gwyn Albyn Davis | Claudio Luzatti | Leanne Togher |
| Michael Dickey | Edwin Maas | Connie Tompkins |
| Neila Donovan | Nadine Martin | Julie Wambaugh |
| Patrick Doyle | Sharon Mauszycki | Brendan Weekes |
| Melissa Duff | Lisa Milman | Linda Worrall |
| Yasmeen Faroqi Shah | Gloria Olness | Heather Wright |
| Alison Ferguson | J. B. Orange | Greig de Zubicaray |
| Valerie Fleming | Emma Power | |

# APHASIOLOGY

## SUBSCRIPTION INFORMATION

Subscription rates to Volume 24, 2010 (12 issues) are as follows:
To institutions (full subscription): £1,419.00 (UK); €1,874.00 (Europe); $2,354.00 (Rest of the world).
To institutions (online only): £1,349.00 (UK); €1,780.00 (Europe); $2,236.00 (Rest of the world).
To individuals: £597.00 (UK); €789.00 (Europe); $991.00 (Rest of the world).
Dollar rate applies to all subscribers outside Europe. Euro rates apply to all subscribers in Europe, except the UK and the Republic of Ireland where the pound sterling rate applies. All subscriptions are payable in advance and all rates include postage. Journals are sent by air to the USA, Canada, Mexico, India, Japan and Australasia. Subscriptions are entered on an annual basis, i.e., January to December. Payment may be made by sterling cheque, dollar cheque, euro cheque, international money order, National Giro or credit cards (Amex, Visa, and Mastercard).
An Institutional subscription to the print edition also includes free access to the online edition for any number of concurrent users across a local area network.
Subscriptions purchased at the personal (print only) rate are strictly for personal, non-commercial use only. The reselling of personal subscriptions is strictly prohibited. Personal subscriptions must be purchased with a personal cheque or credit card. Proof of personal status may be requested. For full information please visit the Journal's homepage.
A subscription to the print edition includes free access for any number of concurrent users across a local area network to the online edition. ISSN 1464-5041.
Print subscriptions are also available to individual members of the British Aphasiology Society (BAS), on application to the Society.
*Aphasiology* now offers an iOpenAccess option for authors. For more information, see: www.tandf.co.uk/journals/iopenaccess.asp

For a complete and up-to-date guide to Taylor & Francis's journals and books publishing programmes, visit the Taylor & Francis website: http://www.tandf.co.uk/

*Aphasiology* (USPS 001413) is published monthly by Psychology Press, 27 Church Road, Hove, BN3 2FA, UK. The 2010 US Institutional subscription price is $2,354.00. Airfreight and mailing in the USA by Agent named Air Business, C/O Worldnet Shipping USA Inc., 155-11 146th Avenue, Jamaica, New York, NY 11434, USA. Periodicals postage paid at Jamaica NY 11431. US Postmaster. Send address changes to *Aphasiology* (PAPH), Air Business Ltd, C/O Worldnet Shipping USA Inc., 155-11 146th Avenue, Jamaica, New York, NY 11434, USA.

Orders originating in the following territories should be sent direct to the local distributor.
**India:** Universal Subscription Agency Pvt. Ltd. 101–102 Community Centre, Malviyn Nagar Extn. Post Bag No. 8, Saket, New Delhi 110017.
**Japan:** Kinokuniyna Company Ltd, Journal Department, PO Box 55, Chitose, Tokyo 156.
**USA, Canada, and Mexico:** Psychology Press, a member of Taylor & Francis, 325 Chestnut St. Philadelphia, PA 19106. USA
**UK and other territories:** Psychology Press, c/o T&F Customer Services, Informa UK Ltd. Sheepen Place, Colchester, Essex, CO3 3LP, UK. Tel: +44 (0)20 7017 5544; Fax: +44 (0)20 7017 5198. E-mail: tf.enquiries@tfinforma.com

The online edition can be reached via the journal's website: http://www.psypress.com/aphasiology

**Back issues:** Taylor & Francis retains a three-year back issue stock of journals. Older volumes are held by our official stockists: Periodicals Service Company, 11 Main Street, Germantown, NY 12526, USA, to whom all orders and enquiries should be addressed. Tel: +1 518 537 4700; Fax: +1 518 537 5899; E-mail: psc@periodicals.com; URL: http:www.periodicals.com/tandf.html

Typeset by H. Charlesworth & Co. Ltd., Wakefield. UK

APHASIOLOGY, 2010, 24 (6–8), 669

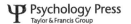

# Introduction

This year's special issue contains papers presented at the 39th Clinical Aphasiology Conference held in Keystone, Colorado in May, 2009. The issue contains another excellent mix of articles, demonstrating the depth and breadth of issues covered in clinical aphasiology at the present time. Exploration of everyday discourse continues to increase, while findings in the important area of neuroplasticity and the effects of early treatment are increasingly being addressed in clinical aphasiology studies and are represented in this issue. A report on the excellent research resource of Aphasia-Bank is also included, and it will be of great interest to monitor the progress of AphasiaBank as researchers increasingly access and contribute to this valuable international database. Apraxia treatments continue to flourish and are also well represented in this issue. As a venue for the discussion of applied research in aphasia, CAC encourages researchers to explore the ultimate social ramifications of different assessment and treatment protocols, while retaining strong theoretical underpinnings related to both neurological and cognitive factors involved in the impairment. I hope this issue provides a flavour of all of these aspects of aphasia and thank all authors for their wonderful contributions. I also want to acknowledge again this year the ever invaluable contributions of the numerous reviewers who so thoughtfully and efficiently provided excellent reviews that assisted both the Editor in making decisions, but also the authors in reaching their valuable final products.

Beth Armstrong PhD
Guest Editor
*Edith Cowan University, Perth, Australia*

© 2010 Psychology Press, an imprint of the Taylor & Francis Group, an Informa business
http://www.psypress.com/aphasiology     DOI: 10.1080/02687038.2010.496259

APHASIOLOGY, 2010, 24 (6–8), 671–684

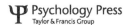

# Individual variability on discourse measures over repeated sampling times in persons with aphasia

Rosalea M. Cameron and Julie L. Wambaugh

*VA Salt Lake City Healthcare System and University of Utah,
Salt Lake City, UT, USA*


Shannon C. Mauszycki

*VA Salt Lake City Healthcare System, Salt Lake City, UT, USA*

*Background*: Although persons with aphasia typically have difficulty with the production of language at the level of discourse, there is a paucity of reliable measurement systems to quantify the characteristics of spoken language. Nicholas and Brookshire (1993) developed one of the few standardised, rule-based systems to quantify the informativeness of spoken language samples. While the authors reported temporal stability for all measures, they also noted variability at the individual level. Because individual data were not reported, it is difficult to determine the nature and extent of that variability.
*Aims*: The aim of the current investigation was to further explore Nicholas and Brookshire's (1993) quantitative linguistic analyses, and to examine individual variability over time in persons with aphasia.
*Methods & Procedures*: Five fluent and six nonfluent persons with aphasia produced language samples over repeated sampling times in response to the 10 stimulus items used by Nicholas and Brookshire (1993). Measurements of mean number of words, mean correct information units (CIUs), percent CIUs, words per minute, and CIUs per minute were calculated, and results from the sessions were compared. To examine factors related to individual variability, correlations between linguistic measures, months post onset of aphasia, and scores on standardised assessment tools were explored.
*Outcomes & Results*: Visual inspection of the data and descriptive statistics suggested that participants were more variable in their repeated productions than previously described by Nicholas and Brookshire (1993). Repeated measures ANOVAs revealed non-significant effects at the group level. There was no pattern of variability uniquely associated with aphasia fluency type. Range of mean number of CIUs was positively and significantly correlated with all test measures; however, the other range correlations were non-significant.
*Conclusions*: The current results suggest greater variability over repeated sampling times in the spoken language of persons with aphasia than previously reported by Nicholas and Brookshire (1993). Clinicians and researchers should consider this variability, and establish stable baselines prior to the initiation of treatment to document meaningful change over time.

*Keywords:* Aphasia; Discourse; Variability.

Address correspondence to: Rosalea M. Cameron, 151A-Building 2, 500 Foothill Boulevard, VA Salt Lake City Healthcare System, Salt Lake City, UT 84148, USA. E-mail: Rosalea.Cameron@va.gov

This research was supported by Rehabilitation Research and Development, Department of Veterans Affairs. Thanks are extended to Christina Nessler and Sandra Wright for their assistance with this project.

http://www.psypress.com/aphasiology       DOI: 10.1080/02687030903443813

Persons with aphasia typically have difficulty with the production of language at the level of discourse; however, clinicians and researchers encounter challenges when measuring behaviours and documenting changes in connected spoken language. Several authors have developed analyses to quantify linguistic markers within language samples (for reviews see Armstrong, 2000; Prins & Bastiaanse, 2004); however, as noted by Prins and Bastiaanse, most tools are devoid of test–retest reliability data necessary to support their use in clinical and research settings. This lack of evidence of temporal stability compromises the potential value of these quantitative analyses to objectively assess both spontaneous recovery and outcomes related to aphasia intervention (Armstrong, 2000; Prins & Bastiaanse, 2004).

To address the need for a reliable discourse measurement tool, Nicholas and Brookshire (1993) described a standardised, rule-based system for quantifying the informativeness of spoken language for persons with aphasia. These authors elicited discourse samples from 20 non-brain-damaged adults and 20 persons with aphasia (14 fluent and 6 nonfluent) using 10 stimulus items. The stimuli included: two requests for personal information ("Tell me where you live and describe it to me", and "Tell me what you usually do on Sundays"), two requests for procedural information ("Tell me how you would go about writing and sending a letter", and "Tell me how you would go about doing dishes by hand"), two picture sequences, and four single pictures. To explore stability of participant performance, two trials were performed on the same day and a third sample was collected 7–10 days later. Language samples were timed and coded for "words" and "correct information units" (CIUs). Words were defined as productions, "intelligible in context to someone who knows the picture(s) or topic being discussed" (p. 348), while CIUs were described as, "words that are intelligible in context, accurate in relation to the picture(s) or topic, and relevant to and informative about the content of the picture(s) or the topic" (p. 348). Measurements of mean number of words, mean CIUs, percent CIUs (%CIUs), words per minute (WPM), and CIUs per minute (CIUs/min) were calculated and results from the three sessions were compared.

Although Nicholas and Brookshire (1993) reported temporal stability for all measures with their groups of participants, they acknowledged that variability was noted at the individual level. Unfortunately, details of individual data were not reported and participant description was limited to information related to age, education, and scores on the *Shortened Porch Index of Communicative Ability* (Disimoni, Keith, & Darley, 1980), and *The Boston Naming Test* (Kaplan, Goodglass, & Weintraub, 1983). Given that aphasia severity has been reported as impacting discourse skills for persons with aphasia (Gordon, 2008), participant characteristics related to this feature warrant further exploration. This will be particularly important if factors related to individual variability are to be examined.

Despite potential limitations in the stability of the linguistic measures developed by Nicholas and Brookshire (1993), the instrument is frequently used in studies of aphasia (Gordon, 2008; Peach & Reuter, in press). Interestingly, the tool is more regularly applied in aphasia research than the well-validated Story Retell Procedure developed by Doyle et al. (1998); perhaps because the stimuli are more readily available. Many researchers have used the Nicholas and Brookshire analyses to gauge effects of treatment within the context of single-participant research designs. There is, however, variability with respect to both the number and requisite stability of baseline sessions that have been completed (Boyle, 2004a, 2004b; Cameron, Wambaugh, Wright, & Nessler, 2006; Peach & Reuter, in press; Wambaugh &

Ferguson, 2007). Given the popularity of the tool, additional data regarding the stability of the analyses would be beneficial, particularly given the need for meaningful measurement of treatment effects.

The purpose of the current project was to further explore individual variability for the mean number of words, mean CIUs, %CIUs, WPM, and CIUs/min produced by persons with aphasia over repeated sampling times. Also of interest were various factors that could potentially influence individual variability in production of discourse. It was theorised that a greater degree of impairment of language, including word-retrieval skills, may serve to restrict flexibility in responding, and as such be associated with reduced variability in discourse measures. The length of time since onset of aphasia was also considered to have potential to influence repeated production of discourse. Specifically, habituated patterns of responding were thought to be more likely to occur with individuals who had had aphasia for a longer period of time. Therefore, correlations between the range values for each of the calculated measures, scores on assessment measures, and months post onset (MPO) of aphasia were also examined.

## METHOD

### Participants

A total of 11 stroke survivors with aphasia (two females and nine males) served as participants. The discourse tasks under investigation were completed as a component of the pre-treatment assessment phase of a treatment study for improvement of word retrieval skills. Participants were enrolled in the order in which they were referred for that protocol. Mean age was 49.27 years (range 22–66 years). All were native speakers of English and had negative histories for neurological problems other than stroke. In addition, all had negative self-reported histories of alcohol/substance abuse and mental illness, were non-hospitalised, and passed vision and pure tone air conduction hearing screenings.

Participant characteristics and assessment results can be seen in Tables 1 and 2. Six individuals presented with Broca's aphasia, four with anomic aphasia, and one with Wernicke's aphasia as classified by *The Western Aphasia Battery* (*WAB*; Kertesz, 1982).

### Stimulus materials and sampling procedures

Spoken language samples were elicited using stimuli described by Nicholas and Brookshire (1993). The responses to the 10 stimuli comprised one complete sample; participants were allowed unlimited time for production of samples. Unlike Nicholas and Brookshire, practice stimuli were not used. In order to evaluate reliability over time, complete samples were repeatedly obtained; five samples were elicited from 10 participants and four samples were elicited from 1 participant. Sessions were completed an average of 7 days apart (range 1–42 days) with no intervening speech or language therapy.

Four ASHA certified speech-language pathologists (SLPs)/research associates collected the samples in a quiet environment. With the exception of two samples (Participant 7: Time 4; Participant 9: Time 1), all sessions for each individual were collected by the same SLP. Participant responses were orthographically transcribed

TABLE 1
Participant characteristics

| Characteristic | Participant 1 | Participant 2 | Participant 3 | Participant 4 | Participant 5 | Participant 6 | Participant 7 | Participant 8 | Participant 9 | Participant 10 | Participant 11 |
|---|---|---|---|---|---|---|---|---|---|---|---|
| Age | 58 | 59 | 61 | 47 | 59 | 52 | 66 | 64 | 22 | 54 | 39 |
| Gender | Male | Female | Male | Male | Male | Male | Male | Female | Male | Male | Male |
| Aetiology | Stroke | Stroke | Stroke | Stroke | Stroke | Stroke | Stroke | Stroke | Stroke | Stroke | Stroke |
| Marital status | Single | Married | Widowed | Married | Married | Married | Married | Widowed | Single | Single | Married |
| Handedness | Left | Right | Right | Right | Right | Right | Right | Right | Right | Right | Right |
| MPO | 126 | 42 | 31 | 187 | 65 | 13 | 65 | 18 | 6 | 9 | 58 |
| Years of education | 14 | 12 | 11 | 13 | 22 | 11 | 16 | 12 | 12 | 12 | 18 |
| Former occupation | Bookkeeper | Bookkeeper | Maintenance | Mechanic | Physicist | Carpenter | Military | Bill Collector | Missionary | Woodcarver | Mortgage Broker |

TABLE 2
Assessment results

| Measure | P 1 | P 2 | P 3 | P 4 | P 5 | P 6 | P 7 | P 8 | P 9 | P 10 | P 11 |
|---|---|---|---|---|---|---|---|---|---|---|---|
| *PICA* (Porch, 2001) | | | | | | | | | | | |
| Overall Percentile | 53rd | 73rd | 63rd | 59th | 35th | 49th | 63rd | 75th | 75th | 38th | 86th |
| Verbal %ile | 51st | 68th | 58th | 56th | 38th | 39th | 63rd | 80th | 74th | 35th | 83rd |
| Auditory %ile | 54th | 64th | 64th | 46th | 28th | 54th | 74/99th | 74/99th | 74/99th | 42nd | 74/99th |
| *TAAWF* (German, 1990) | | | | | | | | | | | |
| Total Raw Score | 17/107 | 48/107 | 36/107 | 67/107 | 8/107 | 27/107 | 39/107 | 101/107 | 74/107 | 0/107 | 90/107 |
| Comprehension | 7 94% | 7 97% | 7 100% | 7 97% | 7 72% | 7 99% | 7 100% | 7 99% | 7 100% | 7 78% | 7 100% |
| *WAB* (Kertesz, 1982) | | | | | | | | | | | |
| Aphasia Quotient | 53.4 | 82.0 | 63.0 | 66.0 | 50.8 | 66.0 | 70.7 | 90.6 | 88.3 | 33.2 | 93.6 |
| Classification | Broca's | Anomic | Broca's | Broca's | Broca's | Broca's | Broca's | Anomi c | Anomi c | Wernick e's | Anomic |
| *Assessment of Intelligibility of Dysarthric Speech* (Yorkston & Beukelman, 1984) | | | | | | | | | | | |
| Word level (transcription format) | 82% | 88% | 94% | 84% | 80% | 90% | 70% | 86% | 84% | 54% | 100% |
| *Test of Nonverbal Intelligence-3* (Brown, Sherbenou, & Johnsen, 1997) | | | | | | | | | | | |
| Percentile Ranking | 7 | 17 | 21 | 26 | 9 | 5 | 24 | 23 | 21 | 5 | 45 |

from audio recordings and were timed in the manner of Nicholas and Brookshire (1993). An SLP other than the one who performed the transcription verified transcript accuracy. Following discussion and resolution of disagreements between the two SLPs, words and CIUs were scored for each transcript using the guidelines of Nicholas and Brookshire.

## Dependent measures

Consistent with the procedures of Nicholas and Brookshire (1993), two measures of verbal productivity: mean number of words and mean WPM for stimulus items were calculated for each sample. Measures of information content included mean number of CIUs, %CIUs, and CIUs/min for each sample.

# RESULTS

## Agreement of scoring

To assess inter-rater agreement, a scorer other than the individual who initially scored the transcripts calculated both words and CIUs for one randomly selected set of stimulus items for each participant (20% of samples). Mean point-to-point inter-rater agreement was 98.21% for words (range 95.01–100%) and 90.27% for CIUs (range 72.41–97.40%). Intra-rater reliability was calculated on an additional randomly selected transcript at least 3 months following the initial scoring. Mean point-to-point intra-rater agreement was 99.26 % for words (range 97.07–100%) and 94.39% for CIUs (range 81.37–100%).

## Inter-session stability of measures

Mean number of words, mean CIUs, %CIUs, WPM, and CIUs/min for Participants 1 to 4, Participants 5 to 8, and Participants 9 to 11 can be found in Tables 3, 4, and 5, respectively. Range of individual performance for each of the five measures on each sample can be seen in Table 6. Participant 1 exhibited the least variability for mean number of words (3.9 words) and mean CIUs (2.6 CIUs) per stimulus item, while Participant 11 demonstrated the largest range for both measures (47.5 words and 36.2 CIUs). Variability for %CIUs was least for Participant 2 (3.11 %CIUs) and most for Participant 9 (18.15 %CIUs). The per-item difference for WPM was least for Participant 11 (6.71 WPM) and greatest for Participant 3 (34.27 WPM). The range for CIUs/min was lowest for Participant 5 (2.30 CIUs/min) and highest for Participant 9 (27.07 CIUs/min). Individual mean %CIUs for each session are displayed in Figure 1. Mean CIUs/min for each session are shown in Figure 2a for Participants 1 to 5, and in Figure 2b for Participants 6 to 11 (data for the two groups are presented separately for visual clarity).

Calculated measures over time for the group of 11 participants are presented in Table 7. Mean CIUs, %CIUs, and CIUs/min over time for the groups of fluent ($N = 5$) and nonfluent ($N = 6$) participants are listed in Table 8.

Repeated measures ANOVAs were calculated to examine differences in mean words, mean CIUs, %CIUs, WPM, and CIUs/min over time at the group level. No significant effects were found. Additional repeated measures ANOVAs yielded no significant main effects of group (fluent versus nonfluent) for mean CIUs, %CIUs, or CIUs/min over time.

TABLE 3

Mean words, mean CIUs, %CIUs, WPM, and CIUs/min per session for 10 elicitation stimuli for Participants 1–4

| Participant | Sampling time | Words | CIUs | %CIUs | WPM | CIUs/min |
|---|---|---|---|---|---|---|
| P1 | Time 1 | 8.2 | 5.5 | 67.07% | 24.48 | 16.42 |
| Broca's | Time 2 | 6.9 | 5.0 | 72.46% | 20.72 | 15.02 |
| | Time 3 | 9.7 | 7.1 | 73.20% | 29.67 | 21.71 |
| | Time 4 | 10.8 | 7.6 | 70.37% | 29.43 | 20.72 |
| | Time 5 | 9.0 | 6.7 | 74.44% | 25.71 | 19.14 |
| P2 | Time 1 | 53.6 | 27.4 | 51.12% | 36.79 | 18.81 |
| Anomic | Time 2 | 65.4 | 31.4 | 48.01% | 39.23 | 18.84 |
| | Time 3 | 86.1 | 43.8 | 50.87% | 41.69 | 21.21 |
| | Time 4 | 92.2 | 46.9 | 50.87% | 49.49 | 25.17 |
| | Time 5 | 82.3 | 41.2 | 50.06% | 54.07 | 22.83 |
| P3 | Time 1 | 51.4 | 24.3 | 47.28% | 99.42 | 47.00 |
| Broca's | Time 2 | 45.4 | 28.1 | 61.90% | 95.58 | 59.16 |
| | Time 3 | 32.4 | 17.9 | 55.25% | 83.51 | 46.13 |
| | Time 4 | 36.2 | 20.8 | 57.46% | 93.54 | 53.75 |
| | Time 5 | 47.7 | 23.9 | 50.10% | 117.78 | 59.01 |
| P4 | Time 1 | 30.7 | 9.3 | 30.29% | 35.57 | 10.78 |
| Broca's | Time 2 | 67.9 | 13.4 | 19.73% | 41.25 | 8.14 |
| | Time 3 | 40.1 | 10.8 | 26.93% | 30.80 | 8.29 |
| | Time 4 | 41.3 | 13.7 | 34.16% | 36.16 | 12.00 |
| | Time 5 | 59.1 | 15.9 | 26.90% | 36.94 | 9.94 |

Session scores represent average performance across 10 stimuli. CIUs = correct information units. WPM = words per minute. CIUs/min = CIUs per minute.

## Correlation of range values to factors potentially associated with variability

Pearson correlation coefficients were computed between the range values for each of the dependent measures and the AQ on the *WAB* (Kertesz, 1982), the overall percentile ranking on the *Porch Index of Communicative Ability* (*PICA*; Porch, 2001), the raw score on the *Test of Adolescent/Adult Word Finding* (*TAAWF*; German, 1990), and MPO of aphasia. With the exception of MPO, the range of mean number of CIUs was positively and significantly correlated ($p < .05$) with all of the test measures (correlations ranged between .72 and .89). The other range correlations were non-significant.

## DISCUSSION

This investigation examined the temporal stability of the communicative performance of persons with aphasia, as assessed using the Nicholas and Brookshire (1993) analysis system. Visual inspection of individual data for mean number of words, mean CIUs, %CIUs, WPM, and CIUs/min (depicted in Tables 3, 4, 5, & 6; Figures 1, 2a, & 2b) suggests relative stability for some participants and marked variability for others. Whereas Nicholas and Brookshire reported that %CIUs changed 3% or less for 75% of their participants with aphasia on repeated presentation of the 10 stimulus items, no participant in the current study demonstrated variability as low as 3%. In a subsequent report, Nicholas and Brookshire (1994) indicated that none of

TABLE 4
Mean words, mean CIUs, %CIUs, WPM, and CIUs/min per session for 10 elicitation stimuli for
Participants 5–8

| Participant | Sampling time | Words | CIUs | %CIUs | WPM | CIUs/min |
|---|---|---|---|---|---|---|
| P5 | Time 1 | 23.4 | 6.4 | 27.35% | 18.65 | 5.10 |
| Broca's | Time 2 | 21.4 | 3.4 | 15.89% | 18.77 | 2.98 |
| | Time 3 | 22.6 | 3.6 | 15.93% | 17.59 | 2.80 |
| | Time 4 | 30.9 | 3.5 | 11.32% | 25.43 | 2.88 |
| | Time 5 | 20.4 | 5.1 | 25.00% | 14.87 | 3.72 |
| P6 | Time 1 | 19.0 | 7.6 | 40.00% | 22.17 | 8.87 |
| Broca's | Time 2 | 32.7 | 11.5 | 35.17% | 28.63 | 10.07 |
| | Time 3 | 44.0 | 17.1 | 38.86% | 41.04 | 15.95 |
| | Time 4 | 34.4 | 13.8 | 40.10% | 32.06 | 12.86 |
| | Time 5 | 36.8 | 13.4 | 36.41% | 36.18 | 13.18 |
| P7 | Time 1 | 30.7 | 13.6 | 44.30% | 22.69 | 10.05 |
| Broca's | Time 2 | 20.3 | 9.8 | 48.28% | 14.55 | 7.03 |
| | Time 3 | 21.9 | 10.7 | 48.86% | 15.05 | 6.03 |
| | Time 4 | 25.9 | 12.7 | 49.03% | 27.79 | 13.61 |
| | Time 5 | 15.3 | 6.6 | 43.14% | 16.02 | 6.91 |
| P8 | Time 1 | 54.5 | 37.9 | 69.54% | 92.37 | 64.24 |
| Anomic | Time 2 | 86.3 | 59.8 | 69.29% | 98.63 | 68.34 |
| | Time 3 | 90.2 | 64.1 | 71.06% | 118.68 | 84.34 |
| | Time 4 | 74.1 | 50.0 | 67.48% | 104.37 | 70.42 |
| | Time 5 | 83.5 | 55.9 | 66.95% | 106.10 | 71.03 |

Session scores represent average performance across 10 stimuli. CIUs = correct information units.
WPM = words per minute. CIUs/min = CIUs per minute.

their 20 participants with aphasia exceeded a 10% CIU difference among the three sessions; however, in the current study four participants (Participants 3, 4, 5, and 9) exhibited a difference of at least 14% CIUs across the five sessions. Nicholas and Brookshire (1993) also reported that 85% of persons with aphasia exhibited a change of 10 WPM or fewer among the sessions. In contrast, the current study showed that the majority of participants displayed > 10 WPM changes, and only Participants 1, 10, and 11 (27%) demonstrated variability of less than 10 WPM. The previous authors also indicated that 90% of their participant scores changed by 10 CIUs/min or fewer with repeated production. Visual inspection of Tables 3, 4, 5, and 6 and Figures 2a and 2b reveals highly variable performance in CIUs/min for Participants 3, 8, and 9. With the exception of Participant 11, the remaining participants produced such limited CIUs/min (fewer than 25 CIUs/min) that variability would necessarily be less than 10 CIUs/min.

Overall, individual participants were more variable in repeated production of spoken language than those described by Nicholas and Brookshire (1993, 1994). The dispersion of scores for mean number of CIUs across the five sampling occasions was positively and significantly correlated with scores reflecting severity of aphasia and severity of word-retrieval deficits, but not with MPO. That is, with less severe aphasia, fewer confrontation-naming errors were associated with a greater range of number of CIUs produced across sessions. When the number of CIUs was adjusted for word production (%CIUs), and time (CIUs/min), the dispersion of scores was no longer significantly correlated with the test scores. The finding that participants with less severe language impairment had more variability in production of number of

TABLE 5
Mean words, mean CIUs, %CIUs, WPM, and CIUs/min per session for 10 elicitation stimuli for Participants 9–11

| Participant | Sampling time | Words | CIUs | %CIUs | WPM | CIUs/min |
|---|---|---|---|---|---|---|
| P9 | Time 1 | 111.3 | 54.2 | 48.70% | 98.50 | 47.96 |
| Anomic | Time 2 | 116.3 | 77.6 | 66.72% | 100.26 | 66.61 |
| | Time 3 | 130.9 | 82.3 | 62.87% | 97.69 | 61.42 |
| | Time 4 | 107.4 | 71.8 | 66.85% | 112.23 | 75.03 |
| P10 | Time 1 | 91.8 | 10.8 | 11.76% | 93.20 | 10.96 |
| Wernicke's | Time 2 | 63.5 | 7.9 | 8.04% | 86.75 | 10.79 |
| | Time 3 | 84.5 | 8.9 | 9.49% | 96.35 | 10.15 |
| | Time 4 | 59.5 | 10.2 | 5.83% | 96.28 | 16.50 |
| | Time 5 | 71.7 | 11.5 | 6.23% | 96.50 | 15.48 |
| P11 | Time 1 | 165.5 | 99.3 | 60.00% | 89.50 | 53.73 |
| Anomic | Time 2 | 170.2 | 105.6 | 62.00% | 92.50 | 57.39 |
| | Time 3 | 176.0 | 121.1 | 68.80% | 87.34 | 60.10 |
| | Time 4 | 187.7 | 123.2 | 65.64% | 85.79 | 56.31 |
| | Time 5 | 213.0 | 135.5 | 63.62% | 89.42 | 56.88 |

Session scores represent average performance across 10 stimuli. CIUs = correct information units. WPM = words per minute. CIUs/min = CIUs per minute.

CIUs suggests that repeated sampling prior to treatment initiation may be warranted with such individuals if number of CIUs is desired as an outcome measure. Participants with more recent onset of aphasia were not more likely to exhibit greater variability in performance.

There was no pattern of variability with respect to the "broad" type of aphasia; however, the unequal numbers of participants in the fluent ($N = 5$) and nonfluent ($N = 6$) groups might have influenced outcomes. It should be noted that the range of aphasia types within the classifications of "fluent" and "nonfluent" was limited in the current study (given that participants were enrolled based on their involvement in a treatment protocol targeting word retrieval). It is possible that differences between more specific subtypes of aphasia would have been detected if more individuals had participated in this study. It would be of value to obtain samples from a greater number of persons with a variety of aphasia types to further explore potential differences in verbal productivity and information content within and between groups.

Nicholas and Brookshire (1993) included the use of trial stimuli (with instruction and feedback) prior to completion of their tasks. Practice stimuli were not used in the current study due to concern that provision of feedback could limit the amount of information produced in the samples. It is therefore possible that the use of trial stimuli could have affected participant variability, and partially account for some of the differences observed. It was interesting to note, however, that five participants (Participants 1, 3, 5, 7, and 10) produced more words, four produced more CIUs (Participants 1, 5, 7, and 10), and six produced a higher ratio of CIUs to words (Participants 2, 4, 5, 6, 8, and 10) in the first administration of the task as compared to the second session (see Tables 3, 4, and 5). This suggests that practice with the task was not the main factor mediating variability for most participants. However, it could be argued that, following repeated trials, participants became more familiar with the task and were reluctant to provide redundant information to their communication partner. If this was the case, it is probable that individuals would provide

TABLE 6
Individual ranges for mean words, mean CIUs, %CIUs, WPM, and CIUs/min for 10 elicitation
stimuli

| Participant | Words | CIUs | %CIUs | WPM | CIUs/min | Aphasia type |
|---|---|---|---|---|---|---|
| P1 | 3.9 | 2.6 | 7.37 | 8.95 | 6.69 | Broca's |
| P2 | 38.6 | 19.5 | 3.11 | 17.28 | 6.36 | Anomic |
| P3 | 19.0 | 10.2 | 14.62 | 34.27 | 13.03 | Broca's |
| P4 | 37.2 | 6.6 | 14.43 | 10.45 | 3.86 | Broca's |
| P5 | 9.5 | 3.0 | 16.03 | 10.56 | 2.30 | Broca's |
| P6 | 25.0 | 9.5 | 4.93 | 18.87 | 7.08 | Broca's |
| P7 | 5.4 | 7.0 | 5.89 | 13.24 | 7.58 | Broca's |
| P8 | 35.7 | 26.2 | 4.11 | 26.31 | 20.10 | Anomic |
| P9 | 23.5 | 28.1 | 18.15 | 14.54 | 27.07 | Anomic |
| P10 | 32.3 | 3.6 | 5.93 | 9.75 | 6.35 | Wernicke's |
| P11 | 47.5 | 36.2 | 8.80 | 6.71 | 6.37 | Anomic |

Session scores represent the range for average performance across 10 stimuli. CIUs = correct information units. WPM = words per minute. CIUs/min = CIUs per minute.

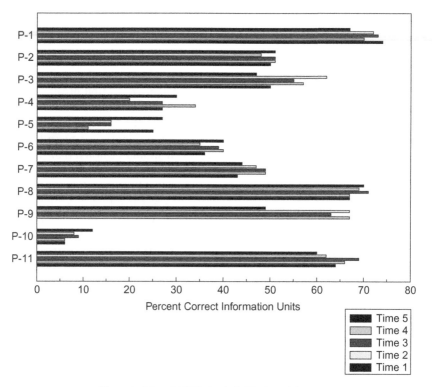

Figure 1. Mean %CIUs for individual participants.

less information during later productions. Conversely, it could be argued that increased familiarity with the task could result in increased production of information. That is, repeated exposure could result in greater numbers of associations made with the stimuli. However, visual inspection of the data reveals no consistent pattern of persons with aphasia providing either more or less information as data collection

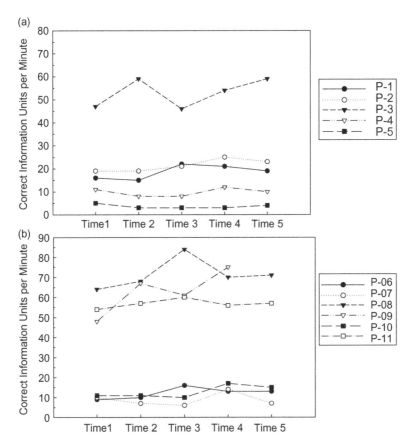

**Figure 2.** (a) Mean CIUs/min for participants 1 to 5. (b) Mean CIUs/min for participants 6 to 11.

progressed. It should be noted that two individuals (Participants 7 and 9) had an alternate SLP collect data for one session due to scheduling issues, and it is possible that this could have influenced their inter-session stability. Examination of the data from those sessions revealed that a few values were lower than the remaining sessions for one participant (Participant 7), but were higher for the other participant (Participant 9). Familiarity with the examiner and variability across examiner are factors that may warrant consideration in future investigations and in clinical application.

Interestingly, when Nicholas and Brookshire (1993) compared the variability of 20 speakers without brain damage to 20 persons with aphasia, they reported that the individuals without brain damage were less variable for %CIUs but more variable for CIUs/min and WPM. Thus, the rate of production of information units was more stable for persons with aphasia but they were more variable in the number of words and CIUs produced over repeated sampling times. The reason for the across-session variability in production of information units in discourse for persons with aphasia remains unclear. It has been suggested that variability is a hallmark characteristic of the disorder and may be related to factors such as processing constraints and executive control of language with variability increasing with task complexity (see Kolk, 2007, for a review). An additional consideration for the variability related to aphasia may be the higher prevalence of depression within this population group. Participants in

TABLE 7

Mean words, mean CIUs, %CIUs, WPM, and CIUs/min over time for the group of persons with aphasia (N = 11)

| Session # | Words | | CIUs | | %CIUs | | WPM | | CIUs/min | |
|---|---|---|---|---|---|---|---|---|---|---|
| | Mean | SD | Mean | SD | Mean | SD | Mean | SD | Mean | SD |
| Session 1 | 58.19 | 47.23 | 26.94 | 28.48 | 45.19 | 17.40 | 57.58 | 35.95 | 26.72 | 21.76 |
| Session 2 | 63.30 | 47.78 | 32.14 | 34.16 | 46.05 | 23.14 | 57.90 | 36.30 | 29.49 | 26.94 |
| Session 3 | 67.13 | 51.88 | 35.21 | 38.48 | 47.49 | 22.19 | 59.95 | 37.11 | 30.74 | 27.61 |
| Session 4 | 63.67 | 50.64 | 34.02 | 36.67 | 46.93 | 22.16 | 62.96 | 35.12 | 32.66 | 25.99 |
| Session 5 | 59.07 | 59.17 | 28.70 | 39.21 | 40.24 | 24.14 | 53.96 | 41.40 | 25.28 | 24.88 |

Session scores represent average performance across 10 stimuli. CIUs = correct information units. WPM = words per minute. CIUs/min = CIUs per minute. SD = standard deviation.

the current study reported a negative history for "major" mental illness; however, they were not screened for depression on a session-by-session basis. It is possible that fluctuating mood could have affected performance on the task and influenced results. It would be of interest to collect additional normative data for persons both with and without aphasia to explore potential differences in verbal productivity and information content on this discourse task, screening for depression on a regular basis.

As both clinicians and researchers strive for evidence-based interventions, the need for meaningful and reliable outcome measures is critical. One methodology frequently used to explore the effects of intervention in aphasia is the implementation of single-participant research designs. Given their logical validity as a tool by which to assess discourse in persons with aphasia, it is likely that the tasks proposed by Nicholas and Brookshire (1993) will continue to be used with relative frequency to measure treatment outcomes in single-participant research designs. In light of the variability in persons with aphasia over repeated sampling times noted in the current study, it is recommended that both clinicians and researchers carefully consider the magnitude of the treatment effect expected when establishing levels of acceptable variability in baseline measurements.

Dispersion of scores is a critical component in the determination of the size of a treatment's effects. Beeson and Robey (2006) defined effect size as, "a quantity that characterizes the degree of departure from the null state" (p. 3) and noted that effect sizes are, "quantified in standard deviation units" (p. 3). Thus, if greater variability were noted in the pre-treatment baseline phase, a larger change following intervention would be required to demonstrate a consequential effect size. As indicated by Beeson and Robey, interventionists should collect a minimum of three pre-treatment baseline probes to allow for an estimation of treatment effect. After the variability of these three baseline probes has been examined, a judgement should be made as to how much change would be required post-treatment in order to suggest a meaningful result from the applied intervention. Given the relationship between variability and the calculation of effect size, if the person with aphasia exhibited unstable performance, it could be necessary to collect additional baseline probes. Thus, without consideration of the variability of individual performance over repeated sampling times, valuable data regarding the effectiveness of interventions could be lost or misinterpreted.

TABLE 8

Mean scores over time for the groups of fluent ($N = 5$) and nonfluent ($N = 6$) persons with aphasia

| Session # | Fluent CIUs | | Nonfluent CIUs | | Fluent %CIUs | | Nonfluent %CIUs | | Fluent CIUs/min | | Nonfluent CIUs/min | |
|---|---|---|---|---|---|---|---|---|---|---|---|---|
| | Mean | SD | Mean | SD | Mean | SD | Mean | SD | Mean | SD | Mean | SD |
| Session 1 | 45.92 | 33.76 | 11.12 | 7.06 | 48.22 | 21.97 | 42.65 | 14.21 | 39.14 | 23.07 | 16.37 | 15.44 |
| Session 2 | 56.46 | 38.27 | 11.87 | 8.82 | 50.87 | 25.33 | 42.03 | 22.70 | 44.39 | 27.47 | 17.07 | 20.99 |
| Session 3 | 64.02 | 41.95 | 11.20 | 5.56 | 52.64 | 25.36 | 43.20 | 20.52 | 47.44 | 30.81 | 16.82 | 15.93 |
| Session 4 | 60.42 | 41.49 | 12.02 | 5.93 | 50.76 | 25.94 | 43.74 | 20.41 | 48.69 | 26.52 | 19.30 | 17.81 |
| Session 5 | 48.82 | 53.38 | 11.93 | 7.26 | 37.37 | 31.98 | 42.64 | 18.23 | 33.24 | 29.65 | 18.65 | 20.47 |

Session scores represent average performance across 10 stimuli. CIUs = correct information units. CIUs/min = CIUs per minute. SD = standard deviation.

In summary, the results of the current study suggest substantial temporal instability/ variability in discourse of persons with aphasia performing the tasks proposed by Nicholas and Brookshire (1993) over repeated sampling times. Clinicians and researchers should consider this variability when measuring effects of treatment and collect a minimum of three baselines prior to initiating therapy. Further study with larger groups of persons presenting with a wider range of aphasia subtypes would be of value to obtain more complete descriptions of individual and group variability.

Manuscript received 2 July 2009
Manuscript accepted 26 October 2009
First published online 25 May 2010

## REFERENCES

Armstrong, E. (2000). Aphasic discourse analysis: The story so far. *Aphasiology, 14*(9), 875–892.

Beeson, P. M., & Robey, R. R. (2006). Evaluating single-subject treatment research: Lessons learned from the aphasia literature. *Neuropsychological Review, 16*(4), 161–169.

Boyle, M. (2004a). *Discourse treatment for word retrieval impairment in chronic aphasia.* Poster presented at the Clinical Aphasiology Conference. Park City, UT, May.

Boyle, M. (2004b). Semantic feature analysis treatment for anomia in two fluent aphasia syndromes. *American Journal of Speech-Language Pathology, 13*, 236–249.

Brown, L., Sherbenou, R. J., & Johnsen, S. K. (1997). *Test of Nonverbal Intelligence* (3rd ed.). Austin, TX: Pro-Ed.

Cameron, R. M., Wambaugh, J. L., Wright, S. M., & Nessler, C. L. (2006). Effects of a combined semantic/phonologic cueing treatment on word retrieval in discourse. *Aphasiology, 20*(2), 269–285.

Disimoni, F. G., Keith, R. L., & Darley, F. L. (1980). Prediction of *PICA* overall score by short versions of the test. *Journal of Speech and Hearing Research, 23*, 511–516.

Doyle, P. J., McNeil, M. R., Spencer, K. A., Goda, A. J., Cotrell, K., & Lustig, A. P. (1998). The effects of concurrent picture presentations on retelling of orally presented stories by adults with aphasia. *Aphasiology, 12*(7/8), 561–574.

German, D. J. (1990). *Test of Adolescent/Adult Word Finding.* Allen, TX: DLM.

Gordon, J. K. (2008). Measuring the lexical semantics of picture description in aphasia. *Aphasiology, 22*(7/8), 839–852.

Kaplan, E., Goodglass, H., & Weintraub, S. (1983). *The Boston Naming Test.* Boston: Lea & Febiger.

Kertesz, A. (1982). *The Western Aphasia Battery.* New York: Grune & Stratten.

Kolk, H. (2007). Variability is the hallmark of aphasic behaviour: Grammatical behaviour is no exception. *Brain and Language, 101*, 99–102.

Nicholas, L. E., & Brookshire, R. H. (1993). A system for quantifying the informativeness and efficiency of the connected speech of adults with aphasia. *Journal of Speech and Hearing Research, 36*, 338–350.

Nicholas, L. E., & Brookshire, R. H. (1994). Speech sample size and test–retest stability of connected speech measures for adults with aphasia. *Journal of Speech and Hearing Research, 37*, 399–407.

Peach, R. K., & Reuter, K. A. (in press). A discourse-based approach to semantic feature analysis for the treatment of aphasic word retrieval failures. *Aphasiology.* Epub ahead of print:doi:10.1080/02687030903058629.

Porch, B. (2001). *Porch Index of Communicative Ability (Vol. 1): Administration, Scoring, and Interpretation* (4th ed.). Palo Alto, CA: Pro-Ed.

Prins, R., & Bastiaanse, R. (2004). Analysing the spontaneous speech of aphasic speakers. *Aphasiology, 18*(12), 1075–1091.

Wambaugh, J. L., & Ferguson, M. (2007). Application of semantic feature analysis to retrieval of action names in aphasia. *Journal of Rehabilitation Research and Development, 44*(3), 381–394.

Yorkston, K. M., & Beukelman, D. R. (1984). *Assessment of Intelligibility of Dysarthric Speech.* Austin, TX: Pro-Ed.

APHASIOLOGY, 2010, 24 (6–8), 685–696

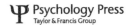

# Describing the experience of aphasia rehabilitation through metaphor

Alison Ferguson

*University of Newcastle, Callaghan, NSW, Australia*

Linda Worrall and Bronwyn Davidson

*University of Queensland, Brisbane St Lucia, QLD, Australia*

Deborah Hersh

*Edith Cowan University, Joondalup, WA, Australia*

Tami Howe

*University of Canterbury, Christchurch, New Zealand*

Sue Sherratt

*University of Queensland, Brisbane St Lucia, QLD, and University of Newcastle,*

*Callaghan, NSW, Australia*

*Background*: Previous research into metaphoric expression has suggested that metaphor offers a window into intra-individual conceptions as well as into socio-cultural understandings of illness and recovery. This study explored how people with aphasia, their family members, and their speech-language pathologists described their experiences of rehabilitation through the linguistic resource of metaphor.

*Aims*: This study aimed to compare the perspectives of five people with aphasia, five of their family members, and their eight treating speech-language pathologists by analysing the way they used the linguistic resource of metaphor to describe their experience of aphasia therapy.

*Methods & Procedures*: Interviews with five people with aphasia, five of their family members, and their eight speech-language pathologists were recorded, transcribed, and coded for metaphoric expressions and concepts.

*Outcomes & Results*: Quantitatively across all participants, the metaphorical concepts of JOURNEY, BATTLE, and PRODUCT were the most frequently used metaphoric

Address correspondence to: Associate Professor Alison Ferguson, School of Humanities and Social Science, University of Newcastle, Callaghan, NSW 2308 Australia.
E-mail: Alison.Ferguson@newcastle. edu.au

This research was supported through a grant from the National Health and Medical Research Council, Australia (NHMRC Project Grant ID: 401532 – "What people with aphasia want: Toward person-centred goal-setting in aphasia rehabilitation") led by Professor Linda Worrall from University of Queensland. The authors wish to acknowledge and thank the participants for their time and contribution, and the Aphasia Registry (Communication Disability Centre, University of Queensland) for assistance with recruitment.

http://www.psypress.com/aphasiology        DOI: 10.1080/02687030903438508

concepts expressed by the participants. Qualitatively within sets of participants, differences in the patterns of use of metaphoric concepts indicated important contrasts in the way they viewed their experiences.

*Conclusions*: The frequent use of JOURNEY metaphor accorded with previous research into recovery, while the identification of BATTLE and PRODUCT metaphor was suggested to point to critical sites reflecting social disempowerment. Attention to the use of metaphoric expression may offer clinicians a window into how others involved in the collaborative therapy process are constructing their experience.

*Keywords:* Aphasia; Rehabilitation; Metaphor; Discourse analysis; Goals.

Metaphor has been of interest to linguists and health professionals since the late 1970s. In 1978 Susan Sontag's influential book on illness and metaphor (Sontag, 1990) critically appraised the potential adverse effects of the way metaphors are used to characterise features of illnesses in ways that do not reflect the reality of the conditions (e.g., characterising repressive personality as a causative factor in cancer), as well as the way illnesses themselves are used metaphorically to describe other events and situations (e.g., a political idea spreading "like a cancer"). Lakoff and Johnson's *Metaphors we live by* (Lakoff & Johnson, 1980) became a cornerstone work in providing the theoretical and methodological framework for analysing metaphoric expressions (e.g., "it was the luck of the draw") in systematic ways in relation to underlying metaphoric concepts (e.g., LIFE IS A GAMBLING GAME—in keeping with Lakoff and Johnson's (1980) conventions, metaphorical expressions are written in lower case, while metaphorical concepts are written in upper case. Lakoff and Johnson argued that metaphor was common in everyday talk, and not simply reserved for literary works, and also suggested that metaphoric concepts formed fundamental cognitive representations that guided both conscious and unconscious thought processes. This cognitive linguistic viewpoint has resulted in much research, but at the same time the socio-cultural origin of metaphors has raised considerable interest (Kovecses, 2005); many metaphoric expressions take "fixed forms" and become so much part of the culture that their metaphoric nature is obscured. For example, expressions such as "I'm feeling down" is metaphoric in its use of location to express emotion, but would rarely be noticed as such.

The windows that metaphor opens on both the inner thoughts of individuals and on socio-cultural influences have meant that the interpretation and manipulation of metaphor have come to be used strategically within the context of counselling (Strong, 1989). For example, the client's use of metaphor may change over time and be used as an index of improvement in response to therapy (Levitt, Korman, & Angus, 2000). In the case studies presented by Levitt and colleagues (2000), BURDEN metaphors changed to include "unloading" the burden in a case study with a positive outcome. Likewise, for those clinicians using narrative reconstruction as a means of countering biographical disruption (Faircloth, Boylstein, Rittman, Young, & Gubrium, 2004; Williams, 1996), metaphors may provide an index of change. For example, Boylstein and colleagues suggest that their data from a study of stroke recovery indicate that the nature of metaphors shifted in relation to changes in reported depression and measures of self-identity (Boylstein, Rittman, & Hinojosa, 2007). Previous case study research by Kirmayer (2000) has illustrated some of the "contested ground" between patient and professional through the analysis of metaphor, and Kirmayer argues for the necessity for professionals to be alert to both their patients' and their own metaphoric concepts and expression as a reflection of the culturally and institutionally derived power relationship (Kirmayer, 2000).

Metaphoric expression used by family members of people with a range of communication disorders including those arising from neurological damage (Mastergeorge, 1999) has been researched previously through analysis of ethnographic interviews. Mastergeorge interviewed 60 family members on two occasions (37 parents of children with communication disorders and 18 spouses of adults with traumatic brain injury; as well as 5 adults who stuttered). The main focus of these ethnographic interviews was their experience of receiving a diagnosis and the researcher was interested in "how family members cope with the ambiguity of diagnosis and disorder" (p. 246). The main metaphors used to describe the experience of the diagnosis were categorised into sleep states ("walking into a dream"), barrier structures ("doors closed"), forces of nature ("we were in rocky waters on a sinking ship") (pp. 248–249, Mastergeorge, 1999) . Metaphors used to describe coping were categorised as religion ("God has a plan"), journeys ("on the same path"), routines and everyday events ("learning how to walk"), and fairy tales ("like the wolf who comes and blows your house down") (pp. 250–251). Metaphors used to personify experiences were categorised as physical ("not like a broken leg"), illness ("like hearing you had AIDS"), and animal metaphors ("like being on a horse", "like the elephant in the living room") (pp. 252–253). Metaphors used to describe ambivalence were described in terms of dilemma ("walk this sort of line or tightrope") (pp. 254–255). Mastergeorge's research focused on assessment issues rather than therapy, and her data were not analysed with reference to disorder types. The present research sought to further explore metaphoric description of aphasia therapy in particular, and to compare the expressions and concepts used across people with aphasia, their family members, and their speech-language pathologists.

This research is part of a larger research project that aimed to find out more about what people with aphasia and their family members wanted during their period of recovery following stroke (Worrall et al., 2007, 2009). In brief, the analyses of this interview data have highlighted areas of dissatisfaction with current services, particularly with the experience of acute hospitalisation in relation to insufficient information about the nature of aphasia and the lack of apparent relevance of the types of assessment and therapy tasks. Inpatient rehabilitation experiences were also reported as lacking these features, along with some dissatisfaction with the amount of therapy services provided. In general, satisfaction with community-based services seemed higher, with a very high degree of satisfaction reported in relation to opportunities for group therapy and group support services. These content analyses and the ongoing investigations of the research group are revealing important areas where there is considerable divergence in the understandings and perceptions of the people experiencing aphasia and their family members with those of their speech-language pathologists. The analysis of metaphor provides another layer to this investigation of the perspectives of people with aphasia, their family members, and their treating speech-language pathologists.

In this paper the interviews of five people with aphasia, their family members, and speech-language pathologists were analysed in order to investigate their use of metaphor to describe their experiences during the course of rehabilitation. The research questions were as follows. What types of metaphoric expressions and concepts were used during the interviews with people with aphasia, their family members, and their treating speech-languagepathologists? Are there differences in the types of metaphoric expressions and concepts used across the types of participants (i.e., people with aphasia, family members, speech-language pathologists), or within the sets of participants (i.e., the person with aphasia, their family member, their treating speech-language pathologist/s)?

## METHOD

The research used a small cohort design, involving consideration of group and single-case results. The analysis of data used descriptive linguistic methods.

### Participants

There were five sets of participant interviews (total of 18 participants) drawn from a larger pool of interviews for a project investigating what people wanted from aphasia therapy (Worrall et al., 2007). See Table 1 for details. There were three male and two female participants with aphasia, aged between 57 and 79 years, whose aphasia resulted from stroke between $1^1/_2$ years and 11 years prior to the interview. The severity of their aphasia was relatively mild, with Aphasia Quotient scores from the Western Aphasia Battery (Kertesz, 2006) ranging between 81.3 and 95.6. All family members were female, aged between 56 and 76 years. All speech-language pathologists were female, aged between 24 and 60 years. Each set of participants comprised a person with aphasia, their family member, and their speech-language pathologist/s. All 18 participants spoke English as their first language, and were living in Australian capital cities at the time of the interview. Research code numbers replaced participants' names in the transcripts, and pseudonyms are used in referring to participants in all presentations and publications, including this paper.

TABLE 1
Participants

| Set | Code (pseudonym) | Participant type | Gender | Age | Months post onset of aphasia | WAB AQ[1] at time of interview |
|-----|------------------|------------------|--------|-----|------------------------------|--------------------------------|
| 1 | Ulysses | PWA | Male | 71 | 134 | 87.3 |
|   | Ursula | Wife | Female | 67 | | |
|   | Uma | SLP | Female | 46 | | |
| 2 | Rose | PWA | Female | 79 | 45 | 89.7 |
|   | Rhonda | Daughter | Female | 56 | | |
|   | Roberta | SLP | Female | 24 | | |
| 3 | Mavis | PWA | Female | 76 | 19 | 81.3 |
|   | Maud | Sister | Female | 76 | | |
|   | Mary | SLP | Female | 39 | | |
|   | Mathilda | SLP | Female | 58 | | |
| 4 | Neville | PWA | Male | 57 | 36 | 95.6 |
|   | Nina | Wife | Female | 57 | | |
|   | Nicky | SLP | Female | 50 | | |
|   | Naomi | SLP | Female | 60 | | |
| 5 | Elton | PWA | Male | 68 | 28 | 86.5 |
|   | Eunice | Wife | Female | 65 | | |
|   | Evelyn | SLP | Female | 24 | | |
|   | Emma | SLP | Female | 49 | | |

[1]Western Aphasia Battery, Aphasia Quotient (Kertesz, 2006).

## Data collection and analysis

Participants were interviewed separately in their home (for people with aphasia and family members), and at their place of work (speech-language pathologists). Family members were interviewed separately, but were often present at the interview with the person with aphasia. All 18 interviews were recorded (video recording for people with aphasia and their family members, audio recording for speech-language pathologists). The interviewers were experienced speech-language pathologists (members of the research team), and had not been involved in the clinical management of the participants with aphasia. The interviews for each set of participants (i.e., the person with aphasia, their family member, and their treating speech-language pathologist/s) were conducted by the same interviewer, and each interview lasted between 1 and 2 hours. The interviews were semi-structured, following a topic guide for participants with aphasia that began with "Tell me a little about yourself", which led to his/her narrative about the series of events surrounding the participant's stroke and subsequent life following the stroke. Prompt questions included: When you first had your stroke what was important to you? What were your concerns? What did you want to work on in speech therapy? Did you work on these areas in speech therapy? If yes, how did you work on them? If no, what did you want to work on? Did speech therapy help? What other services or things did you want at that time related to your aphasia? These prompts were repeated for specified times after the stroke: when they first went home, when they had outpatient speech therapy, later, and at the time of the interview. The interview schedule for family members adopted a similar approach. The interview for speech-language pathologists asked about their experiences of providing therapy to the person with aphasia and his/her family member, their goals of therapy for the person with aphasia and his/her family member, and their perceptions of the goals of the person with aphasia and his/her family member.

Following transcription, the interviews were imported into the qualitative database software program NVivo (QSR).

The initial coding for this study identified metaphoric expressions using Thompson's definition: ". . . the expression of a meaning through a lexicogrammatical form that originally evolved to express a different kind of meaning"( Thompson, 2004, p. 223). Each metaphoric expression identified was then checked, using the steps described by the group of metaphor researchers known as "Pragglejaz" (2007), as follows. For each lexical unit, its meaning in the interview context was reviewed to establish whether it had a contrasting meaning that could be considered as more basic (e.g., more concrete, more precise, or an historically prior meaning). Refer to the Appendix for an example of this stage of analysis. Each expression for which this contrast could be established was confirmed as metaphorical. The next layer of coding described the extent to which metaphoric expressions were drawn from the more fixed forms often used in everyday talk or were novel, i.e., uniquely coined by the speaker (Crider & Cirillo, 1991). Subsequently, all expressions were grouped thematically into metaphoric concepts (Lakoff & Johnson, 1980) that refer to the underlying or core meaning being variously expressed. Initial coding provided for the categorisation of metaphoric expressions across more than one metaphoric concept. For example, the expression "throw in the towel" was initially coded within both BATTLE and SPORT, since the more basic meanings are associated most recently with "giving up", and more historically with boxing. Where expressions were categorised across more than one concept, the more contemporary basic meaning determined which metaphoric concept was used in subsequent reliability checks, and for report-ing the results of the analysis in this paper. All data were analysed by the first author. Inter-judge agreement was established between the first author and two other analysts (one member of the research team, Davidson; and one experienced speech-language pathology researcher with experience in linguistic analysis who was inde-pendent of the research team). Agreement was established for the three interview transcripts for set 1 (three of 18 transcripts, 17% of the data). Agreement was only considered to have been reached when both reliability analysts agreed with the first author as to both the identification of the metaphoric expression and the categorisa-tion into the metaphoric concept. The total number of metaphoric expressions in the reliability set was 42, agreement was present for 34, with disagreement for 8, i.e., 81% (point-to-point agreement).

## RESULTS

### Metaphoric concepts

Quantitatively, 256 metaphoric expressions were identified across the 18 interviews, and these were grouped into 13 metaphoric concepts. (Cell size was insufficient for inferential statistics.) As can be seen from Table 2, the most frequently occurring metaphoric concepts were JOURNEY, PRODUCT, and BATTLE (and examples of these are discussed below). Table 2 includes the metaphoric expressions used by Interviewers (35/256, 13.7%). In all cases, Interviewers' use of metaphoric expres-sions echoed those used by the participants, as they explored the participants' perspectives, and so their use of metaphor did not "lead" the participants' use of this resource.

One finding of importance to note is that the participants with aphasia were observed to make use of metaphoric expressions, which reflects their relative pre-served access to this aspect of language use in the context of mild severity of aphasia. By way of example (example 1), the person with aphasia rejected the notion of goal formation as his experience up until the point of discharge as an inpatient. Instead he characterised his experience up until that point as a "journey" and one that was about to "end". While this instance is more clearly "more metaphoric" it is a com-monplace metaphor, and one that in this instance was contributing mainly to the ide-ational meanings in the discourse.

> Example 1. JOURNEY – Neville (PWA)
> INT: Did you have a goal?
> Neville: Not at all. No.
> INT: No goals?
> Neville: I was, for me, going to [name of rehabilitation hospital] was, **that's a journey** to go back to work. To me **the journey was going to end there** and let's run with it, get along with life. There was no, to me there was no, no.

Throughout the interviews, and across all types of participants, metaphoric expressions were used that invoked more basic meanings of war, fighting, and viol-ence, and these were grouped within the metaphoric concept of BATTLE. In the fol-lowing example (example 2), this speech-language pathologist (Naomi) was describing the therapy process involved with the goal of attempting to identify strate-gies that the person with aphasia could use to deal with the impact of cognitive fatigue. As was commonly found throughout the data, this example came from an

TABLE 2
Metaphoric concepts (in order of frequency)

| METAPHORIC CONCEPTS | Examples | Person with aphasia metaphoric expressions | | Family member metaphoric expressions | | Speech-language pathologist metaphoric expressions | | Interviewer metaphoric expressions | | TOTAL |
|---|---|---|---|---|---|---|---|---|---|---|
| | | # | % | # | % | # | % | # | % | |
| JOURNEY | They've identified that that's where they want to go, you set them on the track (SLP) | 9 | 18.4 | 8 | 42.1 | 54 | 35.3 | 8 | 22.9 | 79 |
| PRODUCT | ...and it would be an add-on. It's not a take-away (SLP) | 11 | 22.4 | 2 | 10.5 | 38 | 24.8 | 13 | 37.1 | 64 |
| BATTLE | ...he will face it full on like a Sherman tank (SLP) | 8 | 16.4 | 4 | 21.1 | 20 | 13.1 | 5 | 14.3 | 37 |
| BODY | But, I think in the end he began to feel as though there was something he could stand on. (SLP) | 10 | 20.4 | 0 | 0.0 | 12 | 7.8 | 3 | 8.6 | 25 |
| SPORT | Um. . . . It's a bit like going to gym, sometimes you don't want to do anything except sit in the spa. (FAM) | 3 | 6.1 | 3 | 15.8 | 3 | 2.0 | 3 | 8.6 | 12 |
| SIGNIFICANT IS BIG | Cognitive fatigue was absolutely "gi-normous" for him. (SLP) | 0 | 0.0 | 0 | 0.0 | 10 | 6.5 | 0 | 0.0 | 10 |
| PRISON | ..you will find things different when you get outside.(PWA) | 4 | 8.2 | 0 | 0.0 | 5 | 3.3 | 0 | 0.0 | 9 |
| NATURAL ENVIRONMENT | ..the cold hard truth can dawn (SLP) | 1 | 2.0 | 1 | 5.3 | 4 | 2.6 | 2 | 5.7 | 8 |
| MADNESS | I think they'd go crazy otherwise (FAM) | 3 | 6.1 | 0 | 0.0 | 0 | 0.0 | 1 | 2.9 | 4 |
| CHILD, PARENTHOOD | ...she didn't try to mother him (SLP) | 0 | 0.0 | 1 | 5.3 | 2 | 1.3 | 0 | 0.0 | 3 |
| EVOLUTION | ...it's an evolving sort of process (SLP) | 0 | 0.0 | 0 | 0.0 | 2 | 1.3 | 0 | 0.0 | 2 |
| MARRIAGE | Just the fact that I really like the marrying of the individual and the group context (SLP) | 0 | 0.0 | 0 | 0.0 | 2 | 1.3 | 0 | 0.0 | 2 |
| RELIGIOUS | ...that glory period (SLP) | 0 | 0.0 | 0 | 0.0 | 1 | 0.7 | 0 | 0.0 | 1 |
| TOTAL | | 49 | 100 | 19 | 100 | 153 | 100 | 35 | 100 | 256 |

extended chain of lexical metaphor. This reiteration served to intensify the expression of the speech-language pathologist's judgement of this patient's character trait of determination, and so serves to add interpersonal meanings in the discourse (Martin & White, 2005/2007).

> Example 2. BATTLE – Naomi (SLP)
> Naomi: And we spent a lot of time with helping him and his wife understand what his head. . . how his. . .
>     INT: Having his chance to cry and have a chance. . .
> Naomi: Yeah, and also, that with cognitive, about the cognitive fatigue **pushing him around**. And how to deal with some of that stuff. You know, how to deal with you know, how to recognise it and that it's **not being a wimp**. Because you know he will face it full on **like a Sherman tank**.

## Novel expression of metaphoric concepts

Of the 256 metaphoric expressions, 33 of these (12.9%) were described as using "novel" metaphoric expressions (i.e., uniquely formulated in the situation of their use). Only one of the participants with aphasia (Elton—see Example 3) was identified as using these highly metaphoric expressions.

> Example 3. Novel metaphor – Elton (PWA)
>     INT: So you did a . . . you were . . .worked on a computer program?
> Elton: Yeah.
>     INT: OK can you tell me about that a bit.
> Elton: I was (pause) I was **in a (pause) in a quagmire** as we begin to use it and I got it down to a fine art.

Novel metaphoric expressions are of interest as they represent the "more metaphoric" end of the continuum, and are both likely to be more readily identified for analytic or clinical purposes, but also more likely to be expressing meanings of special significance for the speaker. For example (example 4), Ursula, the wife of the individual with aphasia, described her feelings through the use of highly metaphoric expressions conveying the concept of PRODUCT. These expressions added interpersonal meanings conveying her attitude to the information she had provided about not being able to accompany her husband into therapy.

> Example 4. PRODUCT – Ursula (FAM)
> Ursula: I never, ah only ever saw the woman once I think or.
>     INT: The speech therapist?
> Ursula: yeah yeah, when she took Ulysses into, into the room and ah –. . . . Came back out by himself [laughter]. mm so I don't know . . . so I mean this is not . . . it is not . . . ah . . . mm it makes you feel **like a pound of potatoes** or something you know it's . . . not . . . not a very good relationship. Um **you're just being processed**. (pause) That's a bit harsh isn't it . . .

## Comparison of metaphoric concepts within sets of participants

There were a number of concepts that were shared among all participants within sets, notably BATTLE (sets 1, 4), PRODUCT (sets 1, 2), JOURNEY (set 1), SPORT (set 4), and NATURAL ENVIRONMENT (set 5). The person with aphasia and speech-language pathologist (but not the family member) drew on the concepts of BODY (set 1, 4), PRISON (set 1), and JOURNEY and PRODUCT (set 4). The family member and speech-language pathologist (but not the person with aphasia) drew on the concepts of JOURNEY (sets 2, 5), CHILD/PARENT (set 1), and BATTLE (set 3). There were differences within sets in the ways in which participants predominantly constructed their experience. For example, within sets 1 and 2, the speech-language pathologists' construction of therapy as a step-wise journey contrasted with the other participants' description of struggle.

By way of illustration, in one set of participants (set 1 – Ulysses, Ursula, Uma) the use of metaphors by each participant suggested that there were considerable differences in their perceived experiences. Ulysses (person with aphasia) used BATTLE metaphors as a recurring theme throughout his description of his experience in general, as well as in relation to what he was trying to achieve through therapy, e.g., "fighting" and "overcoming" (see example 1). His wife, Ursula, used PRODUCT metaphors, which were novel and highly metaphoric, e.g., "we'd just been processed" (see example 4) in relation to her experience in the early stages of rehabilitation. In comparison, one of their speech-language pathologists (Uma, who worked with them at a later stage in the rehabilitation process) described the therapy process using primarily JOURNEY metaphoric concepts, e.g., "tracks", "steps", and "building".

A further illustration of the differences observed within sets of participants could be seen in the use of metaphoric expressions relating to the concept of PRISON. In those sets in which the metaphoric concept of PRISON was identified, related expressions were used only by the person with aphasia (see example 5) and the treating speech-language pathologist (see example 6), and not the family member.

Example 5. PRISON – Neville (PWA)

Neville: As far as at the hospital I was glad to get out eventually. That was er, I don't know at times I didn't feel comfortable there, at the hospital. Whether **I was so strapped down, not strapped down, no confined** maybe that was something that subsequently I didn't err feel comfortable.

Example 6. PRISON – Naomi (SLP)

Naomi: So dealing with that emotional aspect in that the response to their current situation. It can really. . . it can be difficult to see you know, the wood for the trees, you know **everything closes in on you**. I think he was a bit like that but . . . yeah from memory, so it was probably more a lot of the emotional stuff.

## DISCUSSION

In summary, a wide variety of metaphoric expressions were identified in the data, supporting the previous literature regarding the typicality of metaphor use. Metaphoric expressions were observed to both provide further information to the discourse (through ideational meaning) as well as to contribute to the expression of the speakers' attitudes (i.e., interpersonal meanings). Also, it was noted that metaphoric expression tended not to occur in isolated instances, but rather in chains of meaning running through the text, which suggests that active listening on the part of clinicians would enable these kinds of threads of meaning to be detected "on-line" within an unfolding session. Novel metaphors were used in the interviews, occurring mainly in the discourse of family members and speech-language pathologists. As could be expected the use of novel metaphoric expression was rare for the participants with aphasia. However, it should be noted that for some people, aphasic word substitutions may promote metaphoric creativity (Alajouanine, 1948; Zion, 2006). Novel metaphors provide marked instances of metaphoric expression, and offer windows into attitudinal stances of the speaker. Comparison of the use of metaphors within a set of participants suggested that consideration of these expressions offers an opportunity to consider alignment or misalignment in the perspectives of participants. Where such different perspectives exist for the person with aphasia, their spouse and their treating speech-language pathologist at a particular stage of rehabilitation, this could potentially cause considerable misalignment in the process of negotiating shared therapy goals. Through on-line monitoring of the communication, the speech-language pathologist has the opportunity to gain insights into the client's perspective, and potentially to align his/her use of metaphor with the person with aphasia and their family members in collaborative goal setting. In this way, awareness of the use of metaphoric expressions and their underlying concepts may provide a useful resource for speech-language pathologists in their reflective practice (Ferguson, 2008b).

Consistent with the findings from the larger study (Worrall et al., 2009), the current study identified contrasting perspectives between people with aphasia, their family members, and their treating speech-language pathologists. In particular, the current findings echoed the tensions previously identified between the roles of client (including family member) and professional, the tensions between caring and professional relationships, and the tensions between hopeful and accepting outlooks for the future. However, the present findings also illuminated important differences in perspectives that did not emerge from the larger study. The findings in relation to the use of the PRISON metaphoric concept indicated a close alignment in the understandings of the consequences of aphasia by people with aphasia and speech-language pathologists. The absence of the use of this concept by family members in these data may indicate a useful area for family counselling in cases where it may be important for family members to recognise this aspect of the impact of aphasia. The present study was able to analyse contrasts within sets of participants as well as across types of participants, and this allowed for more in-depth analysis that points to a potentially valuable way for clinicians to gauge the extent of shared understandings with their clients.

In comparison with previous research on metaphor in the area of communication disorders (Mastergeorge, 1999), the present research found some similar themes (JOURNEY), but some of the more elaborated metaphors discussed by Mastergeorge such as those invoking fairytales were not observed. Mastergeorge's interviews focused on diagnosis experiences whereas the present research focused on the therapy experience, and so differences may well relate to this difference in focus. Also, it is not possible from Mastergeorge's account to distinguish which findings related to those participants who were family members of people with aphasia. Certainly the findings of the present research accord with the general observations made in the studies on metaphor as a reflection of stroke experience (Boylstein et al., 2007), in being both frequently occurring and informative. The present study identified two other metaphoric concepts, BATTLE and PRODUCT, which were frequently used by the participants during these interviews. Both of these concepts invite consideration as to the socio-cultural forces faced by people with aphasia, their family members, and their speech-language pathologist. From a critical discourse perspective (Fairclough, 1995), this finding raises questions regarding their experience of disempowerment within the institutional systems that mediate services following aphasia (Ferguson, 2008a).

The research to date has important limitations to consider. The case study basis of the research necessarily limits its generalisability. Further research could productively explore the sensitivity of metaphoric expression to stages of recovery (Boylstein et al., 2007; Strong, 1989), for example, exploring the nature of the metaphors used when discussing the different stages of the recovery process (acute inpatient, inpatient rehabilitation, community). However, there are some direct clinical implications of the present work, in that consideration of metaphor opens one avenue for reflection by the clinician on the alignment or otherwise between their perspectives of the rehabilitation process and those of their clients and their families.

Manuscript received 17 July 2009
Manuscript accepted 22 October 2009
First published online 15 April 2010

## REFERENCES

Alajouanine, T. (1948). Aphasia and artistic realization. *Brain, 71*(3), 229–241.

Boylstein, C., Rittman, M., & Hinojosa, R. (2007). Metaphor shifts in stroke recovery. *Health Communication, 21*(3), 279–287.

Crider, C., & Cirillo, L. (1991). Systems of interpretation and the function of metaphor. *Journal for the Theory of Social Behaviour, 21*(2), 171–195.

Faircloth, C. A., Boylstein, C., Rittman, M., Young, M. E., & Gubrium, J. (2004). Sudden illness and biographical flow in narratives of stroke recovery. *Sociology of Health & Illness, 26*(2), 242–261.

Fairclough, N. (1995). *Critical discourse analysis: The critical study of language.* London: Longman.

Ferguson, A. (2008a). *A critical discourse perspective on understandings of aphasia.* Paper presented at the Critical Approaches to Discourse Analysis across Disciplines (CADAAD) 2008, University of Hertfordshire, UK, July 10–12.

Ferguson, A. (2008b). *Expert practice: A critical discourse.* San Diego, CA: Plural Publishing.

Kertesz, A. (2006). *Western Aphasia Battery – Revised.* San Antonio, TX: Harcourt Assessment.

Kirmayer, L. J. (2000). Broken narratives: Clinical encounters and the poetics of illness experience. In C. Mattingly & L. C. Garro (Eds.), *Narrative and the cultural construction of illness and healing* (Ch.7, pp. 153–180). Berkeley, CA: University of California Press.

Kovecses, Z. (2005). *Metaphor and culture: Universality and variation.* Cambridge, UK: Cambridge University Press.

Lakoff, G., & Johnson, M. (1980). *Metaphors we live by.* Chicago: The University of Chicago Press.

Levitt, H., Korman, Y., & Angus, L. (2000). A metaphor analysis in treatments of depression: Metaphor as a marker of change. *Counselling Psychology Quarterly, 13*(1), 23–35.

Martin, J. R., & White, P. R. R. (2005/2007). *The language of evaluation: Appraisal in English.* Basingstoke, UK: Palgrave Macmillan.

Mastergeorge, A. M. (1999). Revelations of family perceptions of diagnosis and disorder through metaphor. In D. Kovarsky, J. F. Duchan, & M. Maxwell (Eds.), *Constructing (in)competence: Disabling evaluations in clinical and social interaction* (Ch.11, pp. 245–256). Mahwah, NJ: Lawrence Erlbaum Associates Inc.

Pragglejaz. (2007). MIP: A method for identifying metaphorically used words in discourse. *Metaphor and Symbol, 22*(1), 1–39.

Sontag, S. (1990). *Illness as metaphor; and, AIDS and its metaphors.* London: Penguin. [Reprint: first work originally published New York; Farrar, Straus, & Giroux, 1978. Second work originally published New York: Farrar, Straus, & Giroux, 1989.]

Strong, T. (1989). Metaphors and client change in counselling. *International Journal for the Advancement of Counselling, 12*, 203–213.

Thompson, G. (2004). *Introducing functional grammar* (2nd ed.). London: Hodder Education.

Williams, S. (1996). The vicissitudes of embodiment across the chronic illness trajectory. *Body and Society, 2*, 23–31.

Worrall, L., Davidson, B., Ferguson, A., Hersh, D., Howe, T., & Sherratt, S. (2007). *What people with aphasia want: Towards person-centered goal-setting in aphasia rehabilitation.* Paper presented at the ASHA (American Speech-Language-Hearing Association) Annual Convention, Boston, MA, November 15–17.

Worrall, L., Davidson, B., Hersh, D., Ferguson, A., Howe, T., & Sherratt, S. (2009). *Meeting the needs of people with aphasia, their families and speech-language pathologists: Tensions in the goal-setting process.* Paper presented at the Clinical Aphasiology Conference, Keystone, CO, May 26–30.

Zion, L. (2006). Out of aphasia a poet emerges. *ASHA Leader, 11*(8), 47.

# APPENDIX

### Example: Metaphorical expressions described within the metaphorical concept of BATTLE

| Examples of metaphorical expression (lexical unit in **bold italics**) | Source | Meaning in context | More basic meaning |
|---|---|---|---|
| Yes she definitely made an **impact** in my life (2 instances) | PWA/INT | affected | hit |
| **overcome** (6 instances) | PWA | recover | win |
| I'd like to help with people **throw the towel in** (2 instances) | PWA/INT | give up | indicate fight is over (also boxing SPORT) |
| **marched** her up to the bedroom | FAM | walked, led | regular step – soldier |
| (if she had to stay home with PWA all day) I'd **kill** him. | FAM | feel angry, frustrated | murder |
| She's very much a **fighter** | FAM | keeps trying | person who fights |
| These people are discharged from hospital – **bang** – get a bit of therapy and that's it | FAM | suddenly | explosion |
| So we just kept **tackling** little things (4 instances) | SLP | attempting | physically bringing to the ground |
| and have a **stab** at it | SLP | trying | thrust, pierce |
| I think that is always a **struggle** (3 instances) | SLP | difficult, requires effort | fight |
| but I don't often **bombard** them with information | SLP | provide quantity | attack with gun-fire or bombs |
| But, it was just that **wrestling** | SLP | doing something difficult | fight |
| so kind of **struck** down | SLP | unable to act | hit to the ground |
| He was **grabbing** at life himself | SLP | taking action | take hold |
| how the stroke had **pushed** him around (3 instances) | SLP | harmed | physical force |
| and **tramples** on their emotions | SLP | disregarded | step heavily, crush |
| he will face it full on like a **Sherman tank** (2 instances) | SLP | take direct action | vehicle used for war |
| You know you can't deal with cognitive fatigue because it stands up and just **blows you** (out of the) **to smithereens.** | SLP | has a major effect | explosion |
| You were **under orders**? | INT | told what to do | soldier's instructions |
| I suppose the brain has had just a **blast** from the inside (2 instances) | INT/SLP | damaged | explosion |
| He hasn't been completely **destroyed** | INT | hurt | damaged beyond repair |

APHASIOLOGY, 2010, 24 (6–8), 697–708

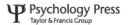

# "Let me tell you the point": How speakers with aphasia assign prominence to information in narratives

Gloria Streit Olness, Samuel E. Matteson, and Craig T. Stewart

*University of North Texas, Denton, TX, USA*

*Background*: A central purpose of narration is to convey one's point of view about a narrated event. One's expressed evaluation of a narrated event (modalising behaviour) is often differentiated from one's expression of the sequence of events proper (referential behaviour). Modalising and referential language may be dissociated in aphasia, with modalising language relatively preserved. Use of narrative evaluative devices is one way to modalise, transmit significance, or assign prominence to information in narratives.

*Aims*: This study examines the frequency of use, co-occurrence, and distribution of multiple evaluative devices in the personal narratives of speakers with aphasia, as compared to that of narratives produced by demographically similar speakers without aphasia.

*Methods & Procedures*: Participants were 33 demographically matched, English-speaking, middle-aged adults. Of these, 17 had aphasia, and 16 had no neurological disorder. Each group included similar proportions of three demographic subgroups: African-American males, African-American females, and Caucasian females. Each participant told a personal narrative of a frightening experience. Narrative evaluative devices in the narratives were analysed for their frequency, co-occurrence, and distribution in the narrative structure.

*Outcomes & Results*: The frequency of use of narrative evaluative devices, their co-occurrence, and their distribution in the narrative structure were similar for narratives of individuals with and without aphasia, unless narrative structure was compromised, e.g., in narrators with relatively more severe aphasia.

Address correspondence to: Gloria Streit Olness, University of North Texas, Department of Speech and Hearing Sciences, 1155 Union Circle # 305010, Denton, Texas 76203-5017, USA. E-mail: golness@unt.edu

Our sincere thanks to the participant volunteers, and to the facilities, institutions, and individuals who referred them: Ashley Court at Turtle Creek, Dallas; Baylor Institute for Rehabilitation; Callier (Dallas) Aphasia Group; Community Partners Program (a collaborative program of the University of Texas at Dallas and Baylor Institute for Rehabilitation); Department of Assistive and Rehabilitative Services—Division for Determination Services; Friendship West Baptist Church; Harris Methodist Forth Worth Hospital; HealthSouth Dallas Medical Center; HealthSouth Plano Medical Center; Methodist Dallas Medical Center; Mobility Foundation Stroke Center, UT Southwestern Medical School; North Texas Stroke Survivors (P. Boland); Parkland Hospital and Healthcare System; South Dallas Communication Groups Program (UTD Center for Brain Health) with Saint John Missionary Baptist Church, Jubilee UMC, St. Paul AME, and St. Luke's "Community" UMC; The Stroke Center – Dallas; the University of North Texas Speech and Hearing Center Adult Communication Therapy Program; the University of Texas at Dallas, Communication and Learning Center; Barbara Punch, Gina Jackson, and Emily Frisch; and students of the University of North Texas Department of Speech and Hearing Sciences (S. Bilton, C. Whiteside, and A. Winans). We also extend thanks to Ella Jones for her assistance with analysis. This research was supported by grants from the University of North Texas Faculty Research Grant Fund; the NIH/NIDCD (1R03DC005151-01); and the University of Texas at Dallas (Callier Center for Communication Disorders, and Dean of the School of Behavioural and Brain Sciences).

http://www.psypress.com/aphasiology     DOI: 10.1080/02687030903438524

*Conclusions*: The relatively intact ability of individuals with aphasia to assign prominence to information in narratives once again raises questions on the neurological underpinnings of modalising language. The clinical potential for assessment and treatment that incorporates narrative evaluative devices needs to be further explored.

**Keywords:** Aphasia; Discourse; Narrative; Evaluative devices; Modalising.

Narratives are ubiquitous in everyday conversations, as individuals exchange stories of their experiences and life history (Bruner, 1990; Ervin-Tripp & Küntay, 1996; Polanyi, 1989; Sacks, 1992). Personal accounts of life events are so pervasive in conversation that one finds detailed descriptions of how dyads communicate when a speaker's turn is extended for narration (e.g., Schegloff, 1982) and metaphorical reference to the human species as *Homo narrans* (Fisher, 1987, p. 62).

Consideration of the psychological, interpersonal, cultural, and societal driving forces behind narration is beyond the scope of a single study. However, the current study addresses what narratologists propose to be the core function of narrative, its *raison d'être*: to convey a point of view about an event (Labov, 1972; Polanyi, 1989). Specifically, this study examines the linguistic and intonational ways in which narrators with aphasia add prominence to selected information in their stories, to convey the narrator's personal attitude about the narrated event.

In the literature, discussion of reference making or *transmission of information* is often used to contrast with the topic of the current study, namely point-making or *transmission of significance*. For example, Polanyi (1989, p. 22) states that a narrator's two tasks are: (1) to give enough detail to events and to state the events clearly, and (2) to highlight the important information in the narrative, to add salience to it. As already noted, she sees the second of these, i.e., expressing salience or prominence, as the key task that motivates narrative telling in the first place. Likewise, in Labov's seminal work on narrative (1972), he differentiates expression of the narrative event line, i.e., expression of the "*who, what, when,* and *where*", from expression of the narrator's stance on the "*so what*", or "*why the story was told in the first place*". He terms this process of making one's point as (*narrative*) *evaluation*, and the linguistic means of narrative evaluation as *evaluative devices*.

In the aphasiology literature a similar differentiation has been made. Nespoulous, Code, Virbel, and Lecours (1998) contrast *referential behaviour* or *referential aspects of language* with *modalising behaviour* or *modalising aspects of language*. Referential (verbal) behaviour makes reference to "persons, objects, ideas, and so on" (p. 317), while modalising (verbal) behaviour conveys the speaker's personal attitude or the illocutionary force (Austin, 1962). Moreover, Nespoulous et al. propose that referential and modal types of linguistic behaviour display a dissociation in the speech production of individuals with aphasia. Building on the hypothesis that "referential language is represented in the classical language area" (p. 324), i.e., supralimbic, left hemisphere cortex, they consider clinical case evidence to examine the possibility that modalising language may be represented: (1) in the right hemisphere; (2) in the right or left hemisphere; (3) in limbic structures; or (4) some combination of the preceding, e.g., interactions between the right hemisphere and limbic system. In other literature, the notion that modalising functions may be preserved in aphasia in the face of difficulties with referential functions is supported by two studies that examine how narrators with aphasia successfully use two evaluative devices, repetition (Ulatowska,

Olness, Hill, Roberts, & Keebler, 2000) and direct speech (Ulatowska & Olness, 2003), despite the presence of aphasia.

Numerous studies and clinical approaches address referential language in aphasia. For instance, we know that core characteristics of aphasia include poor clarity of reference (Ulatowska, Allard, & Chapman, 1990) and reduced efficiency of information transmission (Nicholas & Brookshire, 1993). Likewise, significant progress has been made in our understanding of how lexical access can be treated using pictured representations of non-affective nouns and verbs. However, less work has been dedicated to understanding modalising language, such as aphasic speakers' access to emotive lexicon (e.g., Armstrong, 2005).

The current study examines the modalising function of language in narratives of speakers with aphasia, as it is manifested in the use of narrative evaluative devices during narration. To review, narrative evaluation is the process by which a speaker transforms a mere report of a sequence of events into a story that conveys the narrator's points of view, and personal and cultural values (Labov, 1972); the use of evaluative devices selectively assigns prominence to information in narrative and engages the listener (Polanyi, 1989). Prior studies of the use of narrative evaluation by narrators with aphasia have detailed use of individual evaluative devices such as repetition or direct speech (Ulatowska et al., 2000, 2003) and have examined the evaluative content of narratives of stroke (Armstrong & Ulatowska, 2007). The current study complements prior studies by examining whether and how narrators with aphasia coordinate the simultaneous use of multiple evaluative devices in narratives on emotive topics. In particular, this study examines the frequency of use, co-occurrence, and distribution of multiple evaluative devices in the personal narratives of speakers with aphasia, as compared to that of narratives produced by demographically similar speakers without aphasia.

## METHOD

### Participants

Participants were 33 English-speaking adults living in urban Texas (southern United States). Of these, 17 had aphasia (APH), and 16 had no history of neurological disorder or injury (non-brain-injured, NBI). While the gender and ethnicity of participants within each clinical group was heterogeneous, each clinical group had similar proportions of representation from three demographic subgroups. Of the 33 total participants, 11 were African-American males, 11 were African-American females, and 11 were Caucasian females. Five or six of the participants in each demographic subgroup had aphasia (APH), and five or six had no aphasia (non-brain-injured, NBI). (See Table 1.)

All were participants in a larger discourse study, from which they were selected into the two clinical groups based on similarity of age, educational background, geographic origins, and religious background, to control for the potential effects of these demographic factors on the use of evaluative devices in narrative. Most were middle-aged with a maximum education level of high school, community college, or trade school. All but five of the participants (each in a different subgroup) were reared for at least a portion of their childhoods in the southern United States, and 96% of these in Texas specifically. All participants reported being reared in the Christian faith (Protestant, Catholic, or non-denominational) and all but five (one African-American male,

TABLE 1
Participant details

| Participant group | n | Age (in years) | | Highest education level attained | | Socioeconomic status (maximum = 7) | |
|---|---|---|---|---|---|---|---|
| | | Median | Range | Median | Range | Median | Range |
| African-American males | 11 | | | | | | |
| With aphasia | 6 | 56 | 47–72 | 3 | 2–4 | 4.5 | 2–7 |
| Without aphasia | 5 | 52 | 44–66 | 3 | 2–4 | 4 | 2–4 |
| African-American females | 11 | | | | | | |
| With aphasia | 6 | 61 | 44–74 | 2.5 | 2–4 | 3 | 2–6 |
| Without aphasia | 5 | 56 | 46–68 | 4 | 1–5 | 4 | 3–7 |
| Caucasian females | 11 | | | | | | |
| With aphasia | 5 | 48 | 43–74 | 3 | 2–4 | 5 | 2–5 |
| Without aphasia | 6 | 55 | 40–67 | 3 | 3–3 | 4 | 3–5 |

Age, highest education level attained, and socioeconomic status of participants (two clinical groups in three ethnic/gender groups). Highest education level attained is specified ordinally by number; 1 = less than 12th grade, 2 = high school graduate, 3 = community college or trade school, 4 = some college, 5 = 4-year college graduate

Socioeconomic rating was adapted from Featherman & Stephens (1980); higher numbers reflect higher socioeconomic status.

one African-American female, and three Caucasian females) reported regular attendance at a place of worship.

The 17 APH participants were recruited through local speech-language pathologists and physicians. All had sustained a left-hemisphere cortical stroke with concomitant aphasia, and all were 1 year or more post onset of stroke. Based on the requirements of the larger study, exclusion criteria were: comprehension skills insufficient to understand task instructions (WAB Comprehension Subscore less than 4) and oral expression consisting of semantically "empty speech" (language ranked as 3 or less on the Boston Diagnostic Aphasia Examination rating of "word finding relative to fluency"; Goodglass, Kaplan, & Barresi, 2001). Scores on the Western Aphasia Battery, Aphasia Quotient (WAB-AQ, Kertesz, 1982) appear in Table 2, with participants ordered within demographic group by WAB-AQ score. Aphasia severity ranged from mild ($n = 5$) to mild-moderate ($n = 5$) to moderate ($n = 6$) to moderate-severe ($n = 1$). WAB-AQ scores of all but one of the NBI participants met the normal cut-off of 93.8 points (Kertesz, 1979). All NBI participants passed a self-reported screening questionnaire for neurological diseases and conditions. All participants passed hearing and vision screenings.

## Data set

*Context of discourse sample.* Participants were asked to relate a personal narrative of a frightening experience in guided conversation with a race-matched middle-aged female interviewer (previously unknown to the narrator), as one of five personal narratives told in the final portion of a larger discourse protocol. Narrators were asked to ". . . think of a time when you were frightened or scared" and to relate that event ("What happened?"). During the narration the interviewer played the role of an interested listener (Labov, 1972).

TABLE 2
APH and NBI participants

| Participants | WAB-AQ (max = 100) | Aphasia severity | Narrative length (in propositions) |
|---|---|---|---|
| African-American males | | | |
| A-APH26 | 50.4 | Moderate | 16 |
| A-APH21 | 53.8 | Moderate | 12 |
| A-APH17 | 74.8 | Mild-moderate | 8 |
| A-APH08 | 77.2 | Mild-moderate | 13 |
| A-APH11 | 89.2 | Mild | 12 |
| A-APH15 | 93.1 | Mild | 49 |
| A-NBI (n = 5) | All > 93.8 | – | 25, 31, 37, 48, 87 |
| African-American females | | | |
| A-APH22 | 50.1 | Moderate | 15 |
| A-APH27 | 52.4 | Moderate | 24 |
| A-APH04 | 59.5 | Moderate | 23 |
| A-APH23 | 80.4 | Mild-Moderate | 30 |
| A-APH03 | 92 | Mild | 32 |
| A-APH28 | 93.4 | Mild | 70 |
| A-NBI (n = 5) | All > 93.8 except one (93.6) | – | 17, 30, 36, 43, 94 |
| Caucasian females | | | |
| C-APH35 | 40.3 | Moderate-severe | 85 |
| C-APH11 | 59.6 | Moderate | 10 |
| C-APH29 | 79.2 | Mild-moderate | 24 |
| C-APH37 | 82.1 | Mild-moderate | 78 |
| C-APH 33 | 87.2 | Mild | 27 |
| C-NBI (n=6) | All > 93.8 | – | 44, 50, 51, 51, 60, 90 |

WAB-AQ scores, aphasia severity, and narrative length for APH and NBI participants, by demographic group. Participant numbers are the actual numbers assigned to participants in the larger research project. This numbering is maintained for continuity of reference to participants across studies.

*Discourse sample processing.* Narratives were audio recorded (Sony TCD-D100 digital audio tape-corder and Sony ECM-F01 omni-directional electret condenser microphone). Recordings were orthographically transcribed. The peak fundamental frequency ($F_0$) in each word was measured using Praat software (Boersma, 2001), and $F_0$ was converted to pitch interval in cents relative to the narrator's lowest $F_0$ (e.g., 1200 cents = 1 octave above lowest pitch), to reflect listener pitch perception ('t Hart, Collier, & Cohen, 1990).

*Narrative length, content, and structure.* Length of narratives in propositions (Mross, 1990) is provided in Table 2. A proposition was defined as a semantic unit consisting of the main predicate with its arguments and all embedded predicates and argument(s) associated with it. Narrative topics across all six groups included crime and threats to personal or family health, life, and safety, such as stories of stroke and heart problems, car accidents, domestic hardship and violence, and severe weather. Also included were stories of phobias, and encounters with pests and wild animals. Basic narrative structure—i.e., temporal-causal organisation, with a setting, complicating event(s), and resolution(s) (Labov, 1972)—was present in 29 of the 33 discourse samples, and of these several included a coda, an optional element (e.g., *And that was that*) which brings a narrative to closure (Labov, 1972). The discourse of three of the individuals with relatively severe aphasia had either no clear mention of a complicating event (A-APH22) or multiple mentions of the same complicating event (C-APH35; A-APH04). A-NBI22 produced a topical exposition (logically organised, non-narrative discourse) on his fear of heights in a work setting.

## Coding

*Evaluative devices per proposition.* Based on a specified list of evaluative devices (see Appendix), instances of each evaluative device were identified in the narrative of each participant. Each occurrence of an evaluative device was further coded for the proposition in which it occurred. For each proposition, the number and type(s) of evaluative devices that co-occurred in each proposition were recorded in a spreadsheet. Notably, it is not necessarily the sheer use of an evaluative device that assigns prominence to information, but rather a departure from the baseline frequency of that device in preceding utterances (Polanyi, 1989, p. 22). One should also note that gesture, facial expression, and expressive phonology, which can be used to evaluate, were not considered in this study because the data were not in a visual format, and were transcribed orthographically only. All evaluative devices considered in this study are listed in the Appendix.

The evaluative devices included in the analysis were gleaned from a subset of key works on narrative evaluation (Berman, 1997; Grimes, 1975; Johnstone, 1990; Labov, 1972, 1997; Longacre, 1996; Polanyi, 1989). To enhance theoretical coherence, the authors adapted from this same literature four categories of hypothesised ways in which evaluative devices function to add prominence to information in narratives. Each device is listed under any functional category (or categories) that the literature suggests may be associated that device. Notably, the literature mentions more than one way in which the device of repetition may function to add prominence to information, so repetition is listed under two different categories. Theoretically, any single instance of repetition may be performing both of these prominence-enhancing functions simultaneously.

One way for a speaker to add prominence to information in a narrative is to slow or suspend the progression of the narrative event line, i.e., the sequence of temporal-causally related narrated propositions that correspond to the series of events as they occurred in real life. In doing so, the speaker calls attention to that part of the narrative. An analogue in film-making is the use of slow-motion (Longacre, 1996, p. 39). For instance, the speaker or a character in the story may add commentary external to the event (*He said, "It's important."*), slow the progression by repeating information (*Uh woman uh um rude. Rude.*), or stop to address the listener directly.

A second way to add prominence to information in narrative is to intensify the information. For example, information can be repeated for emphasis (*It was in church . . . My stroke hit right here in church.*) Likewise, pitch peak contributes to perception of stress, which intensifies the content on which the peak occurs, as does onomatopoeia (*I hear, "Pow!"*). Choice of lexicon (*idiot, crazy, so calm*) as well as explanations for evaluations (*very scared . . . because no communication*) can also serve to intensify information.

A third way to add prominence to information in narrative is to use irrealis forms (Labov, 1997). Irrealis forms (such as negatives, futures, modals) are used to express (as yet) unrealised events or states. Because the number of *possible* unrealised events or states is theoretically infinite, the ones selected by the speaker for inclusion are highlighted by their very mention. For example, a speaker's choice to make a statement in the negative (*I couldn't use none of it*) highlights that an assumption about the speaker's basic abilities (or rights) has been broken. Other irrealis forms highlight assumptions that have yet to be realised, such as the future tense (*It's gonna be hard*). Any number of events or states are possible, so the possibilities that a speaker chooses to express are *de facto* evaluative.

A fourth and final way to add prominence to information in narratives is through the use of comparators. Comparisons of narrative characters, states, or events with other literal or figurative entities highlight the item undergoing comparison. For example, the statement, *the most scariest time of my life* highlights how scary that time was, by comparing it with other times in the speaker's life.

*Boundaries of narrative structural elements.* For all structural elements present in each narrative—setting, complicating event(s), resolution(s), coda; Labov,1972—the first and last propositions of each structural element were identified.

## Comparisons

*Commonality and frequency of evaluative devices.* For each device, the number of narratives that included the device at least once was tallied. Devices were compared to each other for the number of narratives in which each occurred, to distinguish common from uncommon devices. Also, the proportion of use of each device was calculated within participants: number of times a narrator used a given device, divided by the total number of times the narrator used any device. Proportion of use of each device was compared within narrators, to distinguish frequently and infrequently used devices. Both of these analyses and their associated comparisons provide information about the relative ubiquity or rarity of use of each device in these data as a whole. The more ubiquitous the device, the more important its role may be for modalising in general. This information on the relative pervasiveness of multiple devices is not available in the literature, and provides a backdrop against which the clinical group comparisons can be interpreted.

*APH vs NBI narratives.* APH and NBI narratives were compared for the proportions of narratives that included each device. Specifically, two questions were asked: Do the narratives of both groups (APH and NBI) include evaluative devices from all four of the evaluative device categories? For APH and NBI narratives, are the proportions of narratives that include a given device at least once similar or different for the two groups, as measured for each device?

APH and NBI narratives were compared for patterns of device co-occurrence within propositions. Specifically, two questions were asked: Do all narratives in both groups display instances of co-occurrence of evaluative devices within the same proposition? Where in the narrative structure (setting, complicating event, resolution, coda) are instances of device co-occurrence concentrated in the narrative structure in each group (APH and NBI)?

# RESULTS

## Commonality of evaluative devices

The evaluative devices with the highest percentage of at least one use across each of the 33 narratives were: in the category of suspension of event line, external commentary (85% of narratives), direct speech (70%), addressing listener directly (57%), and repetition of any type (97%); in the category of intensification, repetition of any type (97% of narratives), pitch peaks (100%), attributives (86%), and predicate modifiers; and in the category of irrealis, negation (94% of narratives), and modals (79%). All other devices were used in less than 50% of the 33 narratives.

The devices that formed the highest percentage of total device use within participants were repetition (up to 40% of all devices used by any given participant); pitch peak (up to 37%); external commentary (up to 32%); quotes (up to 24%); attributes (up to 20%); and modals (up to 21%). No other devices exceed 20% of the total devices used by any given participant.

## APH vs NBI narratives

*Proportion of use.* All four categories of evaluative device were represented in the narratives of each APH and NBI demographic subgroup. The degree of association between the presence or absence of each evaluative device and the presence or absence of aphasia in the narrator was assessed from data arranged a $2 \times 2$ contingency table for each device (Cramér's Coefficient C; Siegel & Castellan, 1988; $p_{crit} <$ .05). Devices for which the association was significant were: in the category of intensification, expressive lexicon, nominal ($C = 0.35$), attributives ($C = 0.36$), predicate modifiers ($C = 0.41$), and clausal qualification of an evaluation ($C = 0.35$); in the category of irrealis, modals ($C = 0.35$); in the category of comparators, non-figurative comparators with "like" and "as" ($C = 0.49$), superlatives ($C = 0.43$), and idioms ($C = 0.63$). In all instances of significant association the proportion of use was less in the APH group than in the NBI group.

*Patterns of device co-occurrence within propositions.* Narratives of all participants displayed multiple instances of co-occurrence of evaluative devices within the same proposition, e.g., negative in direct speech with pitch peaks, *(He) . . . says, "Son[1586], you don't[1637] need to go out nowhere today.".* For the 29 participants with intact narrative structure (both APH and NBI), the highest numbers of device co-occurrence within propositions were concentrated at or immediately after the complicating event, and if a coda was included, in the coda. Examples of evaluative device co-occurrence at the complicating event are provided as illustrations: (1) C-APH11 used repetition, predicate modifier, and an attributive (number) in a single proposition describing the complicating action of a husband's binge drinking: *Seven days. Seven days straight.* (2) A-NBI03 used direct speech, repetition, and pitch peak in multiple sequential propositions during the complicating action of a story of a friend's shooting: *And then (he) came out, he, "Say[2782] man[2576]! Say, that[2571] dude[2394] shot[2400], say that[2461] dude[2450] just[2371] turn[2319] around[2383] and[2307] shot[2586] John[2302] in[2222] the[2222] head[glottal fry]." And we go, "What[2985]!".* (3) C-APH29 used repetition, external commentary, and pitch peak at the end of this passage, marking the narrator's reaction to the fact that it took doctors 3 days to diagnose her stroke: *So I layed in bed for um three days. And then I had a stroke. Um, um, then they noticed I had stroke. Yeah. Yeah[917]! Oh[629]! "Oh God[749]!*

This pattern of device concentration in the complicating event for both APH and NBI groups, as well as an exception to this pattern, are illustrated in Figure 1. Figure 1 plots the number of evaluative device co-occurring across the sequential propositions of the narratives of three individuals with aphasia and one with no aphasia, relative to the location of these propositions in the narrative structure. A common pattern is seen in the data of the two individuals with relatively less severe aphasia (A and B in Figure 1) and the individual with no aphasia (C in Figure 1): the modes of evaluative device use are concentrated in complicating events, and in the coda when a coda is present. A contrasting pattern is seen in the data of the individual with moderate-severe aphasia (D in Figure 1): there is a multimodal or non-modal distribution. In other words, the mode of evaluative devices in complicating events is the same as the

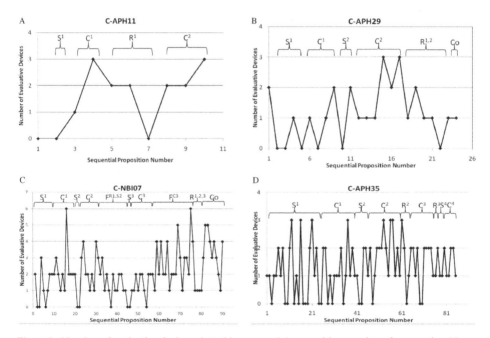

**Figure 1.** Number of evaluative devices plotted by sequential proposition number of a narrative. Narrative structural elements are "S" = Setting; "C" = Complicating event; "R" = Resolution; "Co" = Coda; "F" = Flashback. Structural elements with the same superscript are associated with each other. Flashback superscripts indicate the structural element that is being provided or supplemented by the content of the flashback. (A) Narrative of C-APH11 (moderate aphasia). Modal distribution of evaluative devices, with modes found in complicating event. Mode of evaluative devices in complicating events is greater than the mode of evaluative devices in setting and resolution associated with those complicating events. (Note: First proposition is "Abstract", an optional structural element not considered in this study.) (B) Narrative of C-APH29 (mild-moderate aphasia). Modal distribution of evaluative devices, with modes found in complicating events. Mode of evaluative devices in complicating events is greater than the mode of evaluative devices in settings and resolution associated with those complicating events. (Note: First proposition is "Abstract, an optional structural element not considered in this study.) (C) Narrative of C-NIB07 (no aphasia). Modal distribution of evaluative devices, with modes found in complicating events, in flashback associated with a complicating event, and in coda. Mode of evaluative devices in complicating events is greater than the mode of evaluative devices in settings and resolution associated with those complicating events. A mode is also found in the coda. (D) C-APH 35 (moderate-severe aphasia). Multimodal (i.e., non-modal) distribution. Mode of evaluative devices in complicating events is the same as the mode of evaluative devices in settings and resolutions associated with those complicating events.

mode of evaluative devices in settings and resolutions associated with those complicating events.

## DISCUSSION

Narrators with aphasia transmit the significance ("point") of their stories in ways very similar to narrators without aphasia. This suggests the importance of intact cognitive ability, and potential contributions of the right hemisphere and limbic systems (Nespoulous et al., 1998), to modalise and assign prominence to information in narratives. As compared with narrators with no aphasia, narrators with aphasia use qualitatively similar categories of evaluative devices, and combine and distribute them in similar places in the narrative structure, even though they may use linguistically less complex forms to perform these functions. However, use of evaluative devices may become all-pervasive and undifferentiated in narratives of those with relatively severe aphasia, i.e., when narrative referential function is poor and narrative structure is not intact. The ubiquity of repetition and pitch peaks in narratives suggests their potential importance as evaluative devices. Assessment of evaluative devices and the narrative modalising function may tease apart the relative contributions of cognition and language to narrative point-making, not only for individuals with aphasia, but also for those with clear cognitive and pragmatic involvement, e.g., individuals with traumatic brain injury and right hemisphere syndrome. Given the hypothesis of Nespoulous et al. (1998) that modalising language may be intact in aphasia and represented in the right hemisphere and limbic systems, it may be worthwhile to explore pairing of evaluative language with referential language in treatment approaches for referential language, such as lexical access treatments. This approach would be analogous to approaches such as melodic intonation therapy (MIT, Sparks, Helm, & Albert, 1974), which hypothesise that functions associated with the right hemisphere may facilitate treatment and recovery of language skills associated with the left hemisphere. Finally, relative contributions of gesture and facial expression to narrative evaluation, and the semantic coherence of evaluated information, require further exploration.

Manuscript received 24 July 2009
Manuscript accepted 25 October 2009
First published online 27 April 2010

## REFERENCES

Armstrong, E. (2005). Expressing opinions and feelings in aphasia: Linguistic options. *Aphasiology, 19*, 285–296.
Armstrong, E., & Ulatowska, H. (2007). Stroke stories: Conveying emotive experiences in aphasia. In M. J. Ball & J. S. Damico (Eds.), *Clinical aphasiology: Future directions* (pp. 195–210). New York: Psychology Press.
Austin, J. L. (1962). *How to do things with words*. Cambridge, MA: Harvard University Press.
Berman, R. (1997). Narrative theory and narrative development: The Labovian impact. *Journal of Narrative and Life History, 7*, 235–244.
Boersma, P. (2001). Praat, a system for doing phonetics by computer. *Glot International, 5*(9,10), 341–345.
Bruner, J. (1990). *Acts of meaning*. Cambridge, MA: Harvard University Press.
Ervin-Tripp, S., & Küntay, A. (1996). The occasioning and structure of conversational stories. In T. Givón (Ed.), *Conversation: Cognitive, communicative and social perspectives* (pp. 133–166). Amsterdam: John Benjamins.
Featherman, D. L., & Stevens, G. A. (1980). *A revised socioeconomic index of occupational status. Center for Demography and Ecology Working Paper 79–84*. Madison, WI: University of Wisconsin.

Fisher, W. R. (1987). *Human communication as narration: Toward a philosophy of reason, values and action.* Columbia, SC: University of South Carolina Press.

Goodglass, H., Kaplan, E., & Barresi, B. (2001). *Boston Diagnostic Aphasia Examination* (3rd ed.). Philadelphia: Lippincott, Williams, & Wilkins.

Grimes, J. E. (1975). *The thread of discourse.* The Hague, The Netherlands: Mouton.

Johnstone, B. (1990). *Stories, community, and place: Narratives from middle America.* Bloomington, IN: Indiana University Press.

Kertesz, A. (1979). *Aphasia and associated disorders: Taxonomy, localization, and recovery.* New York: Grune & Stratton.

Kertesz, A. (1982). *The Western Aphasia Battery.* Austin, TX: Pro-Ed.

Labov, W. (1972). *Language in the inner city: Studies in the black English vernacular.* Philadelphia: University of Pennsylvania Press.

Labov, W. (1997). Some further steps in narrative analysis. *Journal of Narrative and Life History, 7,* 395–415.

Longacre, R. E. (1996). *The grammar of discourse* (2nd ed.). New York: Plenum Press.

Mross, E. F. (1990). Text analysis: Macro- and microstructural aspects of discourse processing. In Y. Joanette & H. H. Brownell (Eds.), *Discourse ability and brain damage: Theoretical and empirical perspectives* (pp. 50–68). New York: Springer-Verlag.

Nespoulous, J-L., Code, C., Virbel, J., & Lecours, A. R. (1998). Hypotheses on the dissociation between "referential" and "modalising" verbal behaviour in aphasia. *Applied Psycholinguistics, 19,* 311–331.

Nicholas, L. E., & Brookshire, R. H. (1993). A system for quantifying the informativeness and efficiency of the connected speech of adults with aphasia. *Journal of Speech and Hearing Research, 36,* 338–350.

Polanyi, L. (1989). *Telling the American story.* Cambridge, MA: MIT Press.

Sacks, H. (1992). *Lectures on conversation* (Vol. 2). Cambridge, MA: Blackwell.

Schegloff, E. A. (1982). Discourse as interactional achievement: Some uses of "uh huh" and other things that come between sentences. In D. Tannen (Ed.), *Georgetown University Round Table on Languages and Linguistics. Analysing discourse: Text and talk* (pp. 71–93). Washington, DC: Georgetown University Press.

Siegel, S., & Castellan, N. J. Jr. (1988). *Nonparametric statistics for the behavioural sciences* (2nd ed.). New York: McGraw-Hill.

Sparks, R., Helm, N., & Albert, M. (1974). Aphasia rehabilitation resulting from melodic intonation therapy. *Cortex, 10,* 303–316.

't Hart, J., Collier, A., & Cohen, A. (1990). *A perceptual study of intonation: An experimental-phonetic approach to speech melody.* Cambridge, UK: Cambridge University Press.

Ulatowska, H., & Olness, G. (2003). On the nature of direct speech in narratives of African Americans with aphasia. *Brain and Language, 87,* 69–70.

Ulatowska, H., Olness, G., Hill, C., Roberts, J., & Keebler, M. (2000). Repetition in narratives of African Americans: The effects of aphasia. *Discourse Processes, 30,* 265–283.

Ulatowska, H. K., Allard, L., & Chapman, S. B. (1990). Narrative and procedural discourse in aphasia. In Y. Joanette & H. H. Brownell (Eds.), *Discourse ability and brain damage: Theoretical and empirical perspectives* (pp. 180–198). New York: Springer-Verlag.

Wennerstrom, A. (2001). Intonation and evaluation in oral narratives. *Journal of Pragmatics, 33,* 1183–1206.

# APPENDIX

Lists and examples of narrative evaluative devices included in the analysis, in each of four functional categories. Discussion of categories is found in the text.

## Category 1: Slowing or suspension of the narrative event line

(a) Addition of commentary external to the event: *This is for real!*

(b) Introduction of direct speech. In direct speech, a character may also comment on the events. (See (a) above.) Longacre (1996) states that use of direct speech also increases vividness. *He said, "It's important." I go, "Say man! John sit down!"*

(c) Addressing listener directly: *You know? That let(s) you know . . . they had somethin'!*

(d) Flashbacks or flashforwards, e.g., a mid-narrative flashback to a childhood story, to explain the fear associated with events in the current story.

(e) Repetition. (See also Category 2 below. Note that this list of repetition types excludes repetition associated with cognitive-linguistic processing difficulties, as differentiated in Ulatowska et al., 2000.)
  i. Exact repetition: *Uh woman uh um rude. Rude.*
  ii. Repetition with expansion: *It was in church . . . . My stroke hit right here in church.*
  iii. Paraphrase: *He just talked, talked . . . He was always running his mouth.*
  iv. Syntactic parallelism: *And this car was sitting there. And this guy was sitting there."*
  v. Rhyme and alliteration (not evidenced in the current study).

## Category 2: Information intensification

(a) Repetition of information (see above; also suspends narrative event line).
(b) Pitch peak. Words in which the highest pitch (in cents) was in the top 10% of pitches for a given speaker (Wennerstrom, 2001): *It seem$^{1298}$ like it took$^{1085}$ forever$^{1390}$ to get that plane stopped.* (Note: Pitch in cents is not indicated on words which are not in the top 10% of pitches.)
(c) Profanity, onomatopoeia, and non-linguistic noises: *"I hear, Pow!"*
(d) Expressive lexicon (cf. Armstrong, 2005):
  i. Nominal: *idiot.*
  ii. Verbal: *careened.*
(e) Attributives: *petrified; crazy; You're in a strange theatre . . . and here sit . . . 10, 12 boys . . .*
(f) Predicate modifiers: *so calm; all along the street.*
(g) Clausal qualification of an evaluation: *Very scared for what was going on because no communication.*
(h) Evaluative action (a reaction in the story line to something already evaluated).

## Category 3: Use of irrealis

(a) Negation: *I couldn't use none of it.*
(b) Future tense: *It's gonna be hard. It's gonna be some sick days. But we're gonna pray.*
(c) Modals: *They could've killed her; And they had to come get me.*
(d) Imperatives: *Load (th)em up.*
(e) "If/then" conditionals: *If he hit me, I was goin(g) be run o(ver) by the traffic.*
(f) Questions: *And then, why?* ('Why did I have a stroke?')
(g) Adversatives (e.g. "but"): *I was tryin(g) to wake up. But I couldn't get up.*
(h) Disjunctives (e.g., "or"): *I just didn't know . . . a good man or a bad man?*

## Category 4: Use of comparators

(a) Non-figurative comparators with "like" and "as": *"I knew that my son had not been as active as he had been before."*
(b) Superlatives: *". . . the most scariest time of my life."*
(c) Similes: *"My son looked like the elephant man."*
(d) Metaphor: *"It's a crapshoot."* (referring to life).
(e) Idioms *"Freeze on that."* (*"don't do that"*).

APHASIOLOGY, 2010, 24 (6–8), 709–724

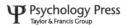

# Content analysis of the fairy tale *Cinderella* – A longitudinal single-case study of narrative production: "From rags to riches"

Jacqueline Ann Stark

*Austrian Academy of Sciences, Vienna, Austria*

*Background*: With regard to spontaneously produced speech and the oral production of a narrative, the content of the message(s) being conveyed by a person with Broca's aphasia with severe agrammatic sentence production must often be inferred from the telegraphic speech output. The clinician's inferences must often be revised to capture the intended meaning of a single utterance or sequence of utterances. When performing a formal analysis of such telegraphic utterances, researchers strive to provide an adequate reconstruction that approximates the speaker's intended meanings.

*Aims*: In this single-case study, multiple oral (re)tellings of the fairy tale *Cinderella* are analysed in terms of the *content* of the produced narratives. The aim of this study is to trace and determine how the *content* of a person with aphasia's production of this fairy tale changes over time, and to tease apart the contribution of various linguistic domains in the production of a narrative.

*Methods & Procedures*: Participant TH suffered a massive left hemisphere CVA at the age of 40 and was initially diagnosed as globally aphasic. By 36 months post onset his language impairment had evolved into Broca's aphasia characterised by agrammatic sentence production (oral and written language), mild apraxia of speech, and asyntactic auditory comprehension. He performed the task of orally (re)telling the fairy tale *Cinderella* eleven times over a 4½-year period, beginning 36 months post onset and extending to 93 months post onset of aphasia. His narratives were video- and audio-taped and the recordings were transcribed. The fairy tale *Cinderella* was interpreted in terms of its propositional content and its superstructure: orientation, development (episode 1, 2a, 2b, 3), complication (= 4), solution (episode 5), coda, and evaluation of the narrative (Labov, 2000; Labov & Waletzky, 1967). The content of TH's narratives was evaluated independently by three clinicians.

Address correspondence to: Jacqueline Ann Stark PhD, Department of Linguistics and Communication Research, Neuropsycholinguistics and Aphasia Research Unit, Austrian Academy of Sciences, Kegelgasse 27/3rd floor, 1030, Vienna, Austria. E-mail: jacqueline.stark@oeaw.ac.at

My special thanks go to Susan C. Etlinger PhD for her constructive feedback and valuable comments. This paper is dedicated to her—to a very good friend who passed away two days before I resubmitted this manuscript.

I am indebted to Heinz Karl Stark MA and Christiane Pons PhD for their assistance at various stages of this study. Márta Sarolta Viola's contribution to the first part of this study (which was published in Stark & Viola, 2007) is gratefully acknowledged. I am very grateful to TH for his time, patience, and willingness to (re)tell the fairy tale *Cinderella* preceding and following an intensive therapy protocol. I would like to thank Márta Sarolta Viola MA and Melissa Akin MA for transcribing TH's language data across time. I would also like to thank the two reviewers for their constructive comments, as well as Professor Gloria Olness PhD for her valuable feedback and suggestions on the poster presented at the 39th CAC meeting on which this study is based.

http://www.psypress.com/aphasiology                    DOI: 10.1080/02687030903524729

*Outcomes & Results*: A marked increase in the number of explicitly produced content units was observed across test times. Longitudinally, TH produced more informative narratives as evaluated in terms of propositional content units, elaborations, and evaluations. These changes in performance are attributed to TH's improved lexical retrieval for both nouns and verbs, and also to his improved syntactic skills.

*Conclusions*: Qualitative and quantitative changes in producing the *Cinderella* narrative mirror TH's improved language processing, in particular his verb retrieval and oral sentence production skills. Longitudinally, analysis of the content of narratives provides insight into the evolution of text production with reference to the influence of several linguistic domains on narrative production. In summary, content analysis of orally produced narratives provides a departure point for examining the complex roles of various linguistic domains in the process of transforming ideas into articulated sentences and narratives.

*Keywords:* Oral narrative production; Fairy tale; *Cinderella*; Content analysis; Longitudinal case study.

"What is necessary for the story of *Cinderella* to be the story of *Cinderella*? Between the traditional fairy tale and King Lear, when does the story of *Cinderella* stop being *Cinderella* and start being something else? Is a magical transformation of *Cinderella* necessary? Is the ball necessary? Is the Prince's search for *Cinderella* necessary? Is the happy ending necessary?"

(Porter Abbott, 2005, p. 19)

The above questions refer to the *content* of the fairy tale *Cinderella*. They indirectly address general and specific themes basic to verbal communication. These, according to Labov (2000), relate to being able to answer underlying questions such as: What was something about? Who? When? What? Where? So what? And then what happened? The final question being: What happened at the end? (see Labov, 2000, p. 234.) The story of *Cinderella* is just one example of a narrative that provides an opportunity to assess how well one's recollections of a past childhood experience—being told this fairy tale—can be recapitulated. Porter Abbott's (2005) questions directly address the issue of how much of the *content* of the fairy tale must be present in order for the produced narrative to still be considered the story of *Cinderella*. And although knowing the content is important, (re)producing a narrative such as a fairy tale requires a complex interaction of various processing components and linguistic levels. Ideally, the content of the fairy tale must be conceptually available and the chronological order of the series of events must be activated. Then it must be produced in the correct sequence of content units, i.e., propositions, in syntactically correct sentences consisting of semantically adequate lexical items in the correct verb tenses. The resulting narrative should be informative, coherent, and cohesive (deBeaugrande & Dressler, 1981).

When considering the oral language production of persons with a severe sentence production deficit, namely agrammatism, the cited questions become even more relevant. The intended message, or content of their messages, must often be inferred from their highly telegraphic speech output. With particular regard to text production by severely impaired agrammatic aphasic patients, the gap lessens in the process of recovery as the content of their utterances and narratives becomes richer. Assuming that the content of the fairy tale *Cinderella* is conceptually accessible, the increasing availability of information and the accessibility of word forms provide insight into *how* the processes of coordinating word forms with syntactic plans changes over time (Bock, 1987) and also how narrative production—i.e., the oral productions of the fairy tale *Cinderella*—improve across time.

In this paper the content and superstructure of 11 (re)tellings of the fairy tale *Cinderella* produced by a person with Broca's aphasia are analysed for a period of 4 years.

The main unit of analysis in this study is the *proposition*. The proposition was selected because it is a basic unit of meaning (Clark & Clark, 1977) and it is close to the conceptual level of language processing. Propositional content constitutes the *substance* of a narrative. The propositional content of the orally produced narratives was analysed with reference to the implicit or explicit production of the propositions or the omission of the propositions assumed to make up the story of *Cinderella*. The superstructure postulated for the fairy tale *Cinderella* was based on Labov and Waletzky's overall structure of a narrative. It includes the elements: abstract, orientation, complicating action, evaluation, result or resolution, and coda. The superstructure represents the "schematic organisational pattern" (van Dijk, 1989, p. 3) for the narrative. It is the more or less conventionalised hierarchically organised form of the knowledge in question. In this case it refers to the narrative *Cinderella*, i.e., the overall structure of the story of *Cinderella*. The abstract is a summary of the narrative preceding its production. The orientation corresponds to the setting for the story. In the development, the story unfolds and is broken down into the complication and solution. The complicating action is further broken down into separate episodes. The episodes constitute the main sequences of events in the story. The ordering of the episodes is fixed for certain events; however, it can also vary with regard to other episodes. The evaluation encompasses the speaker's remarks concerning specific events. The solution refers to the end of the story, and it can be followed by the coda that brings everything together and can include a final evaluation: "... and they lived happily ever after".

Labov and Waletzky's framework encompasses the overall structure of a narrative and the propositional analysis addresses the content of the individual propositions, whereby providing a means for a comprehensive assessment of story retelling. In combination, both reflect a participant's skills for using language to communicate the critical elements that are needed for a story to be a story. Thus, such an analysis comprises basic text-level elements that go beyond counting correctly produced words or analysing syntactic forms.

## METHOD

### Participant

TH is a 47-year-old, English-speaking, right-handed male, who suffered a massive left hemisphere CVA at the age of 40. His initial global aphasia evolved into Broca's aphasia. Although language data produced by TH from 36 to 93 months post onset of aphasia form the data for this study, various other language skills have been investigated starting 14.5 months post onset. At 36 months post onset, his speech was characterised by agrammatic sentence production in both the oral and written language modalities, mild apraxia of speech, and asyntactic auditory comprehension. His initial severe degree of impairment evolved into a moderate degree of impairment. (Excerpts from the transcripts of the narratives produced at 36 months post onset and at 93 months post onset are given in Appendix 1.)

## Procedure

Over a 4-year period beginning 36 months post onset, the task of orally (re)telling the fairy tale *Cinderella* was administered to TH 11 times as part of the routine language testing performed pre and post therapy.

Longitudinally the routine language testing also included the Boston Naming Test (BNT) (Kaplan, Goodglass, & Weintraub, 1983), Action Naming Test (ANT) (Obler & Albert, 1979), and an oral sentence production (SPT, *n* = 80 items) (Stark, 1997). All tasks were videotaped and simultaneously taped on an Olympus digital voice recorder (VN3100PC).

## Data analysis

The digital audio recordings of the narratives were transcribed. Several parameters of the Quantitative Production Analysis (QPA) (Berndt, Wayland, Rochon, Saffran, & Schwartz, 2000) were applied for segmenting and characterising the produced narratives in terms of the narrative words, fillers, repetitions, and false starts (initial phonemes, whole words, and short phrases).

Based on the Labov and Waletzky schema (1967; Labov 2000)—consisting of the elements: orientation, development (episode 1, 2a, 2b, 3), complication (= 4), solution (episode 5), evaluation, and coda of the narrative—a superstructure for the fairy tale *Cinderella* was determined. With regard to this schema, the abstract is not included because for the task of (re)telling a fairy tale an abstract at the beginning of the narrative is not expected. Whereas an evaluation could be produced at any point in the narrative, the coda marks the end of the fairy tale. Each of these narrative elements was further broken down into respective content units or "propositions". For the fairy tale *Cinderella*, a total of 41 possible propositions was postulated to cover the whole story. Episodes 2a and 2b are considered not to have a fixed order—they can be interchanged. Verbatim match with a proposition listed in Table 1 was not required for a proposition to be counted as explicitly produced. Rather the intended meaning of the utterance was interpreted and considered to be equivalent to the content of the proposition being scored. When the content of a proposition was incomplete, it was scored as implicitly produced. In this case the meaning of the utterance approximated the content of the proposition in question. Each of the produced narratives was evaluated independently by three clinicians with regard to the propositions that were omitted, or implicitly or explicitly produced. The inter-rater reliability was at 90%. For the units rated differently, the original transcripts were discussed to arrive at a uniform decision. The list of content units or propositions for *Cinderella* is given in Table 1 according to its overall structure.[1]

---

[1]A different source of information was used to arrive at consensus of the information healthy control participants consider to be crucial for the (re)telling of this fairy tale. Ten healthy control participants were asked to analyse the list of propositions and to determine which propositions were necessary for a summary narration of the fairy tale *Cinderella*. On a second pass, the participants were asked to slim down their initial selection to the most essential, indispensable propositions. Those propositions agreed upon by (almost) all evaluators in this second-pass analysis are considered to be the *constituent* events (Porter Abbott, 2005). The constituent elements are preceded by an asterisk in Table 1. In several cases the healthy speakers' selection of a single proposition within a section of the superstructure differed. When two or three propositions were equally important the propositions are marked by {*}. For these propositions, any one of the two or three is considered to be crucial. Actual comparison of the retelling of the narrative by healthy control participants is required, as judging which information is crucial is an entirely different task. Thus this preliminary analysis was performed to gather more information regarding the propositions in the list.

TABLE 1
List of content units or "propositions" for the fairy tale *Cinderella**

---

*Setting / Orientation*

{*} P 1 be [Cinderella]: Once upon a time // A long time ago there was a girl/woman called Cinderella

{*} P 2 live [Cinderella, with stepfamily]: Cinderella lived with her stepmother and her stepsisters

P 3 do [Cinderella, housework]: Cinderella has to do the housework

* P 4 boss around/be mean [stepsisters, Cinderella]: The (spoiled) stepsisters boss Cinderella around/ are mean to Cinderella

*Episode 1*

* P 5 invite [prince, single women, ball, palace]: The prince invites all young single women to his ball in the palace

P 6 work [Cinderella, hard] Cinderella has to work hard

* P 7 cannot go [Cinderella, to ball]: that she cannot go to the ball

P 8 dress [stepsisters /stepmother, for ball]: The stepsisters and the stepmother dress for the ball

* P 9 be sad/cry [Cinderella]: Cinderella is sad/cries

P10 leave [stepsisters/stepmother, for ball]: The stepsisters and stepmother leave for the ball in a coach

*Episode 2a*

* P11 arrive/enter [stepsisters/stepmother, at palace]: The stepsisters and stepmother arrive at/enter the palace

P12 greet [prince, guests]: The prince greets all the guests

P13 dance [guests]: (At the ball) the guests dance

P14 eat [guests]: The guests eat

*Episode 2b*

* P15 appear/be here [fairy godmother]: The fairy godmother appears/is here

P16 see/find [fairy godmother, Cinderella (crying/sad)]: The fairy godmother sees/finds Cinderella (crying/sad)

* P17 perform [fairy godmother, magic]: The fairy godmother performs magic

* P18 turn into [fairy godmother, Cinderella, enchanting woman]: The fairy godmother turns Cinderella into an enchanting woman (dressed up in a gown with glass slippers)

P19 turn into [fairy godmother, pumpkin, coach and driver]: The fairy godmother turns a pumpkin into a coach and/with a driver

P20 turn into [fairy godmother, (two) mice, horses]: The fairy godmother turns (two) mice into horses

* P21 warn [fairy godmother, Cinderella, about midnight]: The fairy godmother warns Cinderella about leaving the ball by midnight

P22 leave [Cinderella, for ball, in coach]: Cinderella leaves for the ball in the coach

*Episode 3*

P23 be/arrive [Cinderella, at palace]: Cinderella is/arrives at the palace

* P24 see [prince, with Cinderella]: The prince sees Cinderella

* P25 dance [prince, with Cinderella]: The prince/He dances with her

P26 watch [guests, Cinderella and prince]: The stepsisters/All the guests are watching them

*Episode 4 = Complication*

* P27 strike [clock, midnight]: The clock strikes midnight

P28 leave/run out of [Cinderella, palace]: Cinderella leaves/ runs out of the palace

* P29 lose [Cinderella, glass slipper]: Cinderella loses a glass slipper

* P30 find [Prince, glass slipper]: The prince finds the glass slipper

P31 be transformed into [Cinderella/coach and driver, original state]: Cinderella /the coach and the driver are transformed (back) into their original state

*Episode 5 = Solution*

P32 want [Prince, find owner]: The prince wants to find the owner of the glass slipper/Cinderella

* P33 go [Prince (and servant), from town to town/door to door]: On the following days the prince (and his servant) go from town to town/door to door

---

(Continued)

TABLE 1
(Continued)

---

\* P34 look for [Prince and servants, Cinderella]: Prince (and servant) looks (look) for Cinderella/the person whose foot fits into the glass slipper

P35 try on [stepsisters, glass slipper]: (At Cinderella's house) The stepsisters try on the glass slipper

P36 not fit [glass slipper, stepsisters]: The glass slipper does not fit the stepsisters

\* P37 try on [Cinderella, glass slipper]: Cinderella tries on the glass slipper

\* P38 fit [glass slipper, Cinderella]: The glass slipper/It fits Cinderella

*Coda*

{\*} P39 be happy/together [prince and Cinderella]: The prince and Cinderella are happy/together again

{\*} P40 marry/get married [prince and Cinderella]: The prince and Cinderella marry/get married

{\*} P41 live [prince and Cinderella, happily]: They live happily ever after

---

*Those propositions preceded by an asterisk are considered by healthy control participants to be the constituent events on a second pass analysis. In the case of two or three successive propositions marked by {\*}, one of them is considered to be a constituent event by a majority of the control participants.

After determining the presence/omission of the propositions, the transcripts of the narratives were assessed in terms of whether evaluative devices were present (cf. Olness, 2010 this issue). These devices included *information intensification, a slowing or suspension of the progression of the event line to call attention to that part of the narrative, using irrealis forms* and *the use of literal* or *figurative comparisons.*

## RESULTS

An analysis of the content units or "propositions" with respect to the number of omitted, or implicitly and explicitly produced content units for 11 recitations of *Cinderella* is given in Table 2.

For the *Cinderella* narratives produced at 36 months post onset until 56 months post onset, the number of omitted content units was high: 22, 16, 13, 14, respectively out of a possible total of 41 target units. The number of implicitly produced and explicitly produced units was comparable. As of 62 months post onset, the number of explicitly produced units showed a marked increase ($n = 20, 24, 32, 33, 28, 34,$ and 35) from an initial 12% explicitly produced units to 85%. Initially 54% of the possible target units were omitted and 34% implicitly produced. At 93 months post onset only 7.3% of the propositions were omitted and 7.3% were implicitly produced. TH's last two narratives represent his best performance. For the retelling produced at 90 months post onset, TH omitted 3, implicitly produced 4, and explicitly produced 34 out of the possible 41 target propositions. A similar performance was observed for the most recent (re)telling of *Cinderella* version at 93 months post onset: 3 were omitted, 3 implicitly, and 35 explicitly produced content units.

In terms of the number of propositions produced, although a steady improvement was observed, at 82 months post onset TH's performance was not as good as it was for the retellings at 72 and 79 months post onset. A rank ordering of the 11 (re)tellings in terms of overall performance is given in Appendix 2. At 82 months post onset he implicitly stated the propositions for Episode 2b; namely, the propositions regarding the magical transformations. Across time, the scores for the BNT, ANT, and orally produced sentences (Sent.Prod./SPT) depicted in Figure 1 show a steady increase in

TABLE 2
Content analysis

| Structure / Months post onset | Setting/Orientation (n = 4 Prop.)* | | | Development Episode 1 (n = 6 Prop.) | | | Development Episode 2^a (n = 4 Prop.) | | | Development Episode 2b (n = 8 Prop.) | | | Development Episode 3 (n = 4 Prop.) | | | Complication Episode 4 (n = 5 Prop.) | | | Solution Episode 5 (n = 7 Prop.) | | | Coda (n = 3 Prop.) | | | Total propositions (n = 41) [percent] | | |
|---|---|---|---|---|---|---|---|---|---|---|---|---|---|---|---|---|---|---|---|---|---|---|---|---|---|---|---|
| | Om | Imp | Expl | Om | Imp | Expl | Om | Imp | Expl | Om | Imp | Expl | Om | Imp | Expl | Om | Imp | Expl | Om | Imp | Expl | Om | Imp | Expl | Om | Imp | Expl |
| 36 | 2 | 1 | 1 | 6 | 0 | 0 | 1 | 2 | 1 | 3 | 5 | 0 | 1 | 1 | 2 | 2 | 3 | 0 | 5 | 2 | 0 | 2 | 0 | 1 | 22 [53.7] | 14 34.1 | 5 12.2 |
| 41 | 1 | 2 | 1 | 1 | 4 | 1 | 4 | 0 | 0 | 2 | 6 | 0 | 2 | 2 | 0 | 3 | 1 | 1 | 3 | 3 | 1 | 0 | 1 | 2 | 16 [39.0] | 19 46.3 | 6 14.6 |
| 48 | 1 | 2 | 1 | 3 | 2 | 1 | 2 | 0 | 2 | 2 | 5 | 1 | 2 | 1 | 1 | 1 | 3 | 1 | 2 | 5 | 0 | 1 | 1 | 1 | 14 [34.1] | 19 46.3 | 8 19.5 |
| 56 | 1 | 2 | 1 | 2 | 3 | 1 | 2 | 0 | 2 | 2 | 4 | 2 | 2 | 2 | 0 | 1 | 2 | 2 | 3 | 2 | 2 | 0 | 3 | 0 | 13 [31.7] | 18 43.9 | 10 24.4 |
| 62 | 1 | 1 | 2 | 0 | 4 | 2 | 2 | 0 | 2 | 0 | 1 | 7 | 3 | 0 | 1 | 2 | 2 | 1 | 2 | 1 | 4 | 0 | 1 | 2 | 10 [24.4] | 10 24.4 | 21 51.2 |
| 69 | 0 | 1 | 3 | 0 | 1 | 5 | 2 | 1 | 1 | 1 | 1 | 6 | 1 | 0 | 3 | 3 | 1 | 1 | 2 | 1 | 4 | 0 | 2 | 1 | 9 [22.0] | 8 19.5 | 24 58.5 |
| 72 | 0 | 1 | 3 | 0 | 1 | 5 | 0 | 1 | 3 | 1 | 0 | 7 | 0 | 0 | 4 | 2 | 0 | 3 | 2 | 0 | 5 | 1 | 0 | 2 | 6 [14.6] | 3 7.3 | 32 78.0 |
| 79 | 0 | 1 | 3 | 0 | 1 | 5 | 0 | 0 | 4 | 0 | 1 | 7 | 0 | 1 | 3 | 1 | 1 | 3 | 2 | 0 | 5 | 0 | 0 | 3 | 3 [7.3] | 5 12.2 | 33 80.5 |
| 82 | 0 | 1 | 3 | 0 | 2 | 4 | 0 | 0 | 4 | 1 | 3 | 4 | 0 | 0 | 4 | 1 | 1 | 3 | 2 | 1 | 4 | 0 | 1 | 2 | 4 [9.8] | 9 22.0 | 28 68.3 |
| 90 | 0 | 0 | 4 | 0 | 1 | 5 | 0 | 0 | 4 | 0 | 0 | 8 | 0 | 1 | 3 | 1 | 2 | 2 | 2 | 0 | 5 | 0 | 0 | 3 | 3 [7.3] | 4 9.8 | 34 82.9 |
| 93 | 0 | 0 | 4 | 0 | 1 | 5 | 0 | 0 | 4 | 0 | 0 | 8 | 0 | 0 | 4 | 1 | 1 | 3 | 2 | 1 | 4 | 0 | 0 | 3 | 3 [7.3] | 3 7.3 | 35 85.4 |

Content analysis of the fairy tale Cinderella for 11 recitations according to the number of omitted, implicitly versus explicitly produced target propositions (Prop.) based on a breakdown of the superstructure into 41 target units. *The notation (n = x Ps) stands the total number of postulated target content units or "propositions" for the particular section of the fairy tale Cinderella. The overall number of postulated target propositions for a complete retelling of the fairy tale Cinderella is 41. For example, four propositions are postulated to make up the setting. At 36 months post onset, 2 out of the 4 propositions were omitted, 1 was implicitly and 1 explicitly produced.

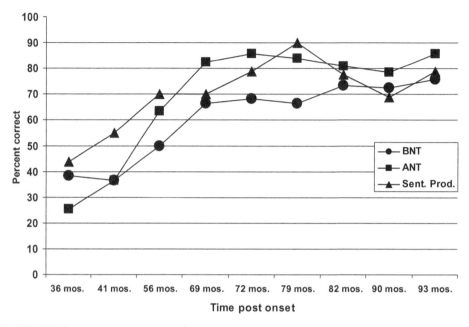

**Figure 1.** Longitudinal language test results for object naming (Boston Naming Test, BNT), verb naming (Action Naming Test, ANT), and for an oral sentence production task (Sent. Prod.) from 36 to 93 months post onset.

TH's abilities to retrieve nouns and verbs, and in producing grammatically correct sentences. As shown in Figure 1, TH's object naming (BNT) increased from 33% to 76% correct. His verb naming performance shows a similar pattern (22% to 86 % correct).

In Figure 2 the overall distribution of narrative words, fillers, repetitions, and false starts (phonemes, whole words, or phrases) is provided over time. The percentage increased from 40% (41 months post onset) of the total produced words to between 65% (93 months post onset) and 68% (at 82 and 90 months post onset). The percentage of fillers decreases over time, but the absolute number is still high even at 93 months post onset. Quantitatively speaking, according to the criteria put forward in QPA (Berndt et al., 2000), the increase in the total number of narrative words produced by TH depicted in Figure 2 highlights the longitudinal changes in lexical retrieval for narrative production. In terms of actual numbers, TH produced 209 narrative words in his first retelling at 36 months post onset. The number of narrative words increased over retellings from 209 to 1660: 209 →180 → 349 → 448 → 450 → 653 → 774 → 962 → 915 → 1202 to 1660 narrative words in his last retelling. The number of fillers remained high. However, the initial lengthy pauses were greatly reduced and his speech output became more fluent. At 41 months post onset TH produced the shortest narrative. With the exception of the first two retellings, a continuous increase in the number of narrative words produced over time was observed. Overall the number of narrative words produced per minute also showed an increase, although the rate showed more variation across retellings. In Table 3 the speaking time for each narrative and the number of narrative words produced per minute are summarised.

To exemplify the overall changes in the word production, the total number of produced words and the number of different words are presented in Table 4 for narrative words, verbs, and nouns for four retellings of *Cinderella* at 36, 56, 72, and 93 months

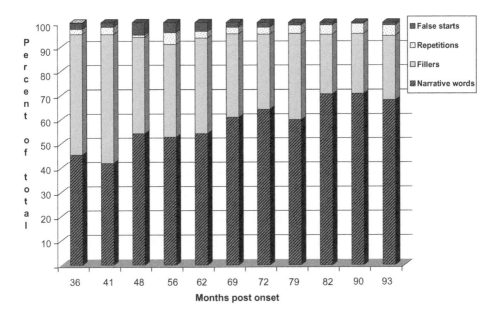

**Figure 2.** Overall distribution of narrative words, fillers, repetitions, and false starts expressed as percentage of the total words/forms produced for 11(re)tellings of the fairy tale *Cinderella* according to months post onset.

TABLE 3
Number of narrative words produced per minute according
to months post onset

| Months post onset | Number of narrative words Produced | Speaking time for narrative (minutes) | Narrative words produced per minute |
|---|---|---|---|
| 36 | 209 | 8.83 | 23.7 |
| 41 | 180 | 9.7 | 18.5 |
| 48 | 349 | 13.12 | 26.6 |
| 56 | 448 | 15.88 | 28.2 |
| 62 | 450 | 16.15 | 27.9 |
| 69 | 653 | 19.5 | 33.5 |
| 72 | 774 | 22.26 | 34.8 |
| 79 | 962 | 29.5 | 32.6 |
| 82 | 915 | 32.0 | 28.6 |
| 90 | 1202 | 34.5 | 34.8 |
| 93 | 1660 | 50.36 | 33.0 |

post onset. In comparison to TH's first Cinderella narrative, he produced 10 times more different verbs in his most recent retelling at 93 months post onset. With reference to nouns, he produced approximately four times more different nouns in his most recent narrative in contrast to his first one at 36 months post onset.

Regarding the content of the narratives, the increased number of produced propositions, the overall number of narrative words, verbs, and nouns produced by TH, as well as the number of different narrative words, verbs, and nouns, illustrate the marked changes in TH's ability to convey the content of the fairy tale *Cinderella* across time.

TABLE 4
Four retellings of *Cinderella*

| Months post onset | Total narrative words | Different narrative words | Total verbs | Different Verbs | Total nouns | Different nouns |
|---|---|---|---|---|---|---|
| 36 | 209 | 59 | 22 | 7 | 70 | 28 |
| 56 | 448 | 115 | 73 | 30 | 119 | 44 |
| 72 | 774 | 158 | 119 | 40 | 169 | 61 |
| 93 | 1660 | 287 | 298 | 69 | 400 | 98 |

Total number of narrative words, verbs, and nouns, and different narrative words, verbs, and nouns produced for four retellings of *Cinderella* at 36, 56, 72, and 93 months post onset.

## DISCUSSION

Longitudinal analysis of the content of narratives provides insight into the evolution of text production with reference to the possible influence of the accessibility of information (e.g., conceptual accessibility, lexical accessibility, and lexical selection) (Bock, 1987). With regard to the production of a fairy tale, the content is constrained by the story on the one hand. (This constraint sets the fairy tale apart from the personal narrative.) On the other hand, as a text-level task, the overall length is not constrained, neither are the possibilities to elaborate on the text and to use evaluative devices. Thus, language data obtained from this task provide an opportunity for observing changes in content and also in form, i.e., syntactic structure. In this context, the ramifications of improved lexical retrieval for both nouns and verbs are most prominent for this text-level task. As performance on both naming tasks improved, it is difficult to determine the main effect of a single grammatical category on TH's narrative production. Taken together, the language data summarised in Figure 1 and Tables 2, 3, and 4 support the assumption that when lexical retrieval improves, the ability to produce a narrative will also show marked changes in content.

Producing a narrative such as a fairy tale without the use of picture elicitation stimuli requires access to and mobilisation of numerous linguistic as well as memory skills. It is a more difficult task than describing what is depicted in a single picture or a sequence of pictures. In this study, prior to the production of the fairy tale, TH was not shown any picture booklet, which might have helped to activate various content units (cf. QPA test booklet or the AphasiaBank test protocol). Thus his performance can be seen as improved language skills on the word to sentence level and possibly better recall of details of the story.[2] TH's first *Cinderella* narrative at 36 months post onset is highly agrammatic, although his lexical retrieval for verbs and nouns improved in the first 35 months, as demonstrated by his language test scores for BNT, ANT, and oral sentence production. TH's most recent narrative (93 months post onset) exemplifies his present performance level in terms of syntactic structure, semantics, text coherence, and cohesion. In his final version, all of the constituent propositions listed in Table 1 were either implicitly or explicitly produced.

The overall structure (i.e., the superstructure) of TH's narratives is intact in all 11 retellings of the *Cinderella* story. The main parts of the narrative are present,

---

[2]TH was tested on the Pointing Span for Noun-Verb Sequences (Task 60 from the PALPA; Kay, Lesser, & Coltheart, 1992). Initially he pointed to two names. His performance improved to five items, i.e., he managed to correctly point to sequences consisting of five names or SVO/SV structures.

although initially in a very telegraphic form. In the first versions, the typical introduction and ending of a fairy tale, i.e., "once upon a time" and "they lived happily ever after" were produced in a "telegraphic" form. In the last versions, TH began the fairy tale with "A long time ago" and "one day in the country". In those versions, he ended the fairy tale with "The new bride and uh prince happy after" or "We are enjoy the rest of the life ... The two people going out in the cart [=coach] and driving a long way. The end". There were only two instances in which all of the postulated propositions for a specific part of the superstructure were omitted: In his first *Cinderella* narrative, all six propositions of Episode 1, and in his second version, none of the content units for Episode 2a were produced.[3] In all of the retellings he did not produce every one of the constituent elements, i.e., those content units considered by the healthy control participants to be essential. However, he did produce a majority of the content units highlighted in Table 1, although the individual units varied across the test times. (Although it is a very different task, healthy control participants show great variation in their judging of the essential content units on a first pass basis. See footnote 1.)

Although TH's first retellings from 36 to 56 months post onset are agrammatic, since elements from each part of the superstructure were present, a primary text-level impairment can be ruled out. A primary text-level impairment would entail a mis-ordering of relevant information, e.g., presenting the solution before the complicating action(s). In contrast, it is difficult to decide whether a *primary* text-level impairment is present when whole parts of the superstructure that contain crucial information are missing. When whole sequences are omitted, e.g., the scene at the ball culminating in the loss of the glass slipper, the source of the problem could be a recall problem or severe word-finding difficulties. However, in this case the textuality criteria including cohesion, coherence, situationality, and informativity are violated (de Beaugrande & Dressler, 1981).

Over time, the content of TH's narratives has become richer, i.e., more informative as evaluated in terms of propositional content units, elaboration of the content of propositions, and the use of evaluative devices. These changes are assumed to be due mainly to his overall improvement in lexical retrieval, in particular his verb retrieval as shown in Figure 1. Although many of TH's utterances are still agrammatic even at 93 months post onset, an improvement in terms of their syntactic structure was observed. Grammatically correct complex sentences in various tenses were observed in the most recent narratives. This is assumed to be the carryover of a therapy effect to the test situation. The intensive therapy provided to TH emphasised lexical retrieval for verbs and nouns in a natural setting of oral sentence production (cf. Stark, 2010). In later protocols the programme was expanded to include work on various tenses (simple past and future) and negation (as of therapy protocol VI), and the development and production of mini-dialogues based on the content of the individual sentences worked on in therapy (as of therapy protocol V). The determining factor for the marked changes in TH's narrative performance is considered to be the long-term build-up and continual improvement of his language skills as a result of the intensive language therapy in which he participated in the chronic phase. This process is discussed in Stark (2010). Often the selection of the picture stimuli and/or topic for the therapy

---

[3]See Footnote 1. Episode 2a was not judged by healthy control participants to be crucial for the story of *Cinderella*. In this regard, TH's produced narratives comply with the control participants' judgement of the most important propositions. It must be stressed that, in contrast to orally producing the narrative *Cinderella,* judging which propositions are crucial for the story of *Cinderella* is a different task.

sessions was based on TH's own suggestions. This made the content of the sessions relevant for his everyday verbal communication. The content of the trained materials stemmed from his life situation and was directly put to use outside the therapy setting. This point is alluded to as it is considered to have an overall effect on TH's verbal communicative abilities.

In terms of the content of the narratives, particular target content units were never produced by TH (e.g., P31, P35, P36) and one important unit was not explicitly produced (P5) even in his most recent version—namely that the prince invites all eligible females to the ball. The implicit formulation encompassed a reference to the ball being given by the prince and that the stepsisters talk about going to the ball. In most cases, when a content unit was omitted in his recitation the initial omission evolved into the implicit production of that content unit in a following version or versions. Further improvement resulted in the explicit mention of the content. One specific aspect of all of TH's versions that differed from the original version was that he systematically referred to three stepsisters. The stepmother was never mentioned. Due to this systematic mention, this departure from the story line was not considered an error. The investigator did not make TH aware that the stepmother was missing, in order *not* to change the test situation for future (re)tellings.

Support for the idea that TH has not overlearned or learned the fairy tale by heart from retelling to retelling is that there is variation in the propositions produced over time and also in the manner in which they are produced: implicitly or explicitly. Although it is difficult to characterise the actual use of gestures and mimics in words, this also varied for the retellings across time. TH's gesturing added to the content of the produced text at very crucial points in the narrative. It functioned as a substitute for specific events that were difficult for TH to formulate in words, and as a way of intensifying the presented information. The intensity of the magic performed by the fairy godmother and the verbal behaviour (i.e., slurred speech) of the inebriated sister at the ball are two of the examples for which TH used gestures to communicate very effectively the content of specific propositions, e.g., in the seventh retelling:

> Oh no! Godmother! Wow! Jesus! Uh . How are you? Fine. Uh um please old jeans and shirt and not funny. Uh maybe new dress and slippers and uh…uh. Hair and uh hat? Yes please, please. Alright wait! [With his eyes closed and waving his left arm as if performing magic, TH makes inarticulate sounds to imitate magical sounds] New dress! Wow! Oh Jesus! Amazing! Fantastic! Wow! You are unbelievable! Wow! And alright.. wait, wait Hooh! [same as above; makes inarticulate sounds to imitate performing magic] Slippers! Wow! Oh you are amazing, wow! Slippers and uh [...] Out in the garden .. uh two mice, alright? Wait [same as above, TH makes inarticulate sounds as if performing magic] Yes, horses! Yes! Wow! And wait, wait. Ah pumpkin, yes, alright [same as above, TH makes inarticulate sounds as if performing magic] Oh, carriage! Wow!

In the process of producing passages such as the above example, TH becomes very emotional and exuberant. He makes use of gestures (i.e., waving his arm), mimics (i.e., closing his eyes), and "language" (i.e., inarticulate sounds) each time he presents the magical scene with the fairy godmother. He also uses direct speech to highlight the roles of the various persons in the narrative (cf. Tannen, 1989). The alternating use of language and gestures demonstrates that the task is a dynamic one and one utterance/ gesture leads to another: "Utterances are not just static verbal objects but ongoing dynamic accomplishments, that is, forms of action" (van Dijk, 1989, p. 3). TH's changes in narrative production illustrate this point very well. Analysis of TH's text production with regard to the relationships among various sign systems in building up predicate-case role(s)—in particular between verbal and nonverbal behaviour—is planned, in particular the parasemantic function of gesturing in text production (see Stark, Bruck, & Stark, 1988).

Several themes or elaborations are repeated throughout the narrative, especially in the later and lengthier versions. For several target units TH produced elaborations for the propositions that reflect his sometimes exaggerated interpretation of the fairy tale. For example, one of the stepsisters was considered to be inebriated as of the seventh retelling of the fairy tale; that is, as of 72 months post onset (retelling at 93 months post onset):

> And the one sister .. 'I had. Uh drinking uh wine and uh yes, very good' [imitates the drunken sister] and one sister: 'Leave it alone alright! I will drink uh champagne, alright [TH laughs] Yes' The sisters had a difficult time at the table with drinking." [...] Uh one sister: 'You will not even uh with Prince, alright! And the Cinderella says: 'You are drinking a lot of wine. Sit down and where's two sisters?' And the one sister: 'You will not even uh talk with .. the prince, alright? [imitates the drunken sister]...

Longitudinal analysis of the narratives also demonstrates how achieved gains in everyday language use are carried over to the task of (re)telling *Cinderella*. TH put his everyday, accessible vocabulary to use by attributing his household activities to Cinderella's daily routine, e.g., ironing, vacuuming, etc. The content units of TH's narratives were adapted to accommodate his more accessible lexical units and a more modern version of the fairy tale. In the last narrative, TH comments that "Then Cinderella and prince both had sex".

At 36 months post onset, TH's narratives were highly agrammatic. Based on the form and content of the narratives, and also on the manner of producing them (e.g., hesitations, filled and unfilled pauses, etc.), it is evident that the task was a difficult one for him (see Figure 2). He searched for the words to capture the content of the story he wanted to tell in the context of his word-finding difficulties for both nouns and verbs. His articulatory difficulties contributed to the overall task difficulty. In later retellings, especially in the last four narratives, TH made use of several evaluative devices. TH became the "storyteller" he had probably been prior to his stroke.[4] In the later versions, evaluation was more prominent throughout the narrative (as of 90 months post onset). Of the four devices discussed by Olness (2010 this issue, and Labov, 2000; see also Tannen, 1989), TH's narrative skills showed a predominance of the use of the second device *information intensification*. That is, by means of repetition of information (e.g., "Waiting and waiting and waiting", "knocking and knocking on the door", "please! please!"), pitch maxima especially for the magical scene, and for the coda, the use of direct speech in asking and answering specific questions, he emphasised parts of his narrative. The first device, *a slowing or suspension of the progression of the event line to call attention to that part of the narrative* was also evident in his later versions, e.g., by means of repetition of information and to a lesser degree by addressing the listener directly (Olness, 2009, 2010 this issue).

---

[4]This assertion is based on his professional background and information from family members and friends. Professionally TH worked as a radio announcer and moderator. He had his own radio programmes for which he was responsible for the entire content. Family members reported that he was the one who could entertain company and hold an audience.

The last two devices of narrative evaluation—*using irrealis forms* and *the use of literal or figurative comparisons*—were not yet observed in his narratives. In the last three versions, approximations were present in his narratives; however, the first two forms were more prevalent throughout the produced narratives. TH has begun to use the future tense, the past tense/past progressive tense, and modals in specific questions, e.g., "Would you ... and me ... uh marry each other?" Examples of metaphor, similes, and real superlatives were not found in the produced narratives. It must be stressed that these two forms of evaluative devices also require a greater command of linguistic skills. Qualitatively speaking, TH's first production of Cinderella at 36 months post onset compared with the latest reveals an increased number of more complete utterances also in direct speech and the use of interrogative pronouns.

Elaborations to the text and evaluations are considered to result from TH's enhanced lexical processing. For the first four retellings (36 to 56 months post onset) it is often difficult to decide whether a proposition is even implicitly produced. This may be an indication that those content units are conceptually inaccessible. Elaborations and repetitions of particular information are made to both relevant content units (e.g., cleaning the house, performing magic) as well as to irrelevant ones ("the guests are eating, drinking, joking, laughing ...").

In summary, longitudinal analysis of the content of TH's narratives provides insight into the complexity of text processing and reveals how the initial gap between the assumed meaning of messages and the actually produced utterances lessens over time as a function of improved linguistic skills (conceptual accessibility, lexical accessibility, lexical retrieval) and syntactic skills that, metaphorically speaking, have evolved "from rags to riches".

Manuscript received 3 August 2009
Manuscript accepted 1 December 2009
First published online 19 April 2010

## REFERENCES

Berndt, R. S., Wayland, S., Rochon, E., Saffran, E., & Schwartz, M. (2000). *Quantitative production analysis*. Hove, UK: Psychology Press.

Bock, J. K. (1987). An effect of the accessibility of word forms on sentence production. *Journal of Memory and Language, 26*, 119–137.

Clark, H. H., & Clark E. V. (1977). *Psychology and language: An introduction to psycholinguistics*. New York: Harcourt Brace Jovanovich.

deBeaugrande, R., & Dressler, W. (1981). *Einführung in die Textlinguistik*. Tübingen: Niemeyer.

Kaplan, E., Goodglass, H., & Weintraub, S. (1983). *Boston Naming Test, second edition*. Philadelphia: Lea & Febiger.

Kay, J., Lesser, R., & Coltheart, M. (1992). *PALPA: Psycholinguistic Assessments of Language Processing in Aphasia*. Hove, UK: Lawrence Erlbaum Associates Ltd.

Labov, W. (2000). The transformation of experience in narrative. In A. Jaworski & N. Coupland (Eds.), *The discourse reader* (pp. 221–235). London: Routledge.

Labov, W., & Waletzky, J. (1967). Narrative analysis: Oral versions of personal experience. In J. Helm (Ed.), *Essays on the verbal and visual arts*. Seattle: University of Washington Press.

Obler, L. K., & Albert, M. L. (1979). *Action Naming Test* (experimental ed.). Boston, MA:VA Medical Center.

Olness, G. (2009, May). *"Let me tell you the point": How speakers with aphasia assign prominence to information in narratives*. Poster presented at the 39th Clinical Aphasiology Conference, Keystone, Colorado.

Olness, G., Matteson. S., & Stewart, C. (2010). "Let me tell you the point": How speakers with aphasia assign prominence to information in narratives, *Aphasiology, 24*(6–8), 697–708.

Porter Abbott, H. (2005). *Narrative*. Cambridge, UK: Cambridge University Press.

Stark, J. (1997). *ELA Sentence Production Task*. Unpublished ms.

Stark, J. (2010). Long-term analysis of chronic Broca's aphasia: An illustrative single case. *Seminars in Speech and Language, 31*, 5–20.

Stark, H. K., Bruck, J., & Stark, J. (1988). Verbal and nonverbal aspects of text production in aphasia. In E. Scherzer, R. Simon, & J. Stark (Eds.), *Proceedings of the First European Conference on Aphasiology*. (pp. 121–129). Vienna: Austrian Workers' Compensation Board.

Stark, J., & Viola, M. S. (2007). Cinderella, Cinderella! – Longitudinal analysis of qualitative and quantitative aspects of seven tellings of Cinderella by a Broca's aphasic. *Brain and Language, 103*(1–2), 234–235.

Tannen, D. (1989). *Talking voices: Repetition, dialogue and imagery in conversational discourse*. Cambridge, UK: Cambridge University Press.

Van Dijk, T. A. (1989). *Handbook of discourse analysis: Volume 2. Dimensions of discourse*. London: Academic Press.

# APPENDIX 1

Excerpts from the original transcripts of the *Cinderella* narratives.

*Retelling at 36 months post onset*

*Setting:* Uh...the...house is...uh...two...uh...too...uh...s...uh s...[ ]spe// uh sep...[J: step-]

T: step uh...uh...sep...sep...sisters, yes. [..] And uh...uh..the uh...uh.. (sighs) uh the uh Cindererra is...uh washing... and ironing... and uh mop and uh... uh.. sweeping, yes? And uh... and the step- sisters.. in the big big uh..uh...big palace, yes?

*Episode 2b:* And um.. uh...and um.. the..f.. f uh... the... fairy..fairy g//.godmother.. is...wish and..uh...uh...Cindererra is..here... and uh.. uh... dress and shoes...and earrings. and.. yes! And uh..uh...mouse and uh...horse: ah yes! And uh..uh...carriage and um.. uh...man, yes?

*Solution and Coda:* Land, yes! And uh...uh...pl uh...hm... uh...uh...uh...palace uh no... um...pi uh...pl...oh...sorry...oh...and uh...uh..guy..no! Yes! Uh...the...shoe is..here! And.. Cill// uh Cillelella is...no! Oh! Yes! Thank you! And uh...the.. uh...pl// uh plink? No....prince is here and uh...and uh... Cinelella and..prince happy. Yes!

*Retelling at 93 months post onset*

*Setting:* One day in the country uh .. three sisters and wonderful uh Cinderella in the uh farm. And Cinderella asked one sister about uh. going to the big uh.. palace. Alright?

*Episode 2b:* And.. one minute later.. god fairy uh prise "Wow!" [7] Cinderella was shocked. And "you! Wow! How are you?" "Good!" The godmother was wa- waving and uh. the.. godmother asked "How are you? Good? You will uh..You will uh clean out with uh.. uhm..." Wait! "You will change.. the dress uh [8] amazing dress. And slippers and earrings and crown. Alright? Very nice with wonderful dress. And and! Then you will uh go out in the uh coach and uhm.. nice. uh. uh. mouses and uh nice uhm uh.. pumpkin. Yes. And and horses! Wooah! Very good. And two uh- two coaches with uh.. [9] two coaches with uh guys. Alright? Very good." And Cinderella was shocked and uh.. shocked and uh.. surprise. "Me? Me? Uh thank you for the wonderful dress and new uh.. uh.. crown and slippers and wonderful earrings and oh! Thank you for the wonderful moment. Yes." and the godmother is uh [10] standing up and she was uh...making a wish and (strange noises imitating magical sounds) ooooh! Beautiful dress! Woah! Yes! Alright! Wohoo! And the Cinderella was unbelievable with uh. new clothes. Wow! Hohoho! Amazing. Uh.. and the godmother.. uh says "Go up and uh.. uh and uh.. and. d- get dressed, alright? [11] And uh one- four five minutes.. you will uh.. you will uh.. be uh wonderful prince yes? Princess. And uh…uh.. out in the uh.. yard uh.. you will uh go out in the garden and see. Alright?" And the uh.. Cinderella was upstairs cleaning and bathroom and uh uh wonderful uh..[12] uh time uh.. with wonderful dress and slippers and earrings and crown. And.. then.. they were out in the garden and…unbelievable coach. What…with uh.. uh.. coat.. coat? No. Coat? J: Coach. T: Coach yes. And new horses and new uh.. wonderful guys. Wooah! Nice. And the uh uh…the [13] godmother says "Come here. Uh.. you will go out in the town and uh beautiful princess. Alright? And and.. uh.. midnight.. you will uh.. go…uh. out in the uh here. Alright? Alright? Don't be long. Alright?"

*Coda:* Then Cinderella and prince both had sex. (laughs) And [48] uh.. the three sisters "Oh.. oh.. uh.. no! No! Please! No! I want to uh.. try with uh…one slipper, please!" and the prince "No. Sorry. You and two sisters go and uh.. in the kitchen in the barn uh.. have a wonderful day. Alright?" and.. uh…"We are enjoy the rest of the life, alright? [49] and uh.. Cinderella please, marry me? Yes?" Oh no! And the Cinderella is tall and handsome and the.. two uh.. two.. people.. going out in the cart and driving.. a long way. [] Oh Jesus! …They…was.. they did uh.. wonderful [50] uh.. honey uh.. moon.

## APPENDIX 2

The overall ranking of the *Cinderella* narratives for the 11 (re)tellings based on the omitted, or implicitly or explicitly produced content units

### Descriptive statistics

| Rank order for retelling of the narrative according to months post onset | N (total no. of possible props.) | Minimum (omitted) | Maximum (explicitly) | Mean | Standard deviation |
|---|---|---|---|---|---|
| 36 | 41 | .00** | 2.00** | .5854 | .70624 |
| 41 | 41 | .00 | 2.00 | .7561 | .69930 |
| 48 | 41 | .00 | 2.00 | .8537 | .72667 |
| 56 | 41 | .00 | 2.00 | .9268 | .75466 |
| 62 | 41 | .00 | 2.00 | 1.2683 | .83739 |
| 69 | 41 | .00 | 2.00 | 1.3659 | .82934 |
| 82 | 41 | .00 | 2.00 | 1.5854 | .66991 |
| 72 | 41 | .00 | 2.00 | 1.6341 | .73335 |
| 79 | 41 | .00 | 2.00 | 1.7317 | .59264 |
| 90 | 41 | .00 | 2.00 | 1.7561 | .58226 |
| 93 | 41 | .00 | 2.00 | 1.7805 | .57062 |

**The variables for this ranking were: 0 = omitted proposition, 1 = implicitly produced proposition, and 2 = explicitly produced proposition. The ranking is based on the values for the 41 possible propositions listed in Tables 1 and 2. Thus the minimum score for an omitted proposition is 0 and the maximum score of 2 is given for an explicitly produced proposition.

APHASIOLOGY, 2010, 24 (6–8), 725–736

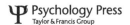

# Constraint induced language therapy in early aphasia rehabilitation

Melanie Kirmess

*University of Oslo, Norway*

Lynn M. Maher

*University of Houston, TX, USA*

*Background*: Constraint induced language therapy (CILT) focuses on improving acquired expressive language deficits after stroke by applying intensive, use-dependent treatment with constraint to spoken verbal expression. Most CILT research has utilised individuals with chronic aphasia, and previous results indicated improvement on the language assessments after intervention that was largely retained at follow-up.

*Aims*: The purpose of this study was to explore the applicability and outcome of a programme of CILT in individuals in the early phase of recovery from aphasia (1–2 months post onset) in an inpatient rehabilitation hospital setting.

*Methods & Procedures*: A 10-day/3 hours a day pre–posttest CILT intervention case series was carried out 1–2 months post onset with three Norwegian rehabilitation inpatients with aphasia following left CVA. Procedures involved card activities using high- and low-frequency picture stimuli with communicative relevance at four levels of complexity, either in a small group or one-to-one with a trained SLP.

*Outcomes & Results*: Results suggested an overall improvement on the language assessments post CILT intervention, as well as at the follow-up. A greater degree of improvement in performance on expressive speech tasks compared to receptive and written tasks suggested a treatment-specific effect of CILT for early aphasia rehabilitation. Participant evaluation of the CILT intervention reflected positive feedback for the treatment experience and satisfaction with individual gains. Challenges in the application of CILT to this phase of recovery were the need to accommodate the demands of the inpatient rehabilitation setting and the decreased stamina of the participants.

*Conclusions*: The results of this study support the applicability of CILT in early aphasia rehabilitation, with some modifications of the original protocol.

*Keywords:* Aphasia; Constraint induced language therapy (CILT); Early rehabilitation.

Address correspondence to: Melanie Kirmess, Department of Special Needs Education, University of Oslo, PO Box 1140 Blindern, NO-0318 Oslo, Norway. E-mail: melanie.kirmess@uv.uio.no

Preliminary results of this study were presented as poster presentations at the 46th Academy of Aphasia, Turku, Finland, 2008, and Clinical Aphasiology Conference, Keystone, CO, USA, 2009. The study is supported by the Faculty of Education, University of Oslo, Norway.

We are grateful for the participation of the persons with aphasia and the speech and language pathologists involved in the data collection.

http://www.psypress.com/aphasiology     DOI: 10.1080/02687030903437682

Aphasia is defined as an acquired neurological multimodality language disorder following focal brain injury (McNeil & Pratt, 2001). Demographic studies across countries indicate that approximately 30–50% of stroke survivors will experience aphasia. With the number of elderly and older people in Western countries projected to grow over the next few decades (Truelsen et al., 2006), the incidence of stroke will increase and the need for effective aphasia treatment will increase simultaneously. Previous reviews on the effect of aphasia treatment have been somewhat contradictory (Greener, Enderby, & Whurr, 1999; Robey, 1994, 1998); however, more recent reports seem to support the importance of intensive treatment (Bhogal, Teasell, & Speechley, 2003; Raymer et al., 2008). Increasing knowledge about brain plasticity and behavioural-dependent neuronal change and recovery invites exploration of new or improved treatment methods (Nudo, 2006b; Robertson & Murre, 1999; Thompson, 2000).

Constraint induced language therapy—CILT, also referred in the literature as constraint induced aphasia therapy (CIAT)—emphasises improving impaired spoken language production following acquired brain injury based on the principles of brain plasticity. In accordance with experience-dependent learning theory, it is assumed that the general use of compensatory strategies exploits healthy brain functions but at the same time reduces stimulation opportunities for the impaired regions. Reduced stimulation opportunities often result from effortful activation, which in turn induces a negative cycle of decreased use resulting in the phenomenon referred to as "learned non-use" of a function (Taub, Uswatte, Mark, & Morris, 2006). CILT represents an expansion of constraint induced movement therapy (Taub & Uswatte, 2006) to language; theoretically targeting the negative effects of learned non-use of spoken verbal communication. In speech, learned non-use is believed to be related to an overuse of compensatory strategies exemplified by gestures, drawing, and writing to the detriment of spoken language recovery (Pulvermüller & Berthier, 2008; Pulvermüller et al., 2001). The theoretical model for CILT relates further to Kleim and Jones's (2008) principles of experience-dependent brain plasticity, in which function-specific activation is presupposed in order to maintain or improve a function or skill, i.e., the "use it or lose it" principle. CILT explicitly utilises a number of these principles in the construction of the treatment setting and treatment characteristics (Pulvermüller et al., 2001): intensive, use-dependent treatment (intensity), 3 hours a day for 10 days; constraint to spoken verbal expression by the use of visual barriers between communication partners, thereby preventing the use of compensatory strategies such as gestures (specificity); massed practice (repetition); shaping of the required response to match individual skill; and stimuli material based on communicative relevance for the person with aphasia (both salience).

Previous CILT research suggested positive results for increased language test scores for persons with *chronic* aphasia. Pulvermüller et al.'s (2001) seminal study compared CILT to distributed, general speech and language therapy, with a significantly better outcome for the CILT group. Meinzer, Djundja, Barthel, Elbert, and Rockstroh (2005) replicated and extended those initial results, comparing CILT and CILT+, where CILT+ included written material as well as involving significant others to extend speech production training beyond the laboratory and into a home setting. To control for the possible effect of intensity alone, Maher et al. (2006) conducted a study comparing CILT to PACE therapy (Davis & Wilcox, 1985), where the group treatments solely differed by either constraint to spoken output (CILT) or the use of total communication facilities (writing, gestures, speech, drawing). Results showed positive outcomes for both groups, but with significant gains for spoken output in the CILT group.

Barthel, Meinzer, Djundja, and Rockstroh (2008) assessed possible factors accounting for the positive outcome of CILT in chronic aphasia by comparing and reviewing CILT, CILT+, and a modality-based treatment (MOAT), specifically tailored for treatment adaptation to individual aphasic deficits for communicative improvement. Everyday training of individual needs yielded positive outcomes across groups, while intensity, shaping, specificity, and the involvement of significant others should be further explored. Recently, Pulvermüller and Berthier (2008) proposed that the communicative relevance and natural communication setting within the treatment structure might be the main reasons for increased verbal production and implicit language changes, based on Wittgenstein's philosophy of the direct relationship of language to action (e.g., language games). The authors introduced "intensive language-action therapy" (ILAT), reflecting those relevant treatment structures and indicating that the role and influence of the actual constraint in constraint induced language therapy (CILT) should be explored further.

Raymer et al. (2008) emphasised the need for research on the impact of time post onset and intensity treatment outcomes within CILT research. Further, Linebaugh, Baron, and Corcoran (1998) discussed the paradox between the methodological claims of efficacy studies in aphasia based on chronic patients, and their applicability and appropriateness in the clinical reality of acute and early rehabilitation services for people with aphasia as is typically seen by the speech and language pathologist (SLP). Hillis and Heidler (2002) described several neural mechanisms as possible causes for variations in the timeline of spontaneous or rapid recovery. Their model supports treatment that targets the structural and functional reorganisation of the brain in the subacute or early aphasia rehabilitation phase, consistent with the theoretical underpinnings of CILT. While general research articles point to a better outcome the earlier intensive treatment is started—addressed by, e.g., Poeck, Huber, and Willmes (1989) and Robey (1998)—such results should be tempered with the possible negative consequences of interventions begun too early. Results from selected animal studies indicated an extension of the stroke area with too-early intervention. However, these findings were mostly connected to intensive treatment occurring within the hyper-acute phase (first 24 hours) and were not replicated in later studies (Kleim & Jones, 2008; Nudo, 2006a).

Despite the increased understanding of brain neuroplasticity, the importance of early rehabilitation for stroke survivors, and encouraging outcomes from chronic studies, there are so far no known studies investigating CILT in early recovery from aphasia (Cherney, Patterson, Raymer, Frymark, & Schooling, 2008). The purpose of this study was therefore to explore the applicability and outcome of a programme of CILT in individuals in the early phase of recovery from aphasia. If it could be shown with some modifications to be effective, clinicians could more easily justify their use of CILT at that time. The term *early aphasia rehabilitation* in this paper refers to the rehabilitation phase after the acute care hospital setting, beginning at about 1–2 months post onset. This time frame also respects the possibility for the stroke survivor to establish a more medically stable condition and aphasia pattern, as well as to adjust somewhat to the life-changing situation.

## METHOD AND PROCEDURE

### Participants

A pre–posttest intervention study was conducted with three right-handed, highly educated (> 12 years) native Norwegian speakers (named HP, FOT, and GA) with aphasia and right-side hemiparesis following first-time CVA. HP was an 89-year-old woman with mild to moderate aphasia following a left MCA CVA, which had evolved to non-fluent speech with limited intelligibility and significant apraxia of speech (AOS) by the time she participated in the study 40 days post stroke. FOT was a 43-year-old male with non-fluent aphasia following a left medial/anterior CA CVA. He received acute thrombolytic treatment as well as a hemi-craniectomy prior to beginning the study. FOT's expressive language was marked by severe anomia without AOS by the time he participated in the study 58 days post stroke. GA, a 68-year-old male, sustained a left intracerebral haemorrhage with midline shift, resulting in severe receptive and expressive aphasia, apraxia of speech (AOS), and dysphagia. GA's language production was limited to yes/no, monosyllabic words, and neologisms at the start of the study, 42 days post onset.

## Intervention

For each participant, CILT was scheduled for 3 hours a day for 10 days, replicating previous studies (Barthel et al., 2008; Maher et al., 2006). However, the acute hospital setting and stamina of the clients required modifications to the original protocol. In some instances the treatment dose needed to be modified, i.e., administered in multiple shorter sessions of 45 minutes rather than in a 3-hour block. Also, in this phase the scheduling of treatment needed to be flexible to accommodate other rehabilitation treatments and medical issues, making the scheduling of group intervention problematic at times. In other instances it was necessary to deliver the intervention at bedside because of physical fatigue. Therefore the number of therapy hours given daily ranged from 1.15 to 3 hours, resulting in a total number of therapy hours of 20 (HP), 24.5 (GA), and 30 (FOT).

The treatment (TX), modelled after Pulvermüller et al. (2001) and Maher et al. (2006), involved constrained spoken output with shaping of the targeted responses in the context of card activities with visual barriers between the participants. The paired cards presented coloured pictures in 10 categories based on assumed communicative relevance for daily living within two frequency rates, and at four complexity levels (see appendix for a detailed description). Hand movements for individual support were neither prohibited nor encouraged. Videotaped samples from all training sessions were checked by the first author to ensure TX fidelity. TX was conducted in a group setting with a second person with aphasia and an SLP (FOT), or individually, with the SLP acting as the communication partner (HP and GA).

The CILT treatment carried out in this study does not involve constraints outside the training sessions, as there are in some constraint motor studies, and therefore we could not control for the use of compensatory strategies for the remaining hours of the day. However, as all three participants were in-patients the environmental surroundings are relatively similar, with typical hospital conversations as the main communication activity. Hospital professionals and significant others were informed about the study but were not informed about specific training items, nor were they encouraged to involve the participants in more communicative action than any other patient. However, individual motivation to practise independently outside the treatment sessions cannot be ruled out, and personal characteristics should be considered as influential factors for outcome in such cases.

## Assessment

The presence and nature of the aphasia were assessed with the Norwegian Basic Aphasia Assessment (NGA) (Reinvang & Engvik, 1980b; Reinvang 1985), which is based on the Lichtheim-Wernicke model and similar to the Boston Diagnostic Aphasia Examination (Goodglass & Kaplan, 1972) and the Western Aphasia Battery (Kertesz, 1982). In addition, the Norwegian versions of the Test for Reception of Grammar (TROG-2) (Bishop, 2009), the subtest 7 (sentence construction) of the Verb and Sentence Test (VOST) (Bastiaanse, Lind, Moen, & Gram Simonsen, 2006), the experimental version of subtest 54, (naming frequency) from the Psycholinguistic Assessments of Language Processing in Aphasia (PALPA) (Kay, Lesser, & Coltheart, 2009), the Cookie Theft (CT) picture description (Goodglass & Kaplan, 1972), and CILT-baseline measures were administered pre and post treatment. The CILT baseline consisted of independent productions of five trained and five untrained high-frequency level 3 requests and low-frequency level 4 requests (total number of items = 20, see appendix). AOS was clinically assessed based on Reinvang and Engvik's form (1980b). In addition to these specific language measures of performance, a questionnaire was developed to evaluate the participants' experience of CILT, including open questions and comments of agreement on a 5-point—2, 1, 0 (neither nor) –1, –2—picture-supported rating scale. Follow-up measures were conducted at 3 months (HP) and 6 months (FOT) post intervention. Because of medical complications, GA was not tested at 3 months post onset. CILT TX and assessments were carried out by experienced SLPs, all trained in CILT administration by the first author. All measures were scored from videotape by the treating SLP, and subsets were scored by a second SLP for reliability. Inter-rater agreement for all available subtests ranged from 50% to 100%, with an average of 92.9%. The lower agreement scores were the result of the treating clinician scoring more liberally, and in cases of disagreement the more conservative scoring was used. Written informed consent was obtained from all participants before the pre-test and renewed orally at the other assessment points. The study was approved by the Regional Committees for Medical Research Ethics (REK) and the Norwegian Social Science Data Services (NSD).

## RESULTS

All participants completed the CILT TX successfully with an overall pre–posttest average improvement on the five language tests (NGA, TROG-2, VOST, PALPA, CILT baseline) ranging from 5.1% (GA) to 18.7% (HP) and 23.3% (FOT) (see Table 1 for detailed scores).

Descriptive quantitative analysis indicated improvement on the six speech production subtests (CILT baseline, NGA repetition, NGA naming, NGA reading aloud, PALPA, VOST) in all three cases (GA, M = 12%; HP, M = 22%; FOT, M = 23%), with individual variation ranging from 1.5% (GA, PALPA 54) to 40% (HP, VOST) (Figure 1).

In comparison, receptive measures (NGA comprehension, NGA reading comprehension TROG-2) and written output (NGA writing) indicated a change of –0.6% (HP), 3.25% (GA), and 4.4% (FOT) after controlling for the fact that FOT did not receive all of the writing subtests pre-TX. HP and FOT showed the most improvement on the sentence-level tasks, whereas for GA, word-level tasks improved the most.

TABLE 1
Pre-test, post-test, and follow-up scores for all cases in percent correct answers
and words per minute (wpm)

| | HP | | | FOT | | | GA* | |
| --- | --- | --- | --- | --- | --- | --- | --- | --- |
| | Pre | Post | Follow-up | Pre | Post | Follow-up | Pre | Post |
| CILT baseline (180 **) | 39 | 52 | 62 | 47.5 | 85 | 85 | 8 | 15 |
| NGA repetition (40**) | 10 | 15 | 25 | 75 | 85 | 95 | 10 | 27.5 |
| NGA naming (41**) | 53 | 78 | 94 | 66 | 83 | 93 | 11 | 43 |
| NGA reading aloud (26**) | 42 | 69 | 85 | 70 | 85 | 96 | 10 | 20 |
| PALPA 54 naming frequency (80**) | 37.5 | 61 | 81 | 59 | 89 | 95 | 11 | 12.5 |
| VOST sentence construction (20**) | 20 | 60 | 70 | 45 | 75 | 90 | 0 | 5 |
| TROG-2 (80**) | 84 | 93 | 98 | 72.5 | 80 | 80 | 9 | 10 |
| NGA comprehension (71**) | 99 | 97 | 98.5 | 89 | 94 | 100 | 31 | 30 |
| NGA reading comprehension (23**) | 100 | 100 | 100 | 73 | 73 | 100 | 17 | 30 |
| NGA writing (10**) | 80 | 70 | 90 | 20 | 70 | 40 | 0 | 0 |
| Cookie theft (wpm) | 57.3 | 64 | 67.4 | 11.1 | 15.9 | 27 | 39 | 36 |
| Conversational interview NGA (wpm) | 54.4 | 69.8 | 66.1 | 9.8 | 19 | 23.4 | 45 | 47.4 |

*Follow-up results for GA could not be obtained for medical reasons.
** Number of items (N) available for each test.

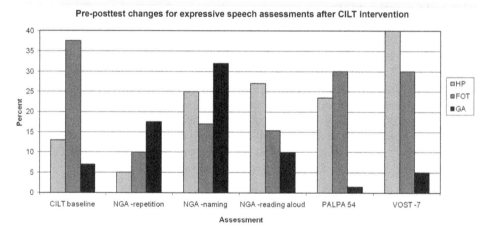

**Pre-posttest changes for expressive speech assessments after CILT Intervention**

Figure 1. Pre- to post-test changes for expressive speech assessments for all three cases.

Typically, when reporting a case series, individual effect sizes would be preferred. However, due to the lack of normative data for many of the Norwegian versions of the tests, effect sizes were calculated within the group, see Table 2.

The effect sizes for expressive oral tasks, while modest, exceed the level of .63 reported by Robey (1998) for untreated recovery and provide support for the treatment effect for speech production tasks.

Analyses of more complex speech production revealed a larger increase of words per minute for the NGA conversational interview (HP = 28%, FOT = 48%, GA = 6%) compared to the Cookie Theft (HP = 12%, FOT = 30%, GA = −1%). These changes suggested an increase in expressive speech output beyond single word naming, indicating a possible impact of CILT on functional communication for at least HP and FOT. Despite limited parametric change in the number of utterances for GA, intelligibility and effort seemed to improve.

TABLE 2
Within-group effect sizes for $N = 3$

| Assessment | M Pre-test (min; max) | M Post-test (min; max) | M Std error Pre-test | SD Pre-test | d* |
|---|---|---|---|---|---|
| NGA (overall) | 110.33 (37; 156) | 132.17 (61.5;180) | 37.03 | 64.14 | 0.34 |
| NGA (naming)** | 17.83 (4.5; 27) | 27.833 (17.5; 34) | 6.82 | 11.81 | 0.85 |
| NGA (aud. comp.) | 51.67 (22; 70) | 52.33 (21; 69) | 14.97 | 25.9 | 0.03 |
| NGA (writing) | 3.33 (0; 8) | 4.67 (0; 7) | 2.40 | 4.16 | 0.32 |
| PALPA subtest54** | 29 (9; 47) | 43.33 (10; 71) | 11.02 | 19.0 | 0.75 |
| VOST subtest 7** | 4 (0; 9) | 9.33 (1; 15) | 2.64 | 4.58 | 1.16 |
| TROG-2 | 34.33 (7; 67) | 38 (8; 74) | 17.52 | 30.35 | 0.12 |
| CILT baseline** | 56.83 (14.5, 85.5) | 91.5 (27.5; 152.5) | 21.61 | 37.42 | 0.93 |

*Within-group effect size ($N = 3$) calculated with the following formula:

$$d = \frac{M_{pre} - M_{post}}{SD_{pre}}$$

** Verbal speech production tasks.

Qualitative evaluation of participation in CILT using the self-report questionnaire revealed mostly positive experiences in all three cases. However, intensity of the intervention was one of the challenges in applying the CILT protocol in this setting. While HP and FOT preferred fewer hours per day, GA preferred more intensive TX. FOT's self-reported evaluation measures did not reflect specific language changes; however, he reported that the experience was positive, and his family members reported better communication on his behalf. FOT was also the most ambivalent about participating at the beginning of the intervention, related to his primary interest in physical therapy, which might be reflected in a more negative performance during the pre-TX evaluation. However, at the follow-up he expressed his appreciation for the study, seeming to have obtained greater understanding of his aphasia and living situation. Follow-up results for both FOT and HP indicate further overall improvement, as expected in early aphasia recovery, as all clients continued with more traditional speech therapy addressing all language modalities after CILT.

## DISCUSSION

Being aware that a pre–post treatment study without a control group has severe limitations and therefore cannot be generalised, we feel the results of this study certainly warrant a larger controlled group study. Taking those methodological concerns into account, the present case series points to some interesting findings. First, all participants completed the study with positive results and continued improvement at follow-up, revealing at least no explicitly negative influences of CILT in early aphasia rehabilitation. Second, the improvement in expressive speech compared to the relatively limited change in receptive language tasks (respecting a likely ceiling effect for some of the comprehension subtests for HP) might indicate a treatment specific outcome. Further, there was also a greater improvement in expressive spoken language compared to expressive written language for HP and GA. Assuming that verbal and written word retrieval activates some of the same language processes in the brain, writing can be viewed as a non-equivalent dependent variable, which should not change with CILT, but which has similar threats to internal validity as spoken language (Shadish, Cook, &

Campbell, 2002). This argues against spontaneous recovery as the overall explanatory factor for the observed positive results. Furthermore, since the emphasis of CILT is primarily on spoken output, the difference in oral versus written production following therapy suggests a predictable treatment-specific response that may be attributed at least in part to the intervention.

One of the challenges in assessing the impact of intervention in acute rehabilitation is the contribution of spontaneous recovery (Poeck et al., 1989). In theory, the influence of spontaneous recovery (or other threats to validity such as a placebo effect) should be observed across all areas of deficit. Results from the Copenhagen aphasia study (Pedersen, Vinter, & Olsen, 2004) support this hypothesis, by finding no explicit difference in the recovery process for comprehension and speech production (spontaneous speech, naming) within the first year post onset. Other studies reported differences in favour of improved comprehension (e.g., Kenin & Swisher, 1972; Vignolo, 1965) or varying results depending on spared comprehension skills (Lomas & Kertesz, 1978), both contrary to the results in this study. While specific changes after a 6-month interval were observed on the NGA by Reinvang and Engvik (1980a), few studies have addressed changes within as short a treatment period as the current study (10 days). The presented TX effects should therefore be considered cautiously.

Another factor that may influence recovery is the type of stroke. In general a better outcome is predicted for haemorrhagic than ischaemic strokes (Murray & Clark, 2006). However, in this case series the participants with ischaemic strokes (FOT and HP) and not the one with a haemorrhagic stroke (GA) had the better outcome, supporting the conclusion of a CILT treatment effect rather than spontaneous recovery. Further, severity of aphasia and size of the lesion are frequently reported as predictors of outcome (Holland, 1989; Kertesz & McCabe, 1977), predicting FOT's positive response based on medical history and absence of AOS. However, while CILT does not particularly emphasise the treatment of AOS, the results on the expressive speech production tasks indicate improvement in the articulatory and speech output levels (HP and GA). The CILT setting with its repetitive pattern and shaping of responses should be further explored for its possible impact on AOS.

Other factors, such as age, pre-stroke physical activity, and motivation are addressed as possible impact factors on treatment outcome, but to varying degrees, (Holland, 1989; Pedersen, et al., 2004). Holland (1989) reported age differences where older persons showed more severe forms of aphasia and fewer effects of spontaneous recovery, predicting a better outcome for the youngest case, FOT. On the other hand, despite her age, HP was an extremely active elderly woman, reinforcing that personal characteristics play a role in treatment intervention. Breitenstein et al. (2009) discussed the influence of cognitive factors on language performance and recovery, arguing for better linguistic prognosis if fewer cognitive deficits are present. From this point of view, additional cognitive tasks would be recommended in future studies.

Pulvermüller and Berthier (2008) addressed the importance of natural speech actions for the best generalisation effect of CILT to daily living, in line with the transfer package as emphasised by Taub et al. (2006) for constraint induced movement therapy, to promote gains beyond the laboratory setting. Using a group setting has previously shown better generalisation effects on communication skills than individual treatment with an SLP (Elmann & Bernstein-Ellis, 1999). However, Barthel et al. (2008) reported no significant differences regarding group or individual treatment. FOT's intervention occurred in a group setting, in contrast to the other two cases. However, the one-to-one settings with the SLPs allowed for more talking time per participant.

Future studies could address differences in individual versus group delivery more systematically. In addition, more detailed functional communication and quality-of-life outcomes should be explored.

Previous CILT research with chronic patients excluded severe aphasia, and GA's positive results encourage exploration of intensive spoken language therapy for severe aphasia. The Pedersen et al. (2004) study indicated a positive prognosis for persons diagnosed with global aphasia within the first weeks post onset by showing an evolution within the first year to a Broca-type aphasia, supporting their therapeutic qualification for aphasia rehabilitation. In the case of GA, changes measured across standardised assessments might partly be limited by the correct/not correct dichotomy of scoring. A more detailed scoring system might reveal more subtle areas of improvement, as observed in functional speech and communication. This notion is supported by the Marini, Caltagirone, Pasqualetti, and Carlomagno (2007) study where small changes on clinical tests were associated with better outcomes on connected speech samples after treatment. Linebaugh et al. (1998, p. 533) also focused on the "magnitude of inaccuracy in changes" as an additional factor in determining efficacy outcomes and in the discussion of the duration of language therapy. Further, the effect of an expressive speech treatment might be different if the goal challenges quality or quantity of speech production, such as increasing fluency using more circumlocutions or decreasing the number of attempts by errorless activation (Bauer & Auer, 2009).

Another consideration is that CILT focuses on expressive speech production, leading to the assumption that it might be more applicable for non-fluent aphasia types as was the case for these three participants. However, extension to fluent aphasia (e.g., Wernicke aphasia) would afford a better assessment of the impact of CILT on (a) comprehension and auditory discrimination, and (b) inappropriate fluency (neologism, paraphasia etc.) based on the structured treatment setting CILT represents. Finally, the influence of memory on recovery of language function after stroke has recently been reinforced, and invites further exploration in the context of CILT.

## CONCLUSION

In conclusion, the results of this study support the applicability of CILT for expressive language production in early aphasia rehabilitation. The strength of this study lies in its real-world clinical setting, applied in typical rehabilitation facilities in Norway, covering the challenges of everyday life in hospitals for patients with acute stroke rehabilitation. Within the overview of research stages as presented by Cherney et al. (2008), this study shows indications for the effectiveness stage; however, exploration in a larger population and control group studies are warranted. Concerning further clinical use, modifications of the original protocol by treating SLPs should be expected based on individual needs.

Linebaugh et al. (1998) suggested criterion-based rehabilitation research in aphasia rather than time-based to assess factors such as generalisation and maintenance. This should be implemented in further studies investigating the optimal time post onset for beneficial intensive treatment outcome, as well as the amount and duration of intensive treatment. Present CILT studies focused mainly on speech production and comprehension in aphasia, and future research should, to a higher degree, extend the treatment-induced intensive training to other language areas such as reading and writing, and investigate the interaction of these language areas.

Manuscript received 17 July 2009
Manuscript accepted 22 October 2009
First published online 25 May 2010

# REFERENCES

Barthel, G., Meinzer, M., Djundja, D., & Rockstroh, B. (2008). Intensive language therapy in chronic aphasia: Which aspects contribute most? *Aphasiology, 22*(4), 408–421.

Bastiaanse, R., Lind, M., Moen, I., & Gram Simonsen, H. (2006). *Verb-og setningstest VOST. Håndbok.* Oslo: Novus forlag.

Bauer, A., & Auer, P. (2009). *Aphasie im Alltag.* Stuttgart: Thieme.

Bhogal, S. K., Teasell, R., & Speechley, M. (2003). Intensity of aphasia therapy, impact on recovery. *Stroke, 34,* 987–993.

Bishop, D. V. M. (2009). *Test for Reception of Grammar. Version 2. TROG-2 Manual. Norsk versjon* (S-A. H. Lyster, Trans.). London: Pearson Education, Inc.

Breitenstein, C., Kramer, K., Meinzer, M., Baumgärtner, A., Flöel, A., & Knecht, S. (2009). Intensives Sprachtraining bei Aphasie. *Der Nervenarzt, 80*(2), 149–154.

Cherney, L. R., Patterson, J. P., Raymer, A., Frymark, T., & Schooling, T. (2008). Evidence-based systematic review: Effects of intensity of treatment and constraint-induced language therapy for individuals with stroke-induced aphasia. *Journal of Speech, Hearing & Language Research, 51*(5), 1282–1299.

Davis, G. A., & Wilcox, M. J. (1985). *Adult aphasia rehabilitation: Applied pragmatics.* San Diego, CA: College Hill Press.

Elmann, R. J., & Bernstein-Ellis, E. (1999). The efficacy of group communication treatment in adults with chronic aphasia. *Journal of Speech, Language, and Hearing Research, 42,* 411–419.

Goodglass, H., & Kaplan, E. (1972). *The Boston Diagnostic Aphasia Examination.* Philadelphia: Lea & Febiger.

Greener, J., Enderby, P., & Whurr, R. (1999). Speech and language therapy for aphasia following stroke. *The Cochrane Database Systematic Reviews* (4).

Hillis, A. A. E., & Heidler, J. (2002). Mechanisms of early aphasia recovery. *Aphasiology, 16*(9), 885–895.

Holland, A. (1989). Recovery in aphasia In F. Boller & J. Grafman (Eds.), *Handbook of Neuropsychology* (Vol. 2, pp. 83–90). Amsterdam: Elsevier.

Kay, J., Lesser, R., & Coltheart, M. (2009). *Psykolingvistisk kartlegging av språkprosessering hos afasirammede (PALPA) (Norsk oversettelse).* Oslo: Novus.

Kenin, M., & Swisher, L. P. (1972). A study of pattern of recovery in aphasia. *Cortex, 8,* 56–68.

Kertesz, A. (1982). *Western Aphasia Battery (WAB).* New York: Grune & Stratton Inc.

Kertesz, A., & McCabe, P. (1977). Recovery patterns and prognosis in aphasia. *Brain, 100*(1), 1–18.

Kleim, J. A., & Jones, T. A. (2008). Principles of experience-dependent neural plasticity: Implications for rehabilitation after brain damage. *Journal of Speech, Hearing, & Language Research, 51*(1), S225–239.

Linebaugh, C. W., Baron, C. R., & Corcoran, K. J. (1998). Assessing treatment efficacy in acute aphasia: Paradoxes, presumptions, problems, and principles. *Aphasiology, 12*(7), 519–536.

Lomas, J., & Kertesz, A. (1978). Patterns of spontaneous recovery in aphasic groups: A study of adult stroke patients. *Brain and Language, 5*(3), 388–401.

Maher, L. M., Kendall, D. L., Swearengin, J. A., Rodriguez, A., Leon, S. A., Pingel, K., et al. (2006). A pilot study of use-dependent learning in the context of constraint induced language therapy. *Journal of the International Neuropsychological Society, 12*(6), 843–852.

Marini, A., Caltagirone, C., Pasqualetti, P., & Carlomagno, S. (2007). Patterns of language improvement in adults with non-chronic non-fluent aphasia after specific therapies. *Aphasiology, 21*(2), 164–186.

McNeil, M. R., & Pratt, S. R. (2001). Defining aphasia: Some theoretical and clinical implications of operating from a formal definition. *Aphasiology, 15*(10/11), 901–911.

Meinzer, M., Djundja, D., Barthel, G., Elbert, T., & Rockstroh, B. (2005). Long-term stability of improved language functions in chronic aphasia after constraint-induced aphasia therapy. *Stroke, 36*(7), 1462–1466.

Murray, L. L., & Clark, H. M. (2006). *Neurogenic disorders of language: Theory driven clinical practice.* New York: Thomson Delmar Learning.

Nudo, R. J. (2006a). Mechanisms for recovery of motor function following cortical damage. *Current Opinion in Neurobiology, 16*(6), 638–644.

Nudo, R. J. (2006b). Plasticity. *NeuroRX: The Journal of the American Society for Experimental Neuro-Therapeutics, 3*(4), 420–427.

Pedersen, P. M., Vinter, K., & Olsen, T. S. (2004). Aphasia after stroke: Type, severity and prognosis. *Cerebrovascular Diseases, 17*(1), 35–43.

Poeck, K., Huber, W., & Willmes, K. (1989). Outcome of intensive language treatment in aphasia. *Journal of Speech and Hearing Disorders, 54*, 471–479.

Pulvermüller, F., & Berthier, M. L. (2008). Aphasia therapy on a neuroscience basis. *Aphasiology, 22*(6), 563–599.

Pulvermüller, F., Neininger, B., Elbert, T., Rockstroh, B., Koebbel, P., & Taub, E. (2001). Constraint-induced therapy of chronic aphasia after stroke. *Stroke, 32*(7), 1621–1626.

Raymer, A. M., Beeson, P., Holland, A., Kendall, D., Maher, L. M., Martin, N., et al. (2008). Translational research in aphasia: From neuroscience to neurorehabilitation. *Journal of Speech, Hearing, & Language Research, 51*(1), S259–S275.

Reinvang, I. (1985). *Aphasia and brain organization.* New York, USA: Plenum Press.

Reinvang, I., & Engvik, H. (1980a). Language recovery in aphasia from 3 to 6 months after stroke. In M. T. Sarno & O. Höök (Eds.), *Aphasia. Assessment and treatment* (pp. 80–88). Stockholm: Almqvist & Wiksell International.

Reinvang, I., & Engvik, H. (1980b). *Norsk grunntest for afasi: Handbok.* Oslo: Universitetsforlag.

Robertson, I. H., & Murre, J. M. J. (1999). Rehabilitation of brain damage: Brain plasticity and principles of guided recovery. *Psychological Bulletin, 125*(5), 544–575.

Robey, R. R. (1994). The efficacy of treatment for aphasic persons: A meta-analysis. *Brain and Language, 47*(4), 582–608.

Robey, R. R. (1998). A meta-analysis of clinical outcomes in the treatment of aphasia. *Journal of Speech, Language, and Hearing Research, 41*(1), 172–187.

Shadish, W. R., Cook, T. D., & Campbell, D. T. (2002). *Experimental and quasi-experimental design for generalized causal inference.* Boston: Houghton Mifflin Company.

Taub, E., & Uswatte, G. (2006). Constraint-induced movement therapy: Answers and questions after two decades of research. *NeuroRehabilitation, 21*(2), 93–95.

Taub, E., Uswatte, G., Mark, V. W., & Morris, D. M. (2006). The learned nonuse phenomenon: Implications for rehabilitation. *Europa Medicophysica, 42*(3), 241–256.

Thompson, C. K. (2000). Neuroplasticity: Evidence from aphasia. *Journal of Communication Disorders, 33*, 357–366.

Truelsen, T., Piechowski-Jozwiak, B., Bonita, R., Mathers, C., Bogousslavsky, J., & Boysen, G. (2006). Stroke incidence and prevalence in Europe: A review of available data. *European Journal of Neurology, 13*(6), 581–598.

Vignolo, L. A. (1965). Evolution of aphasia and language rehabilitation: A retrospective exploratory study. *Cortex, 1*, 344–367.

# APPENDIX

## CILT treatment structure based on the card activity "Go fish"

| Level | Material | Description | Expected request | Expected response |
|-------|----------|-------------|------------------|-------------------|
| 1 | Picture set with pairs of cards | Single word naming. Preferable using intonation for indication of an interrogative phrase. | *Naming* of the pictured object e.g., "Bread?" | "Yes/no + naming" e.g., "Yes, bread" "No bread" |
| 2 | Picture set with pairs of cards | Addressing the other player by name, interrogative phrase including naming of object. | "Name, do you have a *naming*? e.g., "Jane, do you have bread? | "Yes/no, name, I do/don't have a *naming*." e.g., "Yes, Pete, I have bread." |
| 3 | Each object is in addition displayed in two versions | Addressing the other player by name, interrogative phrase including naming of object and differentiating from the other possibility by adding an adjective/adverb. | "Name, do you have a description *naming*?" e.g., "Jane, do you have toasted bread? | "Yes/no, I do/don't have description *naming*." e.g.," Yes, Pete, I have toasted bread" |
| 4 | Each object is in addition to level 3 displayed in two different amounts | Addressing the other player by name, interrogative phrase including naming of object, an adjective/adverb and an amount. | "Name, do you have an amount of description *naming*?" e.g., "Jane, do you have 2 (slices) of toasted bread?" | "Yes/no, I do/don't have an amount of description *naming*." e.g., "Yes, Pete, I have 2 (slices) of toasted bread." |

Change of level or category at about 80% correct.

## Categories: 10 objects each

| High frequency | Example | Low frequency | Example |
|----------------|---------|---------------|---------|
| Persons | Girl | Persons | Physical therapist |
| Home and housing | Radio | Home and housing | Ladder |
| Personal belongings | Dress | Personal belongings | Credit card |
| Food | Bread | Food | Waffles |
| Vehicles | Bus | | |
| Buildings | Restaurant | | |

APHASIOLOGY, 2010, 24 (6–8), 737–751

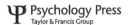

# Treatment-induced neuroplasticity following intensive naming therapy in a case of chronic Wernicke's aphasia

Jacquie Kurland, Katherine Baldwin and Chandra Tauer

*University of Massachusetts, Amherst, MA, USA*

*Background*: Renewed interest in the effects of intensity on treatment has led to development of short-term, intensive treatment protocols, such as Constraint-Induced Language Therapy (CILT), in which participants with chronic aphasia begin to show statistically significant language improvements in as little as 2 weeks. Given its relatively short treatment cycle, CILT is also a good choice of treatment methodology for studying brain/behaviour plasticity in post-stroke aphasia.
*Aims*: This study aimed to examine differences between two short, intensive treatment protocols in a participant with chronic Wernicke's aphasia both in terms of treatment outcomes and changes in patterns of BOLD signal activation.
*Methods & Procedures*: The participant (ACL) participated in language testing and an fMRI overt speech confrontation-naming paradigm pre and post 2 weeks of CILT, post 2 weeks of unconstrained language therapy (PACE), and 6 months post-CILT. He named 48 black/white line drawings from each of four conditions: treated (CILT or PACE), untreated, or consistently correctly named pictures.
*Outcomes & Results*: Naming treated pictures improved, even in the scanner, while naming untreated pictures did not. About one third of PACE and three-fourths of CILT gains were maintained. Rather than a distinct pattern of activation distinguishing treated from untreated or CILT from PACE pictures, ACL recruited a frontal network during naming of all pictures that included left middle and inferior frontal cortex, SMA and pre-SMA, and that varied in spatial extent and degree of activation according to accuracy and performance expectation. In post-hoc analyses of accuracy, this frontal network was most active during incorrect trials. At 6 months post-CILT, compared to controls, incorrect naming recruited a large and significant bilateral network including right Wernicke's area homologue.
*Conclusions*: Results suggest that short, intensive therapy can improve naming and jumpstart language recovery in chronic aphasia, whether responses are constrained to the speech modality or not. Modulation of a left frontal network was associated with accuracy in naming and may represent compensatory adaptation to improve response selection, self-monitoring, and/or inhibition.

*Keywords:* Neuroplasticity; Intensive treatment; Chronic aphasia.

Compared to the century following the earliest recorded observation of recovery in post-stroke aphasia (Gowers, 1888), the past decade has produced considerable growth

Address correspondence to: Jacquie Kurland PhD, Assistant Professor, University of Massachusetts Amherst, Department of Communication Disorders, 358 North Pleasant Street, Amherst, MA 01003-9296, USA. E-mail: jkurland@comdis.umass.edu

The first author would like to thank the University of Massachusetts Amherst Office of the Vice Chancellor for Research for providing MRI-MRS Pilot Finding to acquire this data.

DOI: 10.1080/02687030903524711

in our understanding of the limits and potential for left hemisphere neural map expansion and right hemisphere takeover of function (Price & Crinion, 2005). Still, our knowledge of the precise relationship between therapy and recovery, and how treatment-induced changes are neurally instantiated remains somewhat elusive.

Beyond individual differences inherent in the site and size of lesion, factors known to influence the variability seen in treatment outcomes include the type, amount, and intensity of language therapy. Recently a new model for aphasia therapy has been derived from the work of Taub (2004) and others, based on Constraint-Induced Therapy (CIT) in motor rehabilitation following stroke. Constraint-Induced Language Therapy (CILT) borrows from three CIT principles and is designed to overturn the deleterious effects of "learned non-use" of speech as follows: (1) *Constraint*: do not allow the use of compensatory means for communicating, e.g., drawing, writing, or gesturing; (2) *Forced use*: force use of the speech modality in the context of relevant communicative exchanges; and (3) *Massed practice*: practice therapy in high, concentrated doses. Investigators have devised short-term intensive treatment protocols (e.g., 2–4 hours per day, 4–5 days per week) in which participants with chronic aphasia begin to show statistically significant language improvements in as little as 2 weeks (Maher et al., 2006; Meinzer et al., 2006; Pulvermuller et al., 2001).

Pulvermuller and colleagues (2001) studied two groups with chronic mild-to-severe aphasia. One group ($n = 10$) received CILT in dyads and triads for 3–4 hours per day over 10 days. The second group ($n = 7$) received conventional speech therapy during a less intensive schedule, although total number of therapy hours was the same. The CILT group improved significantly in performance on tests of auditory comprehension, naming, repetition, and following directions, while the control group did not.

Similar outcomes were reported in a replication study (Maher et al., 2006) in which verbal expression was the *only* difference between the two therapy groups. Therapy to both groups was administered in a similar, game-like environment over a short, intensive timeframe. However, only the CILT group was restricted to verbal requests and responses. Pre- and post-therapy and 1 month follow-up testing on standardised tests of aphasia revealed a consistent pattern of improvement in the CILT group ($n = 4$) that exceeded improvements seen in the control group ($n = 5$).

Taub (2004) recently described an "impending paradigm shift in neurorehabilitation" (p. 235) as investigators begin to explore ways to merge basic research in behavioural science and neuroscience. The early returns on CILT suggest that it is a good choice for demonstrating the profound influence that behaviour has on the organisation and function of language networks in post-stroke aphasia.

Unlike vision, hearing, and locomotion, language can only be studied in humans. This has severely limited the methods for elucidating models of functional reorganisation in aphasia recovery. Animal research has shown that cerebral cortex undergoes plasticity, and that effects of reorganisation can be observed in both perilesional tissue and areas remote from the site of injury for months following stroke (Nudo & Friel, 1999). Several recent studies utilising functional neuroimaging to examine patterns of activation in post-stroke aphasia have made similar claims (Crinion & Leff, 2007; Price & Crinion, 2005). However, very few have explored *treatment-induced* recovery using neuroimaging methods before and after treatment to improve word retrieval (but see Meinzer & Breitenstein, 2008).

With so few neuroimaging studies examining treatment-induced neuroplasticity, it is not surprising that the results so far have been equivocal. Moreover, patient performance in the scanner has not often been explicitly addressed in fMRI analyses, in spite of the fact that poor performance may confound interpretation of imaging results. Fridriksson and colleagues (2007) dealt with this issue by using the number of correctly named items as a covariate in examining the neural correlates of anomia treatment in three persons with aphasia. In another study the authors were able to claim treatment-specific changes in their measures of magnetoencephalography (MEG), because they compared correct to incorrect responses in pre- and post-treatment scans (Cornelissen et al., 2003).

Three neuroimaging studies have been published by the groups investigating CILT treatment (Breier, Maher, Novak, & Papanicolaou, 2006; Meinzer et al., 2006; Pulvermuller, Hauk, Zohsel, Neininger, & Mohr, 2005). In a case study of a person with moderate-to-severe aphasia, MEG activation was observed to shift from RH perisylvian language areas pre and post CILT (with increased activation post-therapy), to bilateral activation with significant left temporal lobe activation at 3 months post-therapy (Breier et al., 2006). All changes in activation were correlated with improvements in language function; however, response accuracy during MEG scanning was low. In another case report of an 80-year-old patient with chronic aphasia who was scanned with fMRI pre and post CILT, language improvements correlated with increased activation in right inferior frontal cortex (Meinzer et al., 2006). However, these authors also noted that response accuracy during scanning was low.

Pulvermuller and colleagues (2005) documented bilateral word-specific changes in ERP analyses of lexical decisions in nine patients with chronic aphasia. By analysing correct trials only (on average, approximately 80% of trials), they observed enhanced bilateral neurophysiological activity post-CILT in response to meaningful words. Moreover, a correlational analysis demonstrated a positive relationship between magnitude of the word-evoked enhanced negativity (latency 250–300 ms) and variable patient improvement on the Token Test. The authors suggest that this early word-evoked ERP might represent an "aphasia recovery potential". This intriguing conclusion would be strengthened with a re-examination of their patients after a maintenance period.

Several investigators have recently noted that multiple single-participant longitudinal neuroimaging studies, in conjunction with behavioural tests, may be the most promising method for advancing our understanding of language recovery processes. Maher and colleagues (2006) suggested that their study would have been strengthened by using a multiple baseline design. Such designs have the advantage of controlling confounds, since each participant serves as his or her own control. The present study used a multiple baseline across behaviours design in order to examine treatment-induced neuroplasticity following two different intensive therapies in an individual with chronic Wernicke's aphasia. He underwent testing and participated in an fMRI overt speech confrontation naming paradigm before and after 2 weeks of CILT, then following 2 weeks of unconstrained language therapy (PACE; Davis & Wilcox, 1985), and again 6 months post-CILT. Both phases of therapy were intensive, but only CILT required spoken responses.

CILT necessarily involves strengthening access to the output lexicon, including the phonological representation of words. PACE therapy, which incorporates direct language stimulation and real-life conversation, does not necessarily involve the verbal output channel. Given this difference, it was hypothesised that intensive practice in naming pictures in the CILT condition would elicit greater improvements in picture naming than the PACE condition. It was further expected that experience-dependent learning via massed practice naming pictures (CILT) versus massed practice strengthening a lexical/semantic network that might not include spoken naming (PACE), might recruit different areas within the language network. Specifically, it was hypothesised that functional activation correlated with unsuccessful attempts to name untrained pictures pre-treatment (CILT, PACE, and untrained) would be indistinguishable from one another, but different from the pattern evoked by successful naming of a set of high frequency, consistently correctly named pictures (CORR). Moreover, it was expected that, post-CILT treatment, improvements in naming CILT pictures would evoke a pattern of activation that would begin to resemble the pattern for CORR pictures, and that this would probably involve intact left frontal structures. Given the nature of PACE therapy, i.e., that the participant with aphasia chooses the response modality, a strong hypothesis was not possible. It was, however, hypothesised that post-PACE treatment, improved naming might correlate with a more bilateral pattern of activation, possibly due to the participant's relative strength in, and reliance on, drawing pictures.

## METHOD

### Participant

At study onset, ACL was a right-handed, 55-year-old man with 16 years of education, 3 years post a single left hemisphere MCA stroke. Structural T1-weighted MRI revealed a large, predominantly temporoparietal lesion (Figure 1).

The Institutional Review Board of the University of Massachusetts Amherst approved the study and signed informed consent was obtained prior to assessment

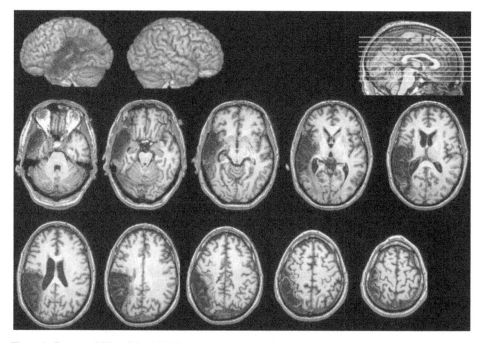

**Figure 1.** Structural T1-weighted MRI. Lesion was present in cortex and subjacent white matter predominantly in left temporal and parietal lobes, including left inferior, middle, and superior temporal gyri from the temporal pole extending back and including Wernicke's area and the transverse temporal gyri; S1 mouth and hand areas; supramarginal and angular gyri; and portions of the inferior and superior parietal lobules. Lesion also extended into the insula and putamen, and minimally to the inferior frontal gyrus, pars opercularis. To view this figure in colour, please visit the online version of the Journal.

TABLE 1
Pre- and Post-Treatment Scores for ACL

| Test or Task [max. score] | Pre-CILT [1] | Post-CILT | Post-PACE | 6 Mos. Post-CILT |
|---|---|---|---|---|
| Aud. Comp. (BDAE-mean %tile)[2] | *9th* | *25th* | *27th* | *31st* |
| Word Comprehension [37] | 24 (65%) | 30 (81%) | 31 (84%) | 29.5 (80%) |
| Commands [15] | 6 (40%) | 10 (67%) | 11 (73%) | 11 (73%) |
| Complex Ideational Material [12] | 2 (17%) | 6 (50%) | 5 (42%) | 7 (58%) |
| Repetition (BDAE) | | | | |
| 1-word [10] | 7 (70%) | 6 (60%) | 8 (80%) | 7 (70%) |
| Sentences [10] | 1 (10%) | 1 (10%) | 1 (10%) | 0 (0%) |
| Naming | | | | |
| Boston Naming Test[3] [60] | 9 (15%) | 10 (17%) | 13 (22%) | 10 (17%) |
| Responsive Naming (BDAE) [20] | 2 (10%) | 5 (25%) | 8 (40%) | 2 (10%) |
| Objects and Actions Naming Test[4] | | | | |
| Object [81] | 31 (38%) | 43 (53%) | 40 (49%) | 49 (60%) |
| Actions [50] | 17 (34%) | 24 (48%) | 29 (58%) | 30 (60%) |
| Treated and Untreated Pictures[5] | | | | |
| CORR [48] | 18 (38%) | 39 (81%) | 35 (73%) | 41 (85%) |
| CILT [48] | 1 (2%) | 22 (46%) | 21 (44%) | 16 (33%) |
| PACE [48] | 1 (2%) | 9 (19%) | 27 (56%) | 9 (19%) |
| UNTR [48] | 2 (4%) | 4 (8%) | 4 (8%) | 3 (6%) |
| Total stimuli [192] | 24 (12.5%) | 74 (39%) | 87 (45%) | 71 (37%) |

[1]Raw scores and (percentages in parentheses) [*percentiles in italics*]
[2]BDAE (Goodglass, Kaplan, & Barresi, 2001).
[3]BNT (Kaplan, Goodglass, & Weintraub, 2001).
[4]Objects and Actions Naming Test (Druks & Masterson, 2000).
[5]Accuracy in the scanner.

and treatment. A full diagnostic assessment of ACL's language included the Boston Diagnostic Aphasia Examination (BDAE 3rd ed.; Goodglass, Kaplan, & Barresi, 2001). He presented with moderately severe Wernicke's aphasia: 9th percentile on the mean of three auditory comprehension tasks; 30th percentile on both word and sentence repetition; and 10th percentile on responsive naming (see Table 1).

## Treatment experimental design

ACL was tested on three occasions to establish a stable baseline. Four sets of 48 black and white line drawings were selected from nearly 800 objects and actions from the International Picture Naming Project (IPNP; Szekely et al., 2005). One set included pictures that were correctly named on two or more occasions, including the last baseline test (CORR); the other three sets were never correctly named. These three sets were matched for word frequency, visual complexity, number of syllables and letters, and randomly selected for treatment (CILT or PACE) or no treatment (UNTR).

A single-participant multiple baseline design across behaviours was used to detect treatment outcomes and correlated changes in functional activation. Probes were administered approximately twice a week over a 6-week period. Prior to and following each 2-week phase of treatment (CILT first; PACE second) and 6 months post-CILT, the BDAE and Object and Action Naming Battery (Druks & Masterson, 2000) were administered. A functional MRI *overt* naming task was also administered.

Treatment consisted of five 3-hour sessions per week for 2 weeks per phase. CILT pictures were trained in accordance with the methods of shaping, reinforcement, and increasing complexity as described by Pulvermuller et al. (2001). During phase two, PACE pictures were trained in a similar manner, except that ACL's responses were no longer constrained to the speech modality.

## Functional MRI data acquisition

High-resolution ($1mm^3$) T1-weighted MPRAGE anatomical scans were acquired on a Siemens Esprit 1.5T MRI scanner, including 160 slices parallel to the anterior commissure–posterior commissure (AC/PC) line (FOV = 240 mm, TR/TE = 2400/4.1 ms, flip angle = 8 degrees). Functional images were acquired in the same plane using a T2*-weighted gradient echo EPI sequence (FOV = 192 mm, TR/TE = 7000/50 ms; flip angle = 90 degrees). Twenty-five 5-mm thick slices were acquired with an effective TR of 7.0 s, including a 4-s delay inserted between acquisitions.

During each of four 8.5-minute fMRI runs, each condition block (CORR, PACE, CILT, UNTR, or X, a control condition) lasted 42 s: six stimuli presented for 4 s, followed by a crosshair (rest/fixation) for 3 s. In order to minimise motion artefact and maximise speech intelligibility in the scanner, the behaviour interleaved gradient technique (Eden, Joseph, Brown, Brown, & Zeffiro, 1999) was employed. Data acquisition was delayed until after the overt responses were captured, the latter occurring during a delay period when the gradients were off, thereby also capitalising on the haemodynamic delay.

## Functional MRI experimental design

Functional MRI scans were acquired while ACL named blocks of (to be) trained (CILT and PACE) and untrained (CORR and UNTR) pictures during four sessions: S1 (pre-CILT); S2 (post-CILT); S3 (post-PACE); and S4 (6 months post-CILT). Each of four runs per session consisted of 48 experimental (6 objects and 6 actions per condition) and 12 control trials presented in blocks in the following order: X, PACE, CORR, X, CILT, UNTR. In the control blocks ACL was trained to just say "pass" when a series of meaningless shapes with squiggly lines appeared. This task was chosen because it requires low-level visual processing and vocalisation of a single word, as does the experimental task, but does not require retrieval or semantic or phonologic processing of unique words. ACL was trained on a different set of pictures to either name the picture aloud—using a one-word response and staying still—or to say "pass" if he was unable to name the picture. He was trained to respond as quickly as possible and before the crosshair (and scanner noise) began.

## Analyses

Overt responses were recorded via a noise-cancelling microphone (OptoAcoustics; http://www.optoacoustics.com/) and analysed by two raters with a digital audio recording and editing software package (Audacity; http://www.audacity.sourceforge.net).

Functional MRI data were processed using Matlab 7.0.4 (The MathWorks, Inc.) and the SPM5 software package (www.fil.ion.ucl.ac.uk). The following pre-processing steps were used: slice-timing adjustment; realignment using the middle scan as a reference; co-registration with the 3D MPRAGE; normalisation to the MNI T1 template;

smoothing (8-mm isotropic FWHM Gaussian kernel). Cost-function masking (Brett, Leff, Rorden, & Ashburner, 2001) was utilised to mask out ACL's lesion, effectively excluding the area of lesion and potential distortions from the normalisation process.

First-level $t$-tests examined task-related activation during the following contrasts: (1) treated vs untreated; (2) experimental vs control; and (3) correct vs incorrect trials. Voxels were regressed against a box-car waveform and convolved with a canonical HRF. A 128-s HPF was applied and a first order autoregressive model utilised to correct for serial correlations in time. A cluster-level threshold for statistical significance ($p < .05$, FWE) corrected for whole brain analysis was utilised.

# RESULTS

## Treatment outcomes

Confrontation naming improved dramatically. Even in the scanner, with minimal allowable response time, ACL improved significantly on trained pictures (Table 1). McNemar tests between accuracy on naming pre-/post-CILT (S1: 1/48 [2%] vs S2: 22/48 [46%] correct) and pre-/post-PACE pictures (S2: 9/48 [19%] vs S3: 27/48 [56%] correct) were statistically significant ($p < .001$).

## Functional MRI results

Issues with timing during Session 1 (pre-treatment) precluded analysis due to overlapping speech during scanning. Efforts to remove motion artifact due to nuisance volumes were unsuccessful, therefore Session 1 data are not reported.

Results of the other three sessions generally did not demonstrate significant differences in direct contrasts between the treated and untreated conditions. In contrasts between all four experimental (CORR, CILT, PACE, and UNTR) conditions and the control task, considerable overlap in the patterns of activation was observed. This was especially true in left (L) frontal/pre-motor regions (see Figure 2 and Table 2). Differences between experimental conditions can be described more as a matter of spatial extent and degree of activation, rather than as unique patterns of activation. All four conditions produced strong pre-motor and pre-supplementary motor (pre-SMA) activation that appeared to be increasingly recruited in direct proportion with task difficulty, i.e., inversely proportional with task accuracy. A post-hoc analysis of contrasts examining correctly and incorrectly named pictures is also considered.

*Consistently correctly named (CORR) pictures.* Pictures named consistently correctly (on at least 2/3 baseline tests) were more accurately named in the scanner during all three sessions than pictures from any other treatment condition. This relative ease of naming was associated on all three occasions with the smallest profile of regional activation. Post-CILT treatment, compared with the control task, naming CORR pictures produced one cluster approaching significance in L middle frontal gyrus (MFG): BA 8 ($Z = 4.64$; number of voxels [$k$] = 36). Similarly, a L MFG cluster—larger and with significant voxels of peak activation—was activated post-PACE ($Z = 6.09$; $k = 207$) and 6 months post-CILT ($Z = 5.15$; $k = 254$). Sub-threshold activation ($p < .001$ uncorrected) was observed in S3 and S4 in L medial frontal gyrus (pre-SMA: BA 6) in an area significantly activated by the treated conditions.

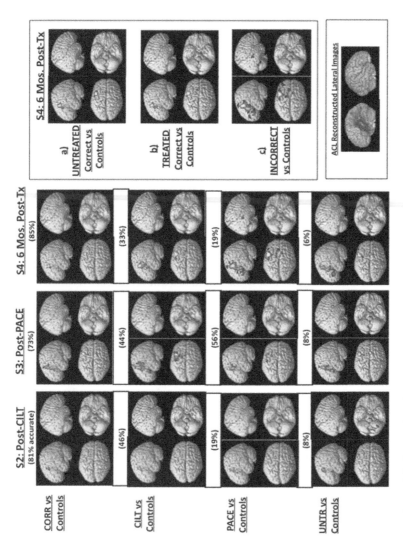

**Figure 2.** BOLD signal increases observed during naming of consistently correct (CORR), trained (CILT or PACE) and untrained (UNTR) stimuli *vs* the control task at three time points: (1) S2: post CILT therapy; (2) S3: post PACE therapy; and (3) S4: 6 months post CILT therapy. Numbers in parentheses indicate accuracy on the task in the scanner. Inset: BOLD signal increases observed in contrasts of: (a) untreated correct, (b) treated correct, and (c) incorrect naming of pictures *vs* the control task during S4. Significant regions of activation (shown here at $p < .001$ uncorrected for display purposes) were rendered onto a standard 3D anatomical template. Lower right: ACL's reconstructed lateral 3D image. To view this figure in colour, please visit the online version of the Journal.

TABLE 2
Mean activation peaks identified during naming of pictures vs. controls

| Session | Contrast<br>Anatomical localization (Brodmann's area) | N voxels | X | Y | Z | Z scores |
|---|---|---|---|---|---|---|
| | *CORR vs. Controls* | | | | | |
| S2 | L middle frontal (8) | 36 | −54 | 9 | 42 | 4.64 |
| S3 | L middle frontal (8,6)[a] | 207 | −48 | 9 | 42 | 6.09 |
| S3 | L inferior frontal (13)[b] | | −51 | 24 | 12 | 3.92 |
| S4 | L middle frontal (6,8)[a] | 254 | −44 | 10 | 50 | 5.15 |
| | *CILT vs. Controls* | | | | | |
| S2 | Left (L) middle frontal (8)[a] | 62 | −48 | 6 | 45 | 4.77 |
| S3 | L middle frontal (6,8)[a] | 659 | −39 | 11 | 49 | 6.75 |
| S3 | L inferior frontal (45)[a] | | −51 | 21 | 15 | 5.43 |
| S3 | L med. frontal/pre-SMA (8,6)[b] | 87 | −3 | 6 | 60 | 4.4 |
| S4 | L middle frontal (6,8)[a] | 1470 | −48 | 4 | 44 | 5.99 |
| S4 | L inferior frontal (44)[a] | | −56 | 16 | 18 | 5.13 |
| S4 | L med. frontal/pre-SMA (6)[b] | 468 | −6 | 14 | 52 | 5.11 |
| | *PACE vs. Controls* | | | | | |
| S2 | L middle frontal (9)[a] | 131 | −51 | 6 | 42 | 4.99 |
| S3 | L middle frontal (6,8)[a] | 147 | −39 | 11 | 49 | 5.41 |
| S3 | L inferior frontal (44)[b] | | −48 | 0 | 21 | 4.22 |
| S3 | L med. frontal/pre-SMA (8,6)[b] | 70 | −3 | 6 | 60 | 4.91 |
| S3 | L middle frontal (9)[a] | 43 | −45 | 15 | 30 | 4.9 |
| S4 | L middle frontal (8,9,6)[a] | 2487 | −48 | 4 | 44 | 7.84 |
| S4 | L superior frontal / cingulate (8,6,32)[a] | 1475 | −6 | 12 | 54 | 7.06 |
| S4 | R lingual / cuneus (18,30)[a] | 324 | 16 | −56 | −2 | 5.23 |
| S4 | R temporal fusiform (37)[b] | 403 | 38 | −48 | −22 | 3.63 |
| S4 | R superior temporal (22)[b] | 180 | 54 | −32 | 2 | 4.34 |
| S4 | R ant cingulate / medical frontal (32,9)[b] | 147 | 22 | 34 | 16 | 4.17 |
| | *UNTR vs. Controls* | | | | | |
| S2 | L middle frontal[a] | 85 | −51 | 6 | 45 | 5.55 |
| S2 | L inferior frontal (47)[b] | 143 | −48 | 21 | 0 | 4.53 |
| S2 | Right (R) occipital fusiform (8,6)[a] | 64 | 27 | −78 | −18 | 4.53 |
| S3 | L middle frontal (8,6)[a] | 275 | −48 | 9 | 42 | 6.51 |
| S3 | L inferior frontal (45)[a] | | −51 | 24 | 13 | 4.87 |
| S3 | L med. frontal/pre-SMA (6)[b] | 101 | −3 | 15 | 51 | 5.7 |
| S4 | L middle/inferior frontal (8,9,6)[a] | 1035 | −52 | 6 | 44 | 5.81 |
| S4 | L med. frontal/pre-SMA/cingulate (6,32)[a] | 364 | −6 | 14 | 52 | 5.28 |
| S4 | L inferior frontal (47)[b] | 331 | −48 | 32 | −4 | 4.75 |
| S4 | L middle/superior frontal (9,46,10)[b] | 141 | −14 | 48 | 26 | 3.97 |

[a]Voxel of peak activation is also significant at $p < .05$ FWE.
[b]Voxel of peak activation is also significant at $p < .05$ FDR.

*CILT pictures.* Post-CILT treatment, naming of CILT pictures (22/48; 46% correct) was associated with a nearly identical pattern of activation as naming of CORR pictures. One significant cluster was activated in L MFG: BA 8 ($Z = 4.77$; $k = 62$). Sub-threshold activation was noted in L pre-SMA. Post-PACE, naming of CILT pictures recruited extensive L frontal activation in L MFG ($Z = 6.75$; $k = 659$), IFG (BA 45; $Z = 5.43$), and pre-SMA ($Z = 4.4$; $k = 87$), although accuracy remained fairly stable (21/48; 44%). At 6 months post-treatment, another increase in cluster size and degree of activation in L MFG ($Z = 5.99$; $k = 1470$), IFG (BA 44; $Z = 5.13$), and pre-SMA ($Z = 5.11$; $k = 468$) was associated with more effortful and less accurate naming of CILT pictures.

*PACE pictures.* Pre-PACE treatment, naming PACE pictures (9/48; 19% correct) recruited a larger and more significantly activated L MFG cluster ($Z = 4.99$; $k = 131$) than those observed during naming of CORR and CILT pictures. Sub-threshold activation was observed in L pre-SMA. Post-PACE, naming accuracy improved significantly (27/48; 56% correct), again with corresponding activation observed in L MFG ($Z = 5.41$; $k = 147$), L IFG ($Z = 4.22$), and pre-SMA ($Z = 4.91$; $k = 70$). Six months later, accuracy returned to 19% correct, but now naming PACE pictures recruited an extensive bilateral (predominantly L frontal) network that included activation in L MFG ($Z = 7.84$; $k = 2487$), and L cingulate and pre-SMA ($Z = 7.06$; $k = 1475$). Large and significant clusters were also activated in right (R) occipital and temporal cortex, including R lingual and cuneus, R temporal fusiform, and R STG (Wernicke homologue).

*Untrained (UNTR) pictures.* Accuracy on the untrained control set of pictures never improved above 8% (4/48), yet it is clear from his responses and the patterns of activation during attempts to name UNTR pictures that ACL's strategy was the same. Post-CILT, UNTR pictures activated a cluster in L MFG very similar to those observed in the trained conditions ($Z = 5.55$; $k = 85$). In addition, activation was present in L IFG (BA 47; $Z = 4.53$; $k = 143$), and R occipital fusiform gyrus. With no improvement 1 month later, and again 6 months post-treatment, similar patterns were observed, each time with greater spatial extent in L MFG (S3: $Z = 6.51$; $k = 275$; and S4: $Z = 5.81$; $k = 1035$), as well as recruitment of L IFG (S3: BA 45; $Z = 4.87$; and S4: BA 47; $Z = 4.75$; $k = 331$) and pre-SMA (S3: $Z = 5.7$; $k = 101$; and S4: $Z = 5.28$; $k = 364$).

*Correct vs incorrect naming.* Since treatment improves performance, examination of *treatment-induced* changes should account for improved response accuracy. Therefore a post-hoc analysis examining untreated correct, treated correct, and incorrect responses at 6 months post-treatment was performed (see Figure 2 inset, and Table 3).

There were no statistically significant differences in direct contrasts examining treated and untreated correct or in those examining correctly vs incorrectly named pictures. Compared to the control task, both treated and untreated correctly named pictures activated ACL's characteristic L IFG/MFG/SFG network with more or less inclusion of IFG and pre-SMA. Specifically, correct naming of untreated pictures (mostly CORR) significantly activated one cluster in L MFG ($Z = 6.24$; $k = 516$), while a cluster in pre-SMA ($Z = 4.65$; $k = 116$) approached significance ($p = .089$). Correct naming of *treated* pictures (CILT and PACE) significantly activated three clusters, including L MFG ($Z = 5.02$; $k = 345$), L pre-SMA/cingulate ($Z = 4.94$; $k = 397$), and L IFG ($Z = 4.25$; $k = 235$). Compared to correct naming of untreated pictures, incorrectly named pictures (collapsed across all four conditions) activated one significant cluster in L pre-SMA ($Z = 4.73$; $k = 137$). Compared to correct naming of treated pictures, incorrectly named pictures activated one significant cluster in L MFG ($Z = 4.19$; $k = 135$). The largest recruitment of this left frontal network was observed in contrasting incorrectly named pictures to the control task. In comparing the least-accurate, most-effortful and the most-accurate, least-effortful task performance, incorrect naming recruited a bilateral network of predominantly left frontal regions that included seven large and significant clusters in: L MFG and IFG ($Z > 8.0$; $k = 3266$), and L pre-SMA ($Z > 8.0$; $k = 1447$). In addition, a number of RH regions were activated,

TABLE 3
Mean activation peaks identified during treated correct,
untreated correct, and incorrect naming

| Contrast | | Coordinates (MNI) | | | | |
|---|---|---|---|---|---|---|
| Session | Anatomical localization (Brodmann's area) | N voxels | X | Y | Z | Z scores |
| *Untreated Correct vs. Controls* | | | | | | |
| S4 | L middle frontal (6)[a] | 516 | −44 | 8 | 50 | 6.24 |
| *Treated Correct vs. Controls* | | | | | | |
| S4 | L middle frontal (6,9)[a] | 345 | −44 | 12 | 45 | 5.02 |
| S4 | L med. Frontal/pre-SMA (6,32)[a] | 397 | −6 | 16 | 47 | 4.94 |
| S4 | L inferior frontal (45,44)[b] | 235 | −48 | 18 | 12 | 4.25 |
| *Incorrect vs. Untreated Correct* | | | | | | |
| S4 | L med. Frontal/pre-SMA (6) | 137 | −6 | 10 | 56 | 4.73 |
| *Incorrect vs. Treated Correct* | | | | | | |
| S4 | L middle frontal (8) | 135 | −48 | 4 | 48 | 4.19 |
| *Incorrect vs. Controls* | | | | | | |
| S4 | L middle frontal (8,6,46)[a] | 3266 | −48 | 4 | 44 | > 8.0 |
| S4 | L med. Frontal/pre-SMA (6)[a] | 1447 | −6 | 14 | 52 | > 8.0 |
| S4 | L middle / superior frontal (10)[a] | 174 | −34 | 47 | 14 | 5.53 |
| S4 | R temporal fusiform (37)[a] | 514 | 36 | −44 | −22 | 5.07 |
| S4 | R ant. cingulate (32)[b] | 243 | 24 | 28 | 20 | 4.58 |
| S4 | R lingual (18,19)[b] | 211 | 16 | −56 | −2 | 4.45 |
| S4 | R sup. Temporal (Wernicke homologue; 22)[b] | 173 | 57 | −23 | 1 | 4.2 |

[a]Voxel of peak activation is also significant at $p < .05$ FWE.
[b]Voxel of peak activation is also significant at $p < .05$ FDR.

including: R temporal fusiform ($Z = 5.07$; $k = 514$), R ant. cingulate ($Z = 4.58$; $k = 243$), R Wernicke's homologue (BA 22; $Z = 4.2$; $k = 173$).

## DISCUSSION

The present study used a multiple baseline across behaviours design in order to examine treatment-induced neural and behavioural changes following two different intensive therapies in an individual with chronic Wernicke's aphasia. He underwent behavioural and fMRI testing before and after 2 weeks of CILT, then following 2 weeks of unconstrained language therapy (PACE), and again 6 months post-CILT. Both phases of therapy were intensive, but only CILT required spoken responses. Both phases resulted in improved naming and auditory comprehension.

Whether constraint or intensity of therapy is responsible for such improvement is still under investigation. Having undergone CILT prior to PACE therapy, ACL exhibited a preference for spoken responses during the PACE phase. This may have minimised differences that might have existed had the two phases been reversed. Nonetheless, evidence increasingly suggests that therapeutic gains are greater, and possibly longer lasting, with intensive therapy schedules (Bhogal, Teasel, & Speechley, 2003). For ACL, the intensive therapy appears to have "kick-started" a progression of recovery that had been stagnant for the previous 2 years of once a week, 1-hour outpatient services. In addition to modest improvements on standardised tests, anecdotal evidence from family and doctors suggests a pattern of increased confidence and functional independence that include making phone calls, independently taking public transportation, meeting with friends, and other measures that can be difficult to capture quantitatively.

## Treatment-induced neuroplasticity

The study of mechanisms supporting language recovery in aphasia is in a relatively nascent stage. Attempts to understand treatment-induced neuroplasticity may be easily confounded due to other treatment-induced changes, namely reduction in task difficulty and improvement in task performance. Measurements in functional neuroimaging may vary due to differences in reaction time, accuracy, and effort, all of which may be modulated by task difficulty. Neuroimaging a successful treatment study targeting domain-specific tasks (such as naming) necessarily involves comparing conditions in which domain-general cognitive processes (such as attention and response inhibition) may also have undergone changes in efficiency or effectiveness. Minimally, such studies require consideration of the role that may be played by these factors.

At first glance, it may appear as if the rapid and somewhat enduring improvements in picture naming were not accompanied by specific changes in neural activation patterns. Direct comparisons between experimental (trained and untrained) conditions did not reach significance, and the same was true of comparisons within condition across time for Sessions 2 and 3. Furthermore, contrasts comparing experimental to the control task all bore a resemblance to a similar frontal network that included MFG (BA 6/8) with more or less extension up to pre-SMA and down to IFG.

If the changes in spatial extent and degree of activation were not tied to varying treatment method, or to treatment vs no-treatment, or to time post-treatment, what is the significance of this change in pattern of activation? Several PET and fMRI studies have demonstrated correlation between the degree of neural activation and the demands of a cognitive task. Increasing sentence complexity in a written comprehension task (Just, Carpenter, Keller, Eddy, & Thulborn, 1996) or re-introducing novelty in a verb generation task (Raichle et al., 1994) increases the magnitude or spatial extent of activation in classical language areas in healthy participants. Conversely, with practice and improved performance, the opposite effect is observed. In patients, increased activation in L and/or R prefrontal cortex has been associated with poor performance, particularly on tasks requiring overt speech responses (Belin et al., 1996; Naeser et al., 2004; Perani et al., 2003). Perani and colleagues, whose patients were retrieving words covertly to semantic cues, suggested that the increased frontal activation might represent mental retrieval *effort*, rather than retrieval *success*.

In ACL's case, given the training schedule and his apparent awareness that some pictures were never trained, task difficulty varied by a combination of training condition and time. Correspondingly, the pattern of neural activation seemed to vary according to a combination of task difficulty and performance expectation. Next to the CORR picture set, CILT pictures post-CILT treatment and PACE pictures post-PACE treatment were the most-practised, least cognitively demanding pictures to name. Over time, ACL increased attempts to name UNTR pictures, but his mostly errorful productions were not accompanied by self-correcting behaviours. On the contrary, when attempting to name *trained* pictures, there was increased self-correction and self-reflection over time. An increase in self-monitoring and self-correcting of CILT pictures post-PACE and CILT and PACE pictures 6 months post-CILT may also have contributed to the greater activation in a frontal network that included medial frontal structures during those sessions.

What about the specific regions that were subject to modulation as a result of task difficulty, accuracy, and performance expectation? The regions activated were not, strictly speaking, the typical cortical regions associated with naming. Of course, many of those regions (e.g., left posterior inferior parietal and lateral temporal) lie within ACL's lesion. However, all of the frontal regions activated across time and condition in this study (left dorsomedial prefrontal, pre-SMA, and inferior frontal) have been implicated in both semantic and phonological processing. For example, lesions in left dorsomedial prefrontal cortex (DMPFC) can cause transcortical motor aphasia, characterised by impaired propositional speech with preserved repetition. Pre-SMA has previously been associated more closely with phonological than semantic aspects of speech, i.e., initiation, planning, and preparation for speech. However, it has recently been suggested that the linguistic deficit preventing fluent semantic retrieval in these patients may be due to DMPFC damage in pre-SMA (Binder, Desai, Graves, & Conant, 2009).

Left inferior frontal cortex (LIFC) has consistently been implicated in both semantic and phonological aspects of naming. Binder and colleagues' (2009) meta-analysis of 120 functional neuroimaging studies unambiguously demonstrates involvement of anterior-ventral LIFC (roughly BA 47) in semantic processing. It is also common knowledge that lesions to LIFC often impair phonological and articulatory planning aspects of spontaneous speech. It is now commonly held that the LIFC may be fractionated into anterior/inferior (roughly BA 47), middle (roughly BA 44/45), and posterior/superior (roughly BA 44/6) sub-regions that correspond more or less to semantic, syntactic, and phonological processing respectively. Each of these regions was subject to graded activation in response to increased task difficulty.

Importantly, this frontal network was active during correct naming *and possibly overactive* during incorrect naming as shown in post-hoc comparisons between treated and untreated correct, and incorrect pictures. While some functional-imaging studies of aphasic individuals still use covert tasks in attempts to avoid motion artefact, the results of the post-hoc analysis of correct/incorrect responses are a reminder that activation maps in the absence of behavioural context may be missing the point in this population. In ACL's case, intensive CILT and PACE treatment did not produce *functional reorganisation* per se. He did not use a different set of cognitive or neuronal strategies when attempting to name CORR vs CILT vs PACE vs UNTR pictures. Rather, as naming improved on trained sets the frontal network was modulated, becoming less active and perhaps reflecting greater efficiency or improved response selection, self-monitoring, and/or inhibition. By contrast, post-hoc analysis of incorrect trials at 6 months post-CILT appears to recruit a much less efficient frontal network and includes activation in areas homologous to his lesion, i.e., in right Wernicke's homologue.

This longitudinal case study adds to a small, but growing, literature that documents neuroplastic changes accompanying treatment-induced language improvements in post-stroke aphasia. It has, of course, limited generalisability. It is further limited to neuroimaging evidence from only one source. Although fMRI data are frequently reported without converging evidence (e.g., from perfusion imaging), future studies may benefit from disambiguation of functional lesions by including other methods.

Future studies may also be improved by lengthening the inter-trial interval (ITI) and utilising a non-canonical haemodynamic response function (HRF) to analyse participants' longitudinal changes in activation patterns. The HRF may not peak 5–6 seconds after stimulus onset in the presence of cerebrovascular disease (Carusone, Srinivasan, Gitelman, Mesulam, & Parrish, 2002). Bonakdarpour and colleagues observed that haemodynamic time to peak (TTP) was delayed in L Broca's area and the posterior perisylvian network in 3/5 aphasic participants (Bonakdarpour, Parrish, & Thompson,

2007). It has also been reported that treatment may induce changes in TTP. Peck and colleagues observed treatment-induced decreases in verbal response time that correlated with decreases in right hemisphere auditory, motor, premotor, and pre-SMA TTP in 2/3 aphasic participants (Peck et al., 2004).

While these studies recommend incorporating individualised time-resolved analyses to optimise detection of BOLD signal changes in stroke recovery, it is also evident that not all of the participants demonstrated delays in or changes to TTP. Moreover, it appears that the long ITI used in these studies may actually affect changes in TTP; i.e., that reducing the time between stimulus onset and response, as often occurs post-therapy, may decrease the TTP. Notably, all eight participants in the above studies were nonfluent. In the current study a fluent aphasic participant was trained to respond within 4 seconds and tended to respond within 2 seconds from the first post-treatment session (S2) onward. This left less room for dramatic treatment-induced decreases in verbal response time. Accordingly it is unlikely, given the design and the participant's strikingly similar patterns of frontal activation across time and treatment conditions, that the canonical HRF was a poor fit. Rather, the similar patterns and lack of results in direct contrasts between conditions suggest this participant's similar cognitive and neural strategy across conditions, in spite of attempts to deliver different treatment methods.

This study documents treatment-induced modulation of a left frontal network tied to task performance, and provides evidence of another case in which RH activation in critical language zone homologues (e.g., Wernicke's area) and LH over-activation may be maladaptive. As Fridriksson et al. (2007) noted, predicting treatment-induced recovery based on neuroimaging data is premature. However, it is reasonable to hope that the accumulation of longitudinal evidence might suggest patterns that could eventually play a role in candidacy for treatment, patient monitoring, or even online biofeedback. Functional neuroimaging studies of patients *who can perform the task* provide information about mechanisms supporting language recovery that is unavailable from structural imaging, behavioural testing, or functional imaging of normal controls (Price, Noppeney, & Friston, 2006). The critical caveat is provision of some do-able tasks in the scanner so that comparisons can be observed between successful and unsuccessful patient performance. Short-term intensive treatment programmes such as CILT (or intensive PACE) can produce quick improvements in naming that allow investigation of treatment-induced neuroplasticity. They may even jumpstart a system wallowing in learned non-use. For more durable language improvements, however, we may need to consider models of learning theory whose criteria for success go beyond a 2-week constraint.

Manuscript received 22 July 2009
Manuscript accepted 1 December 2009

## REFERENCES

Belin, P., Van Eeckhout, Ph., Zilbovicious, M., Remy, Ph., Francois, C., Guillaume, F. S., et al. (1996). Recovery from nonfluent aphasia after melodic intonation therapy: A PET study. *Neurology, 47*, 1504–1511.

Bhogal, S. K., Teasell, R., & Speechley, M. (2003). Intensity of aphasia therapy, impact on recovery. *Stroke, 34*(4), 987–993.

Binder, J. R., Desai, R. H., Graves, W. W., & Conant, L. L. (2009). Where is the semantic system? A critical review and meta-analysis of 120 functional neuroimaging studies. *Cerebral Cortex, 19*, 2767–2796.

Bonakdarpour, B., Parrish, T. B., & Thompson, C. K. (2007). Hemodynamic response function in patients with stroke-induced aphasia: Implications for fMRI data analysis. *NeuroImage, 36*, 322–331.

Breier, J. I., Maher, L. M., Novak, B., & Papanicolaou, A. C. (2006). Functional imaging before and after constraint-induced language therapy for aphasia using MEG. *Neurocase, 12*, 322–331.

Brett, M., Leff, A. P., Rorden, C., & Ashburner, J. (2001). Spatial normalisation of brain images with focal lesions using cost function masking. *NeuroImage, 14*, 486–500.

Carusone, L. M., Srinivasan, J., Gitelman, D. R., Mesulam, M. M., & Parrish, T. B. (2002). Hemodynamic response changes in cerebrovascular disease: Implications for functional MR imaging. *American Journal of Neuroradiology, 23*, 1222–1228.

Cornelissen, K., Laine, M., Tarkiainen, A., Jarvensivu, T., Martin, N., & Salmelin, R. (2003). Adult brain plasticity elicited by anomia treatment. *Journal of Cognitive Neuroscience, 15*, 444–461.

Crinion, J. T. & Leff, A. P. (2007). Recovery and treatment of aphasia after stroke: Functional imaging studies. *Current Opinion in Neurology, 20*, 667–673.

Davis, A., & Wilcox, J. (1985). *Adult aphasia rehabilitation: Applied pragmatics.* San Diego, CA: Singular.

Druks, J., & Masterson, J. (2000). *An Object and Action Naming Battery.* Philadelphia: Psychology Press.

Eden, G. F., Joseph, J. E., Brown, H. E., Brown, C. P., & Zeffiro, T. A. (1999). Utilising hemodynamic delay and dispersion to detect fMRI signal change without auditory interference: The behavior interleaved gradients technique. *Magnetic Resonance in Medicine, 41*, 13–20.

Fridriksson, J., Moser, D., Bonilha, L., Morrow-Odom, K. L., Shaw, H., Fridriksson, A., et al. (2007). Neural correlates of phonological and semantic-based anomia treatment in aphasia. *Neuropsychologia, 45*, 1812–1822.

Goodglass, H., Kaplan, E., & Barresi, B. (2001). *The assessment of aphasia and related disorders* (3rd ed.). Austin, TX: Pro-Ed.

Gowers, W.R. (1888). *A manual of diseases in the nervous system.* (Vol. 1). London, UK: Churchill.

Just, M. A., Carpenter, P. A., Keller, T. A., Eddy, W. F., & Thulborn, K. R. (1996). Brain activation modulated by sentence comprehension. *Science, 274*, 114–116.

Maher, L. M., Kendall, D., Swearengin, J. A., Rodriguez, A., Leon, S. A., Pingel, K., et al. (2006). A pilot study of use-dependent learning in the context of Constraint Induced Language Therapy. *Journal of the International Neuropsychological Society, 12*, 843–852.

Meinzer, M., & Breitenstein, C. (2008). Functional imaging studies of treatment-induced recovery in chronic aphasia. *Aphasiology, 22*, 1251–1268.

Meinzer, M., Flaisch, T., Obleser, J., Assadollahi, R., Djundja, D., Barthel, G., et al. (2006). Brain regions essential for improved lexical access in an aged aphasic patient: A case report. *BMC Neurology, 6*(28), 1–10.

Naeser, M. A., Martin, P. I., Baker, E. H., Hodge, S. M., Sczerzenie, S. E., Nicholas, M., et al. (2004). Overt propositional speech in chronic nonfluent aphasia studied with the dynamic susceptibility contrast fMRI method. *NeuroImage, 22*, 29–41.

Nudo, R. J., & Friel, K. M. (1999). Cortical plasticity after stroke: Implications for rehabilitation. *Revue Neurologique, 155*, 713–717.

Peck, K. K., Moore, A. B., Crosson, B. A., Gaiefsky, M., Gopinath, K. S., White, K., et al. (2004). Functional magnetic resonance imaging before and after aphasia therapy: Shifts in hemodynamic time to peak during an overt language task. *Stroke, 35*, 554–559.

Perani, D., Cappa, S. F., Tettamanti, M., Rosa, M., Scifo, P., Miozzo, A., et al. (2003). A fMRI study of word retrieval in aphasia. *Brain and Language, 85*, 357–368.

Price, C. J., & and Crinion, J. (2005). The latest on functional imaging studies of aphasic stroke. *Current Opinion in Neurology, 18*, 1–6.

Price, C. J., Noppeney, U., & Friston, K. J. (2006). Functional neuroimaging of neuropsychologically impaired patients. In R. Cabeza & A. Kingstone (Eds.), *Handbook of functional neuroimaging of cognition* (2nd ed., pp. 455–480). Cambridge, MA: MIT Press.

Pulvermuller, F., Hauk, O., Zohsel, K., Neininger, B., & Mohr, B. (2005). Therapy-related reorganisation of language in both hemispheres of patients with chronic aphasia. *NeuroImage, 28*, 481–489.

Pulvermuller, F., Neininger, B., Elbert, T., Mohr, B., Rockstroh, B., Koebbel, P., et al. (2001). Constraint-induced therapy of chronic aphasia after stroke. *Stroke, 32*, 1621–1626.

Raichle, M. E., Fiez, J. A., Videen, T. O., MacLeod, A. K., Pardo, J. V., Fox, P. T., et al. (1994). Practice-related changes in human brain functional anatomy during nonmotor learning. *Cerebral Cortex, 4*, 8–26.

Szekely, A., Damico, S., Devescovi, A., Federmeier, K., Heron, D., Iyer, G., et al. (2005). Timed action and object naming. *Cortex, 41*, 7–26.

Taub, E. (2004). Harnessing brain plasticity through behavioral techniques to produce new treatments in neurorehabilitation. *The American Psychologist, 59*, 692–704.

APHASIOLOGY, 2010, 24 (6–8), 752–762

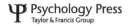

# Verbal and non-verbal working memory in aphasia: What three *n*-back tasks reveal

Stephanie C. Christensen and Heather Harris Wright

*Arizona State University, Tempe, AZ, USA*

*Background*: Researchers have found that many individuals with aphasia (IWA) present with cognitive deficits that may impact their communication, and perhaps underlie their language-processing deficits (e.g., Erickson et al., 1996; Murray et al., 1997; Wright et al., 2003). However, many investigations of cognitive ability in aphasia have included measures that may be considered "language heavy"; they require overt lexical, semantic, and/or phonological processing to follow the task instructions and/or formulate a response. Few have considered the amount of linguistic processing required to perform the task. Subsequently, it is not clear if poorer performance by IWA on cognitive tasks compared to neurologically intact (NI) participants is due to a deficit in the respective cognitive domain or due to the inability of IWA to perform the task because of their language difficulties.

*Aims*: The purpose of the current study was to explore the effect of varying linguistic processing demands in the context of a dynamic working memory task—an *n*-back task for participants with and without aphasia.

*Method & Procedures*: This study compared differences on three different *n*-back tasks within and across groups for individuals with aphasia and NI matched peers. Participants completed three different *n*-back tasks; stimuli for the tasks varied in "linguistic load". For each *n*-back task participants completed two levels of difficulty: 1-back and 2-back.

*Outcomes & Results*: The aphasia group performed significantly worse than the NI participants across the *n*-back tasks. All participants performed significantly better with the stimuli that carried a higher linguistic load (i.e., the fruit), than with the fribbles (semi-linguistic) and blocks (non-linguistic). All participants performed significantly better on the 1-back than the 2-back working memory task. Unlike the NI participants, IWA performed equally poorly with the fribbles and the blocks in the 2-back task.

*Conclusions*: Overall, the performance of individuals with aphasia on working memory tasks that varied in their linguistic load was similar to the control group but reduced. However, unlike the NI participants, IWA were less skilled at rapidly utilising linguistic knowledge to increase performance on the fribbles, demonstrating the further decrement in working memory that results from a decreased ability to utilise a linguistic strategy to increase performance on verbal working memory tasks. The results of this study indicate that language ability has a significant influence on performance on working memory tasks and should be considered when discussing cognitive deficits in aphasia.

*Keywords*: Working memory; Aphasia; *n*-back.

Address correspondence to: Stephanie Christensen, MA CCC-SLP, Department of Speech and Hearing Science, Arizona State University, PO Box 870102, Tempe, AZ 85287-0102, USA. E-mail: Stephanie.Christensen @asu.edu

http://www.psypress.com/aphasiology      DOI: 10.1080/02687030903437690

Performance by adults with aphasia on attention and working memory measures is receiving more attention in the literature. Researchers have found that many individuals with aphasia (IWA) present with cognitive deficits that may impact their communication, and perhaps underlie their language-processing deficits (e.g., Erickson, Goldinger, & LaPointe, 1996; Murray, Holland, & Beeson, 1997; Wright, Newhoff, Downey, & Austerman, 2003). However, many investigations of attention and memory ability in aphasia have included measures that may be considered "language heavy"; they require overt lexical, semantic, and/or phonological processing to follow the task instructions and/or formulate a response. Subsequently, interpretation of the results is limited. It is not clear if poorer performance by IWA on such cognitive tasks compared to NI participants is due to a deficit in the respective cognitive domain or due to the participants' inability to perform the task because of their language difficulties. It has been demonstrated with other populations that disassociations between cognitive and linguistic functions can exist. For example, some individuals with traumatic brain injuries (TBI) present with attention and memory impairments and have relatively preserved language ability (Hagen, 1981). However, it is unclear whether the dissociation is reversible; that is, whether an individual may present with impaired language ability, but relatively preserved attention and memory abilities.

It is well known that linguistic encoding, including phonological and rich semantic encoding, enhances recall of information on short-term memory tasks. Conrad and Hull (1964) demonstrated that short-term memory span is dependent on phonological encoding and subvocal rehearsal of visually presented items. When phonological access or rehearsal is blocked due to articulatory suppression, memory span for visually presented digits significantly decreases (Baddeley, Lewis, & Vallar, 1984).

In addition to phonological encoding, semantic encoding also has an effect on the ability to recall information. It has been well documented that memory is enhanced when information is semantically encoded (e.g., Intraub & Nicklos, 1985; Weldon & Roediger, 1987). For example, Hockley (2008) found that pairs of line drawings were better recalled than when the same pairs were presented verbally, suggesting that pictures receive more extensive semantic processing than words. Semantic information also influences attention, as demonstrated by the cocktail party effect (Moray, 1959). That is, when participants are presented relevant and irrelevant messages, one to each ear via headphones, and asked to attend to the relevant message, they are less able to inhibit the unattended message when it contains semantically meaningful information such as the participant's name (Moray, 1959).

There is a significant body of research demonstrating the linguistic influence on cognitive mechanisms. Craig and Lockhart's (1972) influential levels of processing hypothesis is based on research demonstrating that items processed purely in terms of their physical appearance are not retained as well as items that are verbalised. Further, items that are richly encoded in meaning are those that are best recalled (Baddeley, 2007). It is easily plausible to imagine a negative impact on memory and attention for IWA who may have difficulty accessing verbal and/or semantic representations. Sharing these concerns, Martin and Ayala (2004) cautioned researchers to specify the nature of the task when discussing verbal short-term memory (STM), particularly in IWA. She found a relationship among measures of lexical-semantic and phonological processing and different types of short-term memory tasks and concluded that verbal STM is not a unitary capacity that can be measured in isolation of language abilities.

Martin's measures included digit and word span tasks, and thus were isolated to the capacity of short-term memory. However, working memory takes into account not only storage capacity, but also attention and executive processes (Baddeley, 2007). Impaired performance on measures of working memory has been well documented in IWA (e.g., Caspari, Parkinson, LaPointe, & Katz, 1998; Friedmann & Gvion, 2003; Wright et al., 2003) but minimal consideration has been given to the amount of linguistic processing required to perform the tasks.

Wright, Downey, Gravier, Love, and Shapiro (2007) developed several *n*-back tasks to tap specialised working memory capacities by manipulating the stimulus type as well as the task. The *n*-back task appears ideal for measuring working memory; it requires participants to decide whether each stimulus in a sequence matches the one that appeared *n* items ago. It therefore requires temporary storage and manipulation of information, while constantly updating the contents in working memory (Jonides, Lauber, Awh, Satoshi, & Koeppe, 1997). The *n*-back task is particularly ideal for individuals with aphasia because it requires only a button press for the response. In addition the stimuli can be manipulated to investigate different processes while keeping the working memory load the same.

Although working memory ability in IWA has been extensively investigated in recent years, researchers have done little to consider the amount of linguistic processing required to perform the task. For example, Daneman and Carpenter's (1980) working memory measure, which has been modified and used with individuals with aphasia, requires syntactic, phonological, and semantic processing. It is unknown how participants with aphasia would perform if the linguistic load (see Method section for detailed discussion) of working memory tasks were manipulated. In order to understand the role language plays in working memory tasks, we need to compare the performance of IWA on comparable tasks that vary in their linguistic load.

The purpose of the current study was to explore the effect of varying linguistic processing demands in the context of a dynamic working memory task—an *n*-back task. We were particularly interested in whether IWA performed differently across stimuli that varied in their linguistic load, as well as in comparison to non-language-impaired participants. The *n*-back tasks included three different stimuli that varied in linguistic load. Assuming the working memory deficit in aphasia is specific to and dependent on language, it was hypothesised that individuals with aphasia would be impaired to a greater extent relative to control-matched peers with the *n*-back stimuli that carried a heavier linguistic load (fruit), than on the stimuli with a lighter linguistic load (fribbles). That is, we expected the NI participants to be able to better utilise semantic and phonological encoding on the linguistic and semi-linguistic stimuli than individuals with aphasia. We expected that all groups would have difficulty using a verbal strategy on the non-linguistic stimuli (blocks), therefore we expected no difference between the groups' performance on the blocks. In contrast, if the working memory deficit in aphasia were due to non-linguistic cognitive deficits such as attention or a generalised reduced memory capacity, we expected no interaction between groups, but expected the individuals with aphasia to be depressed in their performance compared with NI participants similarly across stimuli.

# METHOD

## Participants

Participants included 12 IWA and 12 neurologically intact (NI) people who were matched to the IWA by age and education. All participants with aphasia presented with unilateral left hemisphere damage subsequent to cerebrovascular accident. Clinical criteria for participation for individuals with aphasia included (a) presence of aphasia as indicated by performance on the Western Aphasia Battery-Revised (WAB-R; Kertesz, 2006), (b) no history of dementia or other neurological deficits as indicated by self report, (c) at least 6 months post onset of stroke, (d) premorbid right handedness. Inclusion criteria for all participants included self-reported aided or unaided hearing within normal limits; aided or unaided visual acuity within normal limits as indicated by passing a vision screening (Beukelman & Mirenda, 1998); and sufficient dexterity control to make responses using a computer keyboard. NI adults had no history of neurological impairments as indicated by self-report and scores within normal limits on the Mini Mental State Examination (MMSE; Folstein, Folstein, & McHugh, 1975). Demographic information is reported in Table 1.

## Stimuli and tasks

The $n$-back task was presented with three different types of stimuli that varied in their linguistic load. We operationally define "linguistic load" as the degree to which an object could rapidly elicit a consistent name in a confrontation naming task. The term "linguistic load" refers to the semantic and phonological graded differences that are present across the three different types of stimuli included in this study. It does not indicate difficulty level for stimulus types, but rather the ease with which participants can rapidly assign meaning and phonological form to the objects. The stimuli included *fruit*, which carried the greatest linguistic load (easiest to name); *fribbles*,

TABLE 1
Demographic information for the participant groups

| Participant | Age | Level of education | Gender | Months post CVA | WAB-R AQ | WAB-R profile |
|---|---|---|---|---|---|---|
| 1 | 65 | 14 | M | 58 | 76.3 | Conduction |
| 2 | 58 | 13.5 | M | 64 | 86.1 | Anomic |
| 3 | 73 | 12 | M | 39 | 85.2 | Anomic |
| 4 | 55 | 14 | M | 24 | 57.6 | Broca |
| 5 | 66 | 14 | F | 172 | 56.3 | Broca |
| 6 | 34 | 14 | F | 21 | 90.7 | Anomic |
| 7 | 38 | 14 | F | 141 | 57.7 | Broca |
| 8 | 62 | 18 | F | 84 | 61.3 | Broca |
| 9 | 72 | 12 | M | 57 | 64.9 | Anomic |
| 10 | 65 | 11 | F | 119 | 89.4 | Anomic |
| 11 | 65 | 14 | M | 58 | 54.4 | Broca |
| 12 | 76 | 14 | M | 16 | 47.9 | Broca |
| Mean | 60.8 | 13.7 | M = 7, | 70 | 68.82 | |
| (SD) | (12.5) | (1.64) | F = 5 | (46.95) | (15.66) | |
| Mean | 61 | 14.5 | M = 5 | N/A | N/A | Control Group |
| (SD) | (11.20) | (1.89) | F = 7 | | | |

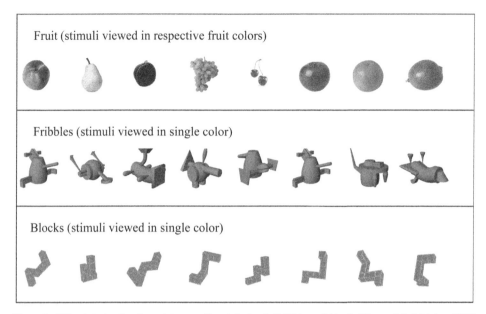

Fruit (stimuli viewed in respective fruit colors)

Fribbles (stimuli viewed in single color)

Blocks (stimuli viewed in single color)

**Figure 1.** N-back task stimuli used to vary linguistic load. Fribble and block (Shepard & Metzler, 1977) stimuli courtesy of Michael J. Tarr, Brown University, http://www.tarrlab.org

which were novel objects and considered the semi-linguistic condition; and *blocks*, which were the non-linguistic stimuli. The fribbles were two-dimensional blue objects easily distinguishable from one another. The blocks were three-dimensional coloured cubes connected to one another in different arrays; they were selections from those used by Shepard and Metzler (1971) in their study of mental rotation. None of the blocks were mental rotations of one another. The fribbles and blocks were maximally distinct objects selected from those provided on the following website: http://www.tarrlab.org/ Stimuli are presented in Figure 1. The fruit stimuli have the heaviest linguistic load because a participant can easily access the phonological form and semantic representation of the stimuli. The fribbles have less of a linguistic load, and the blocks were considered non-linguistic. To verify that the stimuli differed in their linguistic load, five neurologically intact participants viewed each fribble (and block) during task development. They were instructed to assign a name to the item. If participants were not able to generate a name within a reasonable amount of time (15 seconds) the next item was presented. Participants generated meaningful object names for the fribbles; however, there was little agreement across participants. Participants did not generate meaningful object names for the blocks, although some participants were able to come up with lengthy descriptions (e.g., "three blocks down with two across and pointing out").

All participants were administered the tasks at two levels of processing difficulty—1-back and 2-back. For the 1-back and 2-back conditions the participants responded with their non-dominant hand by pressing the spacebar on a keyboard when the current token was the same as the one *n* back. The non-dominant hand was used because some participants were unable to respond with their dominant hand due to hemiparesis. For all tasks, instructions were as follows, *"Push the spacebar when the object you just saw is the same as the one [n] back."* A 0-back task was also administered to all participants to ensure they were able to reliably attend to the task and discriminate between objects. The 0-back level required a response when a specific token was presented (e.g., lime).

Each *n*-back task contained eight different stimuli. In the 1-back task there were 33 target items used for determining performance, and there were 32 targets in the 2-back task. All 1-back tasks included five blocks: one practice block of 10 items with 2 targets; a second block with 26 items and 8 targets; two blocks (blocks 3 and 5) with 24 items and 8 targets; and a fifth block (block 4) with 24 items and 9 targets. All 2-back tasks also consisted of five blocks: one practice block with 10 items and 2 targets; a second and fourth block with 26 stimuli and 8 targets; and a third and fifth block with 24 stimuli and 8 targets. The percentages of tokens that were targets in the 1-back and 2-back tasks were 33% and 32%, respectively. These percentages were selected to be consistent with *n*-back tasks in the literature while also falling within the ability level of the participants, to keep the tasks from being too frustratingly long.

## Experimental procedures

Assessment of participants with aphasia was completed prior to the experimental sessions. During the assessment phase informed consent was obtained, the WAB-R was administered, and vision screening was conducted. The NI participants completed the informed consent, vision, and cognitive screening measures, as well as other experimental tasks that were not related to this study, during their first session. All *n*-back tasks were administered in a second session in a quiet room in the university lab or at the participant's home. All participants were administered the 0-back followed by the 1-back and 2-back tasks. Presentation order for stimuli type was randomised across participants and tasks. Instructions were provided verbally and using paper illustrations prior to each task (0-back, 1-back, 2-back). Instructions were repeated until participants demonstrated understanding by pointing to correct stimuli on the printed sample illustrations. Participants also completed practice items on the computer that were identical to the experimental task. Computer practice items were administered prior to each task for each stimuli type. After completion of the experimental tasks, participants answered open-ended questions regarding their thoughts about the experiment and whether certain tasks or stimuli were easier than others. Additionally, participants completed a confrontation naming task with all stimuli used in the experiment and responses were recorded.

Stimuli were presented using E-prime software with a 3500 ms stimulus onset asynchrony (SOA). The stimulus was presented for 750 ms and the interstimulus interval between tokens was 2750 ms. Accuracy and response times (RT) were recorded by the stimulus presentation software with millisecond precision. Because participants were not specifically instructed to respond with any rapidity—only "quickly, as another item will be coming up soon"—RTs were not viewed as an index of processing time and were not subjected to statistical analyses. Response accuracy, in the form of hit rates and false recognition rates, was recorded and converted to d' values and then subjected to statistical analyses. Signal detection theory advocates for the use of d' as a bias free measure of internal response or sensitivity (Lachman, Lachman, & Butterfield, 1979). D' is valuable because it does not depend on the criterion the participant is adopting. That is, it accounts for the individual's tendency to respond liberally, or in other cases conservatively, in the presence of a signal. D' is calculated by subtracting the *z*-scored false positive rate from the *z*-scored hit rate.

# RESULTS

A mixed analysis of variance (ANOVA) was performed with group as the between-participants factor. The two within-participants factors included stimulus type (fruit, fribbles, or blocks) and working memory load (1-back or 2-back). Descriptive statistics are reported in Table 2. Results of the mixed ANOVA revealed a significant group main effect, $F(1, 22) = 9.28\ p < .01$. The aphasia group had significantly lower d' values compared to the NI group. As expected, there was a significant working memory load main effect within groups, $F(2, 22) = 137.72$, $p < .01$ with d' values for the 1-back being significantly higher than the 2-back. There was also a significant main effect for stimulus type, $F(2, 21) = 24.054$, $p < .001$. Finally, a significant interaction between working memory load and stimulus type was present, $F(2, 21) = 7.51$, $p < .01$. To explore the effect of stimulus type across groups, paired sample $t$ tests controlling for multiple comparisons using Holm's (1979) sequential Bonferroni approach were conducted. Fruit had significantly higher d' values than fribbles, $t(23) = 5.15$, $p < .001$, and blocks, $t(23) = 7.23$, $p < .001$. The d' values for fribbles were also significantly higher compared to d' values for blocks, $t(23) = 3.01$, $p < .01$. Additional analyses to explore the significant interaction revealed that the differences across stimuli types were greater in the 2-back than the 1-back conditions for the comparison between the fruit and fribbles, $t(23) = 3.089$, $p < .01$, and between the fruit and blocks, $t(23) = 3.681$, $p < .01$. There was no significant difference between the fribbles and blocks across the different working memory loads, $t(23) = 1.169$, $p = .26$. No other interaction was significant.

## Aphasia group

Of particular interest was the pattern of performance across the different stimuli types within groups. To explore within-group differences the simple main effects for the aphasia group and the control group adjusting for the multiple comparisons using Holm's sequential Bonferroni approach were analysed. A repeated-measures

TABLE 2
Descriptive statistics for d' scores on 1-back and
2-back tasks with different stimuli

| Task | Group | M | SD |
|------|-------|---|----|
| *1-back* | | | |
| Fruit | Aphasia | 3.23 | .91 |
| | Control | 4.12 | .41 |
| Fribbles | Aphasia | 3.03 | .95 |
| | Control | 3.86 | .53 |
| Blocks | Aphasia | 2.78 | 1.29 |
| | Control | 3.84 | .71 |
| *2-back* | | | |
| Fruit | Aphasia | 1.82 | .85 |
| | Control | 2.55 | .78 |
| Fribbles | Aphasia | 1.09 | .81 |
| | Control | 1.85 | .95 |
| Blocks | Aphasia | 0.86 | .70 |
| | Control | 1.37 | .77 |

$N = 12$.

ANOVA was conducted for the 1-back task with stimulus type (fruit, fribbles, blocks) as the factor. Results indicated no significant differences among stimuli for the aphasia group, $F(2, 10) = 1.12$, $p = .37$. A repeated-measures ANOVA for the 2-back with stimulus type as the factor was also performed. There was a significant main effect for stimulus type in the 2-back, $F(2, 10) = 25.64$, $p < .001$. Planned comparisons indicated the group performed better, with significantly higher d' values, on fruit than fribbles, $t(11) = 3.88$, $p < .01$, and blocks, $t(11) = 6.69$, $p < .001$.

Finally, to explore the relationship between overall language severity and $n$-back performance, a correlation analysis was conducted between WAB-R aphasia quotient (AQ) and the 1- and 2-back tasks for all stimuli. None of the comparisons were statistically significant.

## Neurologically intact group

Similar analyses as performed with the aphasia group were performed with the NI group to determine within-group differences across stimuli type. A repeated-measures ANOVA with stimulus type as the factor revealed significant differences among the stimuli in the 1-back task, $F(2, 10) = 6.36$, $p < .05$. Pairwise comparisons were conducted adjusting for familywise error rate using Holm's sequential Bonferroni approach. Results revealed significant differences between the fruit and fribbles, $t(11) = 3.49$, $p < .01$, but no significant differences between the fruit and blocks, $t(11) = 2.47$, $p = .03$ or the fribbles and blocks, $t(11) = .22$, $p = .83$ were found.

In the 2-back task there was a significant main effect for stimulus type, $F(2, 10) = 23.58$, $p < .001$. Significant differences were found among all stimuli in the 2-back task with fruit having significantly higher d' values than fribbles, $t(11) = 3.12$, $p < .05$, and blocks, $t(11) = 6.77$, $p < .001$; and fribbles having significantly higher d' values than blocks, $t(11) = 3.05$, $p < .05$.

## DISCUSSION

In this study we investigated working memory ability in individuals with and without aphasia. The participants with aphasia performed worse than their NI peers across the working memory measures that varied in linguistic load. The lack of a group interaction demonstrates that the participants with aphasia performed similarly to the NI participants, but with less accuracy across all stimuli. Thus, it appeared that the poorer performance of IWA on the working memory tasks was not solely a result of their language impairment. These results appear to support previous literature indicating that IWA have additional cognitive deficits that may be independent of language (e.g., Erickson et al., 1996; Hula & McNeil, 2008; Tseng, McNeil, & Milenkovic, 1993). Further investigation is warranted to better understand the relationship between cognitive and linguistic deficits in IWA.

Across the three $n$-back task stimuli, both groups performed significantly worse on the 2-back compared to the 1-back tasks. These results are consistent with previous findings indicating that processing load is increased as the number of stimuli to be recalled increases (Jonides et al., 1997; Wright et al., 2007). For the aphasia group, no significant differences were found among stimuli for the 1-back task. However, a significant difference was found for the NI group between the fruit and fribbles $n$-back tasks. The NI group performed significantly better on the 1-back when fruit were the stimuli compared to the fribbles. This was likely a result of the limited within-group variability for these stimuli and may not be particularly meaningful given the relatively high performance of the NI participants on all 1-back tasks (see Table 2). Of interest is how the participant groups performed across the different 2-back tasks.

## NI Participants

In the current study the NI participants performed best on the *n*-back task with fruit stimuli, in comparison to the fribble stimuli; they performed the worst on the task with the block stimuli. Their performance was similar to findings from previous investigations, but with short-term memory (STM) tasks, where the linguistic nature (load) of the stimuli was manipulated (e.g., Baddeley et al., 1984; Conrad & Hull, 1964; Hockley 2008; Intraub & Nicklos, 1985; Weldon & Roediger, 1987). The use of verbal and semantic encoding improves object recall; as linguistic load declines and stimuli are not able to be verbally or semantically encoded easily, then performance declines.

Relatedly, findings from the change-detection literature are relevant for interpreting the results. Change blindness is a phenomenon reported in the visual perception literature, when participants fail to notice overt changes to objects, scenes, or other visual stimuli. For example, Simmons (1996) found that participants were unskilled at detecting changes to objects that were central to a visual scene, even when directly cued to look for such changes. Based on his research, Simons concluded that we are unable to retain information about objects' properties in the absence of verbal encoding. Applying these findings to the current study, possibly the NI participants were unable to accurately recall the blocks because they could not verbally encode the block stimuli.

## Aphasia group

The aphasia group performed differently across the 2-back tasks when the stimuli were manipulated. As the linguistic load declined across stimuli, so did the aphasia participants' task performance. Similar to their age-matched peers, the participants with aphasia performed significantly better on the fruit task compared to the fribbles and blocks tasks. However, no significant difference was found for the aphasia group's performance on the fribbles compared to the block stimuli. One possible explanation for the results is that, similar to the NI participants' performance with the blocks, the participants with aphasia could not easily verbally or semantically encode the stimuli. That is, phonological and/or semantic access was inadequate. According to Baddeley (2007), access to the phonological loop may be unavailable if visual stimuli cannot be converted to images with semantic, and hence phonological, representations, or if participants are blocked from converting semantic representations into phonological codes as is the case during articulatory suppression. After the tasks were completed, several IWA reported that the fribbles reminded them of known objects, but when probed further they were often able to describe, but not verbalise, an object name. In contrast, they were able to recognise and name the fruit. Possibly, the poorer performance by the IWA on the fribbles task compared to the fruit task may be due to their difficulty with rapidly assigning a name to the object that they could subsequently rehearse. Alternatively, it is possible that the participants with aphasia had particular difficulty with the fribbles, not because they were unable to access semantic and phonological information, but that they were unable to do so in a timely manner. The *n*-back task is a timed task that requires a rapid response (3500 ms SOA). To further explore these possibilities, future investigations could include *n*-back tasks where the interstimulus interval is manipulated.

The lack of a correlation between WAB-R AQ and the cognitively demanding *n*-back tasks was interesting, but not entirely surprising. Successful performance on the *n*-back task requires rapid storage and manipulation of semantic and phonological information. The lack of a correlation may be because the WAB-R AQ represents general language function and is not sensitive to the specific phonological and semantic processing demanded by the *n*-back working memory tasks, nor to the additional cognitive demands inherent in the *n*-back task. Additional investigation is warranted to resolve these issues.

## Conclusion

These results demonstrate that working memory is greatly enhanced by verbal encoding, particularly for IWA. Overall, the performance of individuals with aphasia on working memory tasks that varied in their linguistic load was similar to the control group but reduced. However, unlike the NI participants, IWA were less skilled at rapidly utilising linguistic knowledge to increase performance on the fribbles, demonstrating the further decrement in working memory that results from a decreased ability to utilise a linguistic strategy to increase performance on verbal working memory tasks. The results of this study indicate that language ability has a significant influence on working memory performance. Although these findings cannot be generalised to individuals with more severe aphasia, it is apparent that researchers and clinicians interested in cognitive performance in IWA should carefully consider the extent to which language processes influence cognitive function.

Due to the multi-component nature of the *n*-back task, we were unable to distinguish between deficits resulting from a reduced storage capacity and deficits resulting from a more central executive deficit in the ability to rapidly shift attention in order to drop and update the relevant information. Future research should incorporate attention and short-term memory span measures in conjunction with the working memory tasks in order to tease out the primary deficit contributing to the working memory deficits in IWA. In addition, thorough lexical-semantic and phonological testing of individual participants will enable a more concise understanding of the role of phonological and semantic encoding on the working memory process in IWA. Using such measures in combination with cognitive tasks would allow a more precise understanding of the impact of language ability on cognitive task performance.

Manuscript received 25 July 2009
Manuscript accepted 22 October 2009

## REFERENCES

Baddeley, A. (2007). *Working memory, thought, and action*. New York: Oxford University Press.

Baddeley, A., Lewis, V. J., & Vallar, G. (1984). Exploring the articulatory loop. *Quarterly Journal of Experimental Psychology, 36*, 233–252.

Beukelman, D. R., & Mirenda, P. (1998). *Augmentative and alternative communication: Management of severe communication disorders in children and adults* (2nd ed.). Baltimore: Paul H. Brookes.

Caspari, I., Parkinson, S., LaPointe, L., & Katz, R. (1998). Working memory and aphasia. *Brain and Cognition, 37*, 205–223.

Conrad, R., & Hull, A. J. (1964). Information, acoustic confusion, and memory span. *British Journal of Psychology, 55*, 429–432.

Craig, F., & Lockhart, R. S. (1972). Levels of processing: Framework for memory research. *Journal of Verbal Learning and Verbal Behavior, 11*, 671–684.

Daneman, M. & Carpenter, P. A. (1980). Individual differences in working memory and reading. *Journal of Verbal Learning and Verbal Behavior, 19*, 480–466.

Erickson, E., Goldinger, & LaPointe, L. (1996). Auditory vigilance in aphasic individuals: Detecting non-linguistic stimuli with full or divided attention. *Brain and Cognition, 30*, 244–253.

Folstein, J. A., Folstein, S. E., & McHugh, P. R. (1975). "Mini-mental state": A practical method for grading the mental state for the clinician. *Journal of Psychiatric Research, 12*, 189–198.

Friedmann, N., & Gvion, A. (2003). Sentence comprehension and working memory limitation in aphasia: A dissociation between semantic-syntactic and phonological reactivation. *Brain and Language, 86*, 23–39.

Hagen, C. (1981). Language disorders secondary to closed head injury: Diagnosis and treatment. *Topics in Language Disorders, 1*, 73–87.

Hockley, W. E. (2008). The picture superiority effect in associative recognition. *Memory and Cognition, 36*, 1351–1359.

Holm, S. (1979). A simple sequentially rejective multiple test procedure. *Scandinavian Journal of Statistics, 6*, 65–70.

Hula, W. D., & McNeil, M. R. (2008). Models of attention and dual-task performance as explanatory constructs in aphasia. *Seminars in Speech and Language, 29*, 169–187.

Intraub, H., & Nicklos, S. (1985). Levels of processing and picture memory: The physical superiority effect. *Journal of Experimental Psychology: Human Learning and Memory, 11*, 284–298.

Jonides, J., Lauber, E. J., Awh, E., Satoshi, M., & Koeppe, R. A. (1997). Verbal working memory load affects regional brain activation as measured by PET. *Journal of Cognitive Neuroscience, 9*, 462–475.

Kertesz, A. (2006). *Western Aphasia Battery- Revised*. New York: Grune & Stratton.

Lachman, R., Lachman, J., & Butterfield, E. (1979). *Cognitive psychology and information processing: An introduction*. Hillsdale, NJ: Lawrence Erlbaum Associates Inc.

Martin, N., & Ayala, J. (2004). Measurements of auditory-verbal STM span in aphasia: Effects of item, task, and lexical impairment. *Brain and Language, 89*, 464–483.

Moray, N. (1959). Attention in dichotic listening: Affective cues and the influence of instructions. *Quarterly Journal of Experimental Psychology, 11*, 56–60.

Murray, L.L., Holland, A.L., & Beeson, P.M. (1997). Accuracy monitoring and task demand evaluation in aphasia. *Aphasiology, 11*, 401–414.

Shepard, R. N., & Metzler, J. (1971). Mental rotation of three-dimensional objects. *Science, 171*, 701–703.

Simmons, D. J. (1996). In sight, out of mind: When object representations fail. *Psychological Science, 8*, 301–305.

Tseng, C. H., McNeil, M. R., & Milenkovic, P. (1993). An investigation of attention allocation deficits in aphasia. *Brain and Language, 45*, 276–296.

Weldon, M. S., & Roediger, H. L. (1987). Altering retrieval demands reverses the picture superiority effect. *Memory and Cognition, 15*, 269–280.

Wright, H. H., Downey, R. A., Gravier, M., Love, T., & Shapiro, L. P. (2007). Processing distinct linguistic information types in working memory in aphasia. *Aphasiology, 21*, 802–813.

Wright, H. H., Newhoff, M., Downey, R., & Austerman, S. (2003). Additional data on working memory in aphasia. *Journal of International Neuropsychological Society, 9*, 302.

APHASIOLOGY, 2010, 24 (6–8), 763–774

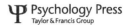

# Perception of visually masked stimuli by individuals with aphasia: A methodological assessment and preliminary theoretical implications

JoAnn P. Silkes

*University of Washington, Seattle, WA, USA*

Margaret A. Rogers

*American Speech-Language-Hearing Association, Rockville, MD, USA*

*Background*: Studies of the automatic processes supporting language processing and dysfunction in aphasia often rely on priming paradigms. However, the ability to confidently interpret these studies in terms of understanding the relative contributions of automatic vs controlled processing depends on the ability to isolate only automatic processes. One way this may be accomplished is through the use of visual masking. The effective use of visual masking, however, depends on verification that there was no task-relevant information consciously available from the prime item.

*Aims*: The study reported here was designed to assess the visibility of visually masked stimuli, for both typical adults and adults with aphasia.

*Methods & Procedures*: This experiment involved 31 typical adults and 21 individuals with aphasia. Visual masking sequences were presented on a computer screen, with 11 different interstimulus intervals assessed. Participants made lexical decisions on the masked stimuli. The two participant groups were compared in terms of their ability to distinguish the word/nonword status of masked stimuli at the various intervals.

*Outcomes & Results*: Participants with aphasia showed an overall poorer ability to discriminate between visually masked words and nonwords than typical adults.

*Conclusions*: The visual masking sequence effectively interfered with task-relevant conscious perception of some masked stimuli for typical adults and all masked stimuli for participants with aphasia. This finding, combined with preliminary data collected on a similar task that involved a simple presence/absence judgement on masked items, suggests that there may be differences in the ability of individuals with aphasia to process rapidly presented masked stimuli, even when there is minimal linguistic processing required.

*Keywords*: Aphasia; Masked priming; Implicit priming; Automatic spreading activation.

Address correspondence to: JoAnn P. Silkes, University of Washington, Department of Speech and Hearing Sciences, 1417 NE 42nd St., Seattle, WA 98105-6246, USA. E-mail: jsilkes@u.washington.edu

This work was completed as part of the first author's doctoral dissertation, and was supported by NIH 5T32DC000033-14 and NIH 1F31DC008736-02. The authors would like to thank two anonymous reviewers who significantly shaped the focus of this paper. We would also like to thank Holly Kavalier and Rebecca Hunting-Pompon for their time and efforts in obtaining pilot data, Laine Anderson, Coralee Choules, and Lina Huang for their work on data reliability, and the members of the University of Washington Aphasia Lab for their insights and support of the study's completion. Finally, we thank the participants, and especially those with aphasia, for their generous contribution of time and energy.

http://www.psypress.com/aphasiology                DOI: 10.1080/02687030903509340

The underlying deficits of aphasia have often been studied with priming tasks, which measure the effect of a prime item on the accuracy or reaction time of a response to a target item. These studies have included, among other things, investigations of the time-course of spreading activation in aphasia (e.g., Prather, Zurif, Love, & Brownell, 1997), assessments of models of the intact and impaired lexical retrieval system (e.g., Martin, Fink, Laine, & Ayala, 2004), and the potential for treating aphasic language deficits through implicit, rather than explicit, language tasks (e.g., Avila, Lambon Ralph, Parcet, Geffner, & Gonzalez-Darder, 2001). Because priming is thought to rely on the automatic spread of activation, rather than strategic processing, these studies have begun to explicate the underlying, implicit mechanisms of language processing, and their breakdown in aphasia.

There is, however, a problem with the interpretation of priming effects as reflective of implicit processing. Most of the priming studies of aphasia reported in the literature confound explicit and implicit language processing by using tasks that allow some level of explicit processing of the prime items. If explicit processing of primes is possible in a task then it is difficult, if not impossible, to attribute priming effects exclusively to automatic, implicit processes (Forster, 1999). One method that has been established for isolating and studying implicit cognitive processes is *masked priming*, which uses very rapid presentation of prime items combined with a visual masking sequence before and/or after the prime items. This technique precludes (or, at the very least, minimises) conscious awareness of the primes, thereby allowing investigation of automatic priming effects ostensibly without the influence of strategic, top-down processing (e.g., Forster, Mohan, & Hector, 2003).

A central issue in masked priming research has been that of how to determine that the masking sequence has effectively eliminated conscious processing of the prime. This is because any conclusions drawn about non-conscious processing of stimuli are only valid if it can be ascertained that the stimuli were *only* unconsciously processed (Erdelyi, 2004; Snodgrass & Shevrin, 2006); that is, that there was no conscious processing of the prime items. In a recent study using masked primes with both typical adults and individuals with aphasia (Silkes, 2009), we were faced with the challenge of addressing this issue in a paradigm that systematically assessed priming at 11 different intervals between primes and targets. This paper presents our approach to determining whether visually masked primes can effectively eliminate conscious processing of primes, both in typical adults and in individuals with aphasia, at these 11 different intervals, which essentially create 11 different masking conditions.

## METHOD

### Participants

Control participants were 31 adults over the age of 21 who reported no history of neurological disorders, substance abuse, or significant psychiatric disorders. Inclusion criteria were a score of at least 20/36 on the Raven's Coloured Progressive Matrices (RCPM; Raven, 1976), which is sensitive to impairments typical of right hemisphere lesions, and at least 50/60 correct on the Boston Naming Test (BNT; Kaplan, Goodglass, & Weintraub, 2001), which is sensitive to impairments typical of left hemisphere lesions. Control participants scored no more than 4/5 on the Depression Intensity Scale Circles (DISC; Turner-Stokes, Kalmus, Hirani, & Clegg, 2005), to rule out severe depression. Vision for all participants was normal or corrected to normal, as per participant report and observed performance on screening tasks. One participant scored 49/60 on the BNT but was still included as a participant because it was determined, on further questioning, that a number of the test stimuli were simply not part of his experience or vocabulary, and he had no other evidence or history suggestive of left hemisphere lesion. Vision for all participants was normal or corrected to normal, as per participant report and observed performance on screening tasks. Control participants ranged in age from 21 to 84 ($\bar{X}$=57.1, $SD$ = 15.26), with an average of 15.97 years of education (range = 12–22, $SD$ = 2.48).

Participants with aphasia were 21 adults over the age of 21 with a diagnosis of aphasia and/or anomia following a unilateral neurological lesion (if there were multiple neurological events, lesions were restricted to the left hemisphere, as per neurology reports). All were at least 9 months post-onset, and native speakers of American English. Participants with aphasia ranged in age from 29 to 82 ($\bar{X}$ = 60.95, $SD$ = 13.28; not significantly different from control participants, $p$ = .34), with an average of 16.33 years of education (range = 12–20, $SD$ = 2.15; not significantly different from control participants, $p$ = .59). Inclusion criteria for the RCPM and the DISC were the same as for control participants and, as with the control participants, individuals with aphasia had no prior history of neurological disorders, significant psychiatric history, or substance abuse, by participant or family report. Diagnosis of aphasia/anomia was made by an experienced, certified speech-language pathologist based on performance on the Western Aphasia Battery (WAB) and the BNT, and/or free conversation (in the case of some participants with mild anomia), in conjunction with otherwise intact cognitive skills, as shown on the RCPM. Aphasia severity ranged from mild to severe (Mean WAB Aphasia Quotient = 62.99/100, range = 7.4–98, $SD$ = 28.77; Mean BNT score = 32.95/60, range = 2–59, $SD$ = 17.5). The BNT could not be conducted with two participants due to severe apraxia of speech. None of the participants had a significant limb apraxia, as measured with the Apraxia Battery for Adults (Dabul, 2000). Participants with aphasia also completed the first four subtests of the Reading Comprehension Battery for Aphasia (LaPointe & Horner, 1979) for descriptive purposes only. This showed combined single-word reading scores from the first four subtests ranging from 7 to 40 ($\bar{X}$ = 34, $SD$ = 8.16). Vision for all participants was normal or corrected to normal, by participant or family report, and no participants showed functional evidence of visual neglect on any of the consent or evaluation procedures.

## Stimuli

Masked stimuli for this task were real words, pronounceable nonwords, or strings of alternating "x"s and "g"s. All stimuli were three to eight letters in length, presented in 30-point, lowercase, black, Arial font, and were forward and backward masked by strings of 12 hash marks (48-point, black, Arial font). Pronounceable nonwords were all phonotactically and orthographically legal in English, and were created by changing each real word used in the study by no more than two letters. Each participant saw only one item from each pair (i.e., either the real word or its derived nonword) over the course of the experiment. In addition, no masked item was presented more than once to a participant. The masking sequence was followed by an unrelated real word, presented in 48-point, uppercase, black, Arial font.

## Procedure

All testing was done in a quiet room, with participants seated at a comfortable distance from a computer screen. Stimuli were presented visually on a 20-inch CRT computer screen with a 100 Hz refresh rate, connected to a personal desktop computer running Microsoft Windows 98, using E-Prime for stimulus delivery (E-Prime version 1.1.4.1, Psychology Software Tools, Pittsburgh, PA). Responses were made using one of two colour-coded keys on a serial response box (Psychology Software Tools, Pittsburgh, PA) interfaced with E-Prime, which collected and recorded response time and accuracy data. Participants wore noise-cancelling headphones (Bose QuietComfort 2) to reduce distraction by ambient noise.

The visibility task involved participants making lexical decisions on the masked stimuli, with responses given by button press when the uppercase real word appeared at the end of the visual presentation sequence (described in detail below). For the participants with aphasia, verbal instructions were simplified and/or supplemented with writing, gesture, and demonstration as needed to maximise comprehension. Participants were given an opportunity to practise this task as many times as they needed to feel comfortable with it. In some cases for participants with aphasia, additional practice runs were specially created with reduced masking or longer stimulus exposure durations to assist them in learning the task. In these cases, once they had learned the task in these special circumstances they then practised in the standard practise condition (which used the same task parameters as the first run of the experiment, as described below) before beginning the experimental conditions.

Visibility was assessed in 11 interstimulus interval (ISI) conditions: 1500, 1000, 750, 500, 250, 200, 150, 100, 70, 50, and 30 ms between the offset of the masking sequence and the onset of the uppercase real word (unrelated to the masked item) signalling the response period. The unmasked real word at the end of the visual sequence had the potential to serve as an additional backward mask to the prime, but its effectiveness as a mask was likely to be reduced at longer ISIs, yielding the possibility that masked items in the longer ISI conditions would be more visible than those in shorter ISI conditions. Thus, assessment of this wide range of intervals (with fixed prime exposure and mask durations) was undertaken to determine whether masking effectiveness varied across the range of ISIs likely to be used in implicit priming paradigms with individuals with aphasia.

Each ISI condition was assessed in a separate run of 16 masked stimuli: 8 real words, 4 XG strings, and 4 pronounceable nonwords. Participants were not told about the two different nonword conditions. They were instructed to make a lexical decision on the masked stimulus in each trial, but not to respond until the unmasked word at the end of the sequence appeared. Responses to the visibility task were made by pressing colour-coded buttons on the serial response box. The control participants were encouraged to respond within 650 ms from onset of the unmasked word, whereas the individuals with aphasia, who had greater difficulty with rapid response, were encouraged to respond within 1000 ms. Every participant began this experimental task with the 1500-ms ISI condition and continued with progressively shortening ISIs. This sequence of presentation, with the easiest-to-discern conditions presented first, was used to maximise the chances of participants being able to detect the masked stimuli so as not to underestimate their visibility.

All visual elements for the masked priming task were presented in the centre of the computer screen, on a white background. The stimulus presentation sequence (see

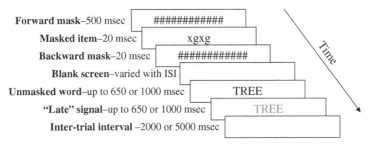

**Figure 1.** Schematic representation of the stimulus presentation sequence.

Figure 1) involved a forward mask (######## in 48-point, black, Arial font) for 500 ms, the masked stimulus (either a real word, a string of alternating "x"s and "g"s, or a pronounceable nonword, in 30-point, black, Arial font, all lowercase letters) for 20 ms, a backward mask (######## in 48-point, black, Arial font) for 20 ms, a blank (white) screen for the duration of the interstimulus interval being assessed, an unmasked word (48-point, black, Arial font, all uppercase letters) for up to 650 ms for typical participants and 1000 ms for participants with aphasia, and (assuming a response was obtained by the end of this interval) a blank (white) screen (2000 ms for typical participants and 5000 ms for participants with aphasia) for an inter-trial interval. If a participant did not respond by the deadline (650 or 1000 ms), an additional screen appeared, containing the same unmasked word in red font. This was a signal to the participants that they had not responded quickly enough. The smaller font size for the masked item compared with all other stimuli in the sequence was used to assure that the masked stimuli were completely covered by the forward and backward masks. The entire protocol took most participants 30–45 minutes to complete.

## Data collection and processing

Each participant completed 16 trials in each of the 11 ISI conditions, for a total of 176 possible responses per participant. Accuracy and reaction time data from the button-press responses in the visibility task were downloaded from E-Prime. All targets were analysed for response accuracy. Responses that were made beyond the response deadline for either group were counted as incorrect, under the assumption that a significant delay was likely to be an indication of difficulty deciding which response to make, which would reflect poor conscious perception of the masked stimulus.

## RESULTS

All control participants successfully learned the experimental task, and completed the entire protocol. Of the participants with aphasia, three were unable to learn the task adequately, even with extended training periods modified extensively to encourage comprehension and success. Therefore, results presented for participants with aphasia are based only on the 18 who successfully learned the task. The one exception to this is the analysis for the 30-ms ISI, in which only 17 participants with aphasia were included due to computer error with data collection for 1 participant. For ANOVA analysis, the missing data point for this participant was replaced by the group average for that ISI.

Visibility of the masked stimuli was assessed using the signal detection measure of d prime (d') (Green & Swets, 1966), based on the proportion of accurate responses and the proportion of false alarms. For each participant, two d' values were calculated at each ISI: one to quantify how well the participant discriminated between real words and XG strings, and one to quantify how well the participant discriminated between real words and pronounceable nonwords. A d' value of zero indicates no discrimination between groups, whereas higher numbers indicate greater degrees of discrimination.

The effectiveness of this masking protocol at preventing conscious perception of the masked items was assessed by comparison of the range of d' values obtained at each ISI against an expected d' of zero, which would reflect no discrimination at all (see Figure 2). One-sample $t$-tests revealed significant differences from zero for the typical adults on Word/ Pronounceable Nonword discrimination in the 30-ms ($t$ = –2.48, $p$ = .019) and 1500-ms ($t$ = 2.983, $p$ = .006) ISI conditions. For Word/XG discrimination, typical adults showed performance significantly different from zero, with positive $t$-values and all $p$ values < .001, in all ISIs from 100 to 1500 ms. A significant difference was also seen in the 70-ms ISI condition ($t$ = 3.022, $p$ = .005). Participants with aphasia showed significant differences from zero on the Word/ Pronounceable Nonword discrimination in the 50-ms ($t$ = –2.484, $p$ = .024), 200-ms ($t$ = –2.505, $p$ = .023), and 250-ms ($t$ = –3.002, $p$ = .008) conditions. For Word/XG discrimination, a significant difference from zero was seen only in the 50-ms ISI condition ($t$ = –2.183, $p$ = .043).

Analysis of individual performance of participants with aphasia was also conducted, to assess the potential impact on this task of single-word reading comprehension and overall aphasia severity. There was no significant relationship revealed with linear regression between overall aphasia severity (as measured by WAB AQ) and average d' value across all ISI conditions ($r^2$ = .0004, $p$ = .94 for the Word/XG and $r^2$ = .02, $p$ = .57 for the Word/Pronounceable Nonword conditions), nor between single-word reading ability (as measured with the first four subtests of the RCBA) and average d' value across all ISI conditions ($r^2$ = .02, $p$ = .54 for the Word/XG and $r^2$ = .10, $p$ = 20 for the Word/Pronounceable Nonword conditions). In addition, the average d' values obtained in both discrimination conditions by the participant with the both the lowest AQ (7.4) and the lowest score on the single-word reading subtests of the RCBA (7) were within 2 standard deviations of the mean for all participants with aphasia. Finally, when all regression analyses were repeated with the two lowest scoring participants' data removed as outliers, relationships continued to be non-significant.

## DISCUSSION

The experiment presented here serves to demonstrate two points. The first is methodological in nature, outlining a method that can be used with individuals with aphasia to assess the visibility of masked primes for the sake of verifying that they are not being consciously processed. This has practical application for future research using masked priming methods with this population. The second point demonstrated here has more theoretical than practical implications—namely, that there are significant differences between typical adults and individuals with aphasia in their ability to perceive masked stimuli. Each of these ideas is discussed in turn below.

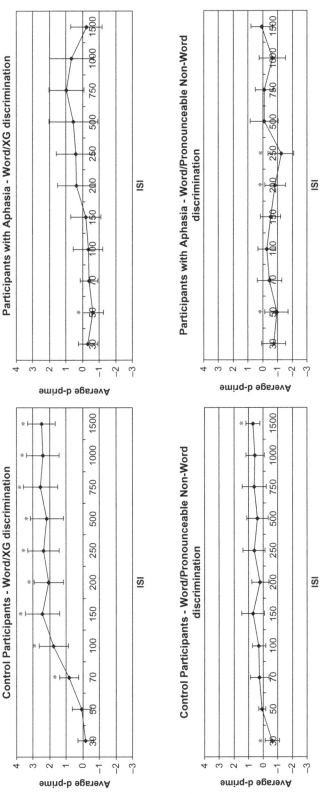

**Figure 2.** Average d' values for each participant group and discrimination condition across all interstimulus intervals. Asterisks indicate values significantly different from zero.

## Methodological analysis

The primary objective in conducting this experiment was to ascertain that masked stimuli were not being processed at a level that would allow them to exert a conscious influence on lexical decision on a subsequent target. Previous research has suggested that ruling out conscious perception of all task-relevant information (if not of all information about the masked item) is adequate to assure that priming effects are not governed by conscious, controlled processing (Snodgrass & Shevrin, 2006). Although the task described here may not definitively rule out all information about masked items, we believe that it does serve to verify that no task-relevant information is being gleaned. Typical participants were largely successful at discriminating between XG strings and real words, but we suspect that their ability to do so may have been based on the conscious perception of single visual features of the XG strings, such as a diagonal line or an x and a g right next to each other. Indeed, after completing this experiment, many of the typical participants reported that they had just looked for single visual features, and used that information to make their decision—if these features were present, they called the masked item a nonword, but if they were not present they called it a word. This level of conscious processing allowed good success on this particular task, but the level of conscious awareness that it demonstrates is not likely to be enough to allow participants to consciously apply information gleaned from masked items to anticipate the lexical status of an upcoming unmasked target. The Word/Pronounceable Nonword discrimination, however, required the processing of masked stimuli at a higher level, and the ability to do this reliably would indicate that the masking was inadequate to prevent conscious application of information from the primes to lexical decision on a subsequent unmasked stimulus. In this task, however, the ability to make judgements based on single visual features was removed. This resulted in much poorer performance, with the typical adults, as a group, showing unreliable discrimination in all but the longest (i.e., most visible) ISI condition. Participants with aphasia showed poor discrimination on both tasks (potential implications of which are discussed below), unrelated to aphasia severity. Based on these results, we conclude that the masking protocol described here was generally effective at eliminating task-relevant conscious processing of the masked primes. In addition, most of the participants with aphasia were able to learn and complete this task, with task success having no apparent relation to aphasia severity (WAB Aphasia Quotients of 34.45, 81, and 21.7 for the three participants who were unsuccessful).

These group data indicate the effectiveness of this protocol at identifying group patterns of visibility, but our hope was to be able to use it to determine visibility on a participant-by-participant basis. This goal arose from the recognition that there are individual differences in the ability to perceive masked primes (McCauley, Parmelee, Sperber, & Carr, 1980) and the desire to be confident that a given individual's priming results were not consciously mediated. We are encouraged that this protocol can be applied to determine visibility on an individual basis, though it was not perfect in its current implementation.

In particular, the task as reported here involved only 16 trials in each ISI condition, with 8 being real words, 4 being pronounceable nonwords, and 4 being XG strings. The decision to use so few trials was the result of an attempt to keep the task short, as it was being completed after a lengthy lexical decision task being used in the larger project with which this task was associated. The imbalance between the number of real words and the other two conditions was implemented because of an initial assumption that the most important analysis would be between real words and both nonword conditions combined, leading us to want an equivalent number of trials for that comparison. However, given that calculation of d′ is dependent on the proportion of hits and false alarms in the lexical decision task, it became evident that, with so few trials, small differences in response accuracy led to large differences in d′, such that random variability seemed to have undue influence on individual d′ values. The results obtained on an individual basis, therefore, led to illogical patterns of performance (such as d′ values reflecting high visibility at a short ISI when visibility was clearly poor at all longer ISIs) due to the large influence of random variability. In order to determine a given individual's likelihood of having consciously processed the masked items in a given ISI condition, therefore, a tripartite criterion of visibility was adopted. This criterion was based on the assumptions that the Word/XG discrimination task was easier than the Word/Pronounceable Nonword discrimination task, and that masked items at longer ISIs are more visible than those at shorter ISIs. A given ISI condition was deemed likely to have yielded conscious perception of masked items if: (1) a d′ of > 1.5 was obtained for Word/Pronounceable Nonword discrimination in that ISI condition; *and* (2) a d′ value of > 1.5 was also obtained for Word/XG discrimination in the same ISI condition; *and* (3) these criteria were met in all longer ISI conditions as well. On the other hand, if large d′ values were obtained without these other criteria being met, it was assumed that they were erroneous.

Using this tripartite criterion allowed us to assess the visibility of the masked items in each ISI condition on an individual basis. When this criterion was applied, 6/31 control participants (19%) showed evidence of conscious perception in at least one ISI condition, but none of the participants with aphasia had discrimination performance reflecting conscious perception of the masked stimuli at any of the ISIs. We then used this information to trim data from the larger project dataset, removing data from conditions in which there was evidence for conscious processing of the masked primes. We are comfortable that this approach gave us a reasonable approximation of the visibility of the masked primes and, if anything, overestimated how visible the masked items had been during the initial task (when participants had not been told of their existence and were focused on the unmasked word at the end of the sequence). We would have preferred, however, to use the d′ values by themselves, without additional interpretive criteria. In future studies using this approach, therefore, we would lengthen the task to include 8–10 trials in each of the three conditions. This increased number of trials would lessen the influence of individual responses, and would allow the d′ values to be interpreted more confidently in their own right.

A further methodological limitation of the task as reported here lies in the wide variety of stimuli used. All masked stimuli in this task were controlled for number of letters (3–8), syllables (1–3), and morphemes (1–2), all pronounceable nonwords were phonotactically and orthographically legal, and all real words had a word frequency of at least 100 words per million (Kucera & Francis, 1967). At the same time, however, there was no control for other lexical factors known to influence lexical decision, such as part of speech, phonological or orthographic neighbourhood density or frequency, age of acquisition, or familiarity. These broad criteria for stimulus inclusion stemmed from the desire to not have any stimuli overlap with the approximately 900 stimuli involved in the larger project with which this experiment was associated, thereby significantly limiting the availability of potential stimuli. It was decided that, for this initial attempt, random assignment of the stimuli to ISI condition would serve to minimise the effects of particular lexical variables on the task outcomes. For future studies, however, it would be beneficial to more closely control the range of lexical variables that might influence performance. In addition, it would be of interest to evaluate the effect on performance of this task of systematically varying these factors.

Finally, further evaluation of this protocol would benefit from inclusion of more detailed analysis of participants' visual acuity and function. The participants here demonstrated adequate visual function for daily activities, with no functional evidence of neglect, and the task involved all stimuli presented in a single, central location. It is possible, however, that subtle differences in visual attention, acuity, or discrimination may impact performance on this task.

## Theoretical implications

The primary purpose of this study was methodological, to ascertain accurate interpretation of priming results in another task. However, the results obtained were surprising, and hold some suggestions for future lines of investigation.

Typical adults showed a consistent ability to discriminate between real words and XG strings at most ISIs under these masking conditions, but a relatively poor ability to discriminate between real words and pronounceable nonwords. As discussed earlier, based on participant reports of their experience with the task, we suspect that this was due largely to their ability to key into small visual features of the masked items, rather than lexical-level information. Adding to this perspective is that gained from the participants with aphasia. When questioned after the experiment was completed, most of them reported that, once they had been told that there were items "hidden" in the visual sequence, they could sometimes identify that there was something there but could not tell anything about what it was. This observation was supported by their poor discrimination not only in the Word/Pronounceable Nonword condition but on the Word/XG discrimination, as well. In addition, many of the participants with aphasia, including the three who were unable to complete the experiment, reported that they were unable perceive anything in the masked position. In all cases, participants demonstrated understanding of the task by successfully completing it when the masked stimuli were presented for longer periods of time.

In spite of our suspicions that differences between groups in this experiment were due to processing at the level of visual perception of basic features (or, perhaps, inter-related factors associated with attention), rather than lexical processing, the task used in this experiment was inherently linguistic, both due to the use of linguistic stimuli and that the participants were doing a linguistic task (lexical decision). It is impossible, based on these data alone, to determine if the differences noted between groups was due to the expected lexical processing differences of the two groups, or whether there may be a deficit that extends beyond linguistic processing evident in the data from participants with aphasia. If we believe that the typical adults in this study were relying on basic visual features, rather than linguistic processing, for their decisions on XG strings, then it is notable that the individuals with aphasia were unable to take advantage of this same cue.

If it could be shown that this pattern of group differences persisted in a non-linguistic task, it would support an interpretation of differences outside of the linguistic processing system, per se. In fact, preliminary data from a similar investigation support this idea. In an effort to determine the prime exposure durations at which individuals show conscious awareness of masked items, we had nine typical adults and eight individuals with aphasia make simple presence/absence judgements to masked stimuli. They were asked to attend to a visual masking sequence that contained a white square on a black background, and to determine whether there was a word present in the square or whether it was empty. This task significantly reduced the need for linguistic processing relative to that needed for the experiment described in this paper, as it asked only for a judgement on whether there was any-thing in the square or not, rather than making a decision on the content of the square. The protocol began with the masked items being exposed for 150 ms, clearly visible to all participants, with a gradual reduction until a participant reached a threshold at which s/he was unable to reliably distinguish the presence vs absence of content in the square. In this preliminary protocol, typical adults all reached thresh-old at 10–20-ms exposure duration, whereas thresholds for participants with aphasia were significantly different, ranging from 10 to 90 ms. Given that this task required no linguistic processing to complete successfully, these results suggest that there may be non-linguistic differences involved. This would be consistent with previous research that has demonstrated non-linguistic, and particularly attention-based, impairments in individuals with aphasia (see, for example, Murray, 1999, for a discussion of these issues). We suggest, therefore, that further investigation of this phenomenon with both linguistic and wholly non-linguistic stimuli is warranted.

## CONCLUSION

The experiment presented here provides a method for assessing the visibility of masked items in individuals with aphasia. The ability to determine visibility is a precursor to confidently using masked priming protocols for the investigation of aphasic language abilities, which is one way to tap into the automatic, implicit mech-anisms underlying language function to the exclusion of explicit, controlled process-ing. The data presented here also indicate that both researchers and clinicians should consider the time course of basic visual perception prior to determining the temporal parameters for stimulus presentation when working with individuals with aphasia. In addition to the methodological report, the visibility results revealed differences between typical adults and participants with aphasia in their ability to consciously perceive masked items. This difference may lie in linguistic processing differences, which would not be surprising, but it may also reveal differences in broader aspects of cognitive processing, warranting further investigation.

Manuscript received 24 July 2009
Manuscript accepted 24 November 2009
First published online 7 June 2010

## REFERENCES

Avila, C., Lambon Ralph, M.A., Parcet, M., Geffner, D., & Gonzalez-Darder, J. (2001). Implicit word cues facilitate impaired naming performance: Evidence from a case of anomia. *Brain and Language*, 79(2), 185–200.

Dabul, B. (2000). *Apraxia Battery for Adults* (2nd ed.). Austin, TX: Pro-Ed.

Erdelyi, M. H. (2004). Subliminal perception and its cognates: Theory, indeterminacy, and time. *Consciousness and Cognition*, 13(1), 73–91.

Forster, K. I. (1999). The microgenesis of priming effects in lexical access. *Brain and Language*, 68(1-2), 5–15.

Forster, K. I., Mohan, K., & Hector, J. (2003). The mechanics of masked priming. In S. Kinoshita & S. J. Lupker (Eds.), *Masked priming: The state of the art* (pp. 3–37). New York: Psychology Press.

Green, D. M., & Swets, J. A. (1966). *Signal detection theory and psychophysics*. New York: John Wiley & Sons, Inc.

Kaplan, E., Goodglass, H., & Weintraub, S. (2001). *The Boston Naming Test*. Philadelphia: Lea & Febinger.

Kucera, H., & Francis, W. N. (1967). *Computational analysis of present-day American English*. Providence, RI: Brown University Press.

LaPointe, L. L., & Horner, J. (1979). *Reading Comprehension Battery for Aphasia*. Tegoid, OR: G.C. Publications, Inc.

Martin, N., Fink, R., Laine, M., & Ayala, J. (2004). Immediate and short-term effects of contextual priming on word retrieval in aphasia. *Aphasiology*, *18*(10), 867–898.

McCauley, C., Parmelee, C. M., Sperber, R. D., & Carr, T. H. (1980). Early extraction of meaning from pictures and its relation to conscious identification. *Journal of Experimental Psychology: Human Perception and Performance*, *6*(2), 265–276.

Murray, L. L. (1999). Attention and aphasia: Theory, research, and clinical implications. *Aphasiology*, *13*(2), 91–111.

Prather, P. A., Zurif, E., Love, T., & Brownell, H. (1997). Speed of lexical activation in nonfluent Broca's aphasia and fluent Wernicke's aphasia. *Brain and Language*, *59*(3), 391–411.

Raven, J. C. (1976). *Coloured Progressive Matrices: Set A, Ab, B*. Oxford, UK: Oxford Psychologists Press.

Silkes, J. P. (2009). *Parameters of implicit priming in aphasia*. Unpublished doctoral dissertation, University of Washington, Seattle.

Snodgrass, M., & Shevrin, H. (2006). Unconscious inhibition and facilitation at the objective detection threshold. Replicable and qualitatively different unconscious perceptual effects. *Cognition*, *101*(1), 43–79.

Turner-Stokes, L., Kalmus, M., Hirani, D., & Clegg, F. (2005). The Depression Intensity Scale Circles (DISCs): A first evaluation of a simple assessment tool for depression in the context of brain injury. *Journal of Neurology, Neurosurgery and Psychiatry*, *76*(9), 1273–1278.

APHASIOLOGY, 2010, 24 (6–8), 775–786

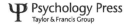

# Melodic Intonation Therapy and aphasia: Another variation on a theme

Monica Strauss Hough

*East Carolina University, Greenville, NC, USA*

*Background*: Melodic Intonation Therapy (MIT) is a therapeutic approach used to increase verbal output in adults with aphasia through combination of melodic intoning and rhythmic tapping with simple phrase production. Although MIT was developed in the 1970s, few studies have been conducted relative to determining the programme's overall effectiveness as well as examining ability to generalise skills to other communicative contexts.

*Aims*: The purpose of the current investigation was to examine the effectiveness of MIT as a means of increasing verbal output in a gentleman with chronic Broca's aphasia.

*Methods & Procedures*: A modified version of MIT without the tapping component was implemented with BR, 69-year-old male with chronic Broca's aphasia of 4 years' duration. BR had tried MIT previously with little success: he had difficulty with the tapping element and the packaged phrases lacked functionality, adversely affecting his motivation. A set of automatic and self-generated phrases were developed and implemented with a multiple baseline design across phrase type with an established criterion of 75% accuracy over two consecutive sessions for both stimulus sets. Generalisation stimuli were presented at the last weekly session. BR attended three hour-long weekly sessions, for 8 weeks. Follow-up probing with all stimuli occurred at 2 and 4 weeks post-treatment. A set of standardised tests and social validation measures were administered pre- and post-treatment.

*Outcomes & Results*: BR reached 75% accuracy on automatic phrases at 4 weeks into the treatment programme, which was retained throughout the maintenance phase and both follow-up sessions. Performance on self-generated phrases was 55% at 8 weeks post-treatment, which was maintained at both follow-up sessions. Separate Welch two sample $t$-tests used to analyse the automatic and self-generated phrase data, yielded highly significant treatment effects for both data sets, with non-significant findings for autocorrelation. Improved performance on standardised tests was observed most notably for auditory comprehension and reading and writing skills, with some improvement in spontaneous speech and naming. Increased perception of communicative effectiveness was reported independently by both BR and his spouse.

*Conclusions*: Overall, BR significantly increased his ability to produce short phrases using MIT without tapping. Thus MIT appears to be a viable option for enhancing verbal output for some individuals with non-fluent aphasia, regardless of time post-stroke. Additional investigations are needed to examine generalisation effects to other linguistic contexts. Efficiency issues (treatment length, intensity) require further exploration relative to MIT efficacy and effectiveness and its variations.

Address correspondence to: Monica Strauss Hough PhD, Communication Sciences & Disorders, East Carolina University, Health Sciences Building, Greenville, North Carolina, USA 27858. E-mail: HoughM @ecu.edu

http://www.psypress.com/aphasiology          DOI: 10.1080/02687030903501941

*Keywords:* Melodic intonation; Chronic aphasia; Tapping; Self-generated phrases; Automatic phrases.

Melodic Intonation Therapy (MIT) is a packaged therapeutic approach developed to increase verbal output in adults with aphasia (Helm-Estabrooks & Albert, 2004; Helm-Estabrooks, Nicholas, & Morgan, 1989; Sparks, Helm, & Albert, 1973, 1974; Sparks & Holland, 1976). The approach combines melodic intoning and rhythmic tapping with simple phrase production to enhance communication.

MIT is based on the premise that increased use of the right hemisphere for the melodic aspect of speech may enhance the role of that hemisphere in the control of language (Goodglass & Calderon, 1977; Marshall & Holtzapple, 1976; Norton, Zipse, Marchina, & Schlaug, 2009; Sparks & Deck, 1994; Sparks & Holland, 1976). Increased right hemisphere stimulation may diminish dominance of the damaged left hemisphere in language output, thus reducing constraints on the left hemisphere to assist in speech production (Gates & Bradshaw, 1977; Goodglass & Calderon, 1977; Schlaug, Marchina, & Norton, 2008; Sparks & Deck, 1994), at least during early post-stroke recovery (Belin et al., 1996). Regardless of whether words/phrases were intoned or spoken, Ozdemir, Norton, and Schlaug (2006) suggested a bi-hemispheric network for vocal output. Based on their fMRI findings with right-handed normal speakers, singing resulted in additional right lateralised activation in the superior temporal gyrus, inferior central operculum, and the inferior frontal gyrus. These observations were more apparent for singing than humming or intoned speaking, and have been supported by others (Hebert, Racette, Gagnon, & Peretz, 2003; Racette, Bard, & Peretz, 2006). Norton et al. (2009) suggested that the reduced rate of articulation and the modulated intonation in singing may increase connections between syllables and words; consequently, there is reduced dependence on the left hemisphere for verbal output. Using diffuse tensor imaging, Schlaug, Marchina, and Norton (2009) found significant increases in the volume and number of fibres of the right arcuate fasciculus of six nonfluent aphasic patients who underwent intensive MIT therapy when comparing pre- and post-treatment assessments. However, functional MRI research by Carlomagno et al. (1997) revealed increased activation of undamaged areas in the left hemisphere, including Heschl's gyrus and the prefrontal cortex, as the physiological mechanisms contributing to improved verbal output as the result of the MIT technique, rather than increased activation of right hemisphere areas.

The MIT technique has been identified as being most beneficial for aphasic patients meeting specific criteria, including non-fluent or Broca's aphasia, good auditory comprehension skills, and the ability to self-correct (Helm-Estabrooks & Albert, 2004; Helm-Estabrooks et al., 1989; Norton et al., 2009; Schlaug et al., 2008, 2009; Sparks & Holland, 1976). Additionally, it is recommended that MIT be administered in frequent sessions during a limited time span, no longer than 8 weeks (Helm-Estabrooks & Albert, 2004; Schlaug et al., 2009).

The traditional MIT programme was designed as a four-level process of progressive stages. In Stage 1 the clinician hums intoned phrases while the patient taps the stress or rhythm of each melodic pattern. In Stage 2 the patient repeats hummed phrases simultaneously with the clinician while tapping the rhythmic pattern. In Stage 3 the patient repeats intoned phrases after the clinician. In Stage 4, a technique called *Sprechgesang*, a type of talking with a singing intonation, is used by the clinician to aid the patient in transitioning constant melodic pitch to the more variable pitch that is typically used in normal conversation (Helm-Estabrooks & Albert, 2004; Sparks & Deck, 1994; Sparks et al., 1974). Modifications in MIT may be made to meet specific patient needs (Norton et al., 2009; Schlaug et al., 2008).

Recent research (Norton et al., 2009; Schlaug et al., 2008) has suggested use of inner rehearsal as an addition to MIT training to aid patients in generating their own phrases using the approach. In inner rehearsal the clinician taps the patient's hand while humming melodic contour, then sings the words; the clinician explains that that they are "hearing" the sung phrase internally. Alterations in MIT, such as inner rehearsal, may be beneficial in making the programme more individualised; however, this particular factor may be one reason why it has been difficult to obtain definitive efficacy results with MIT. Specifically, methodology has not been consistent across reported treatment studies. Furthermore, although MIT methodology was initially developed in the 1970s, few studies have been conducted with aphasic adults who appropriately meet the programme criteria relative to determining the programme's overall effectiveness as well as examining ability to generalise skills to other communicative contexts (Baker, 2000; Bonakdarpour, Eftekharzadeh, & Ashayeri, 2000, 2003; Dunham & Newhoff, 1979; Goldfarb & Bader, 1979; Marshall & Holtapple, 1976; Naeser & Helm-Estabrooks, 1985; Racette et al., 2006; Schlaug et al., 2008). Thus the purpose of this investigation was to examine the effectiveness of a modified version of MIT as a means of increasing verbal output in a gentleman with chronic Broca's aphasia.

## METHOD

A modified version of MIT was implemented with BR, a 69-year-old Caucasian male with chronic Broca's aphasia of 48 months duration and right hemiparesis, resulting from a left cerebro-vascular accident (CVA) 4 years previously. BR specifically presented with a nonfluent aphasia, characterised by one, two, and occasionally three-word utterances. He could follow one-step commands and basic conversation. Speech output was slow and segmented, with some distortion of isolated sounds which he often self-corrected. These latter behaviours are consistent with a moderate-marked apraxia of speech (AOS). BR passed a modified hearing screening for older adults (Ventry & Weinstein, 1983, 1992). He had been a university professor with 22 years of education. Additionally, he was right-handed by self-report and a native English speaker. BR had received traditional speech-language therapy intermittently since his CVA; however, he did not receive any additional therapy during this investigation.

Upon further investigation, it was discovered that MIT had been implemented previously with BR at another facility with little success, although he presented with an appropriate communicative profile for use of the technique. BR's spouse reported that he had difficulty with the tapping element of MIT; attempts at rhythmic behaviour while using the approach interfered with any production of verbal output. It also was reported that the packaged phrases previously used lacked functionality, adversely affecting BR's motivation relative to using the approach.

In preparation for implementing MIT in treatment, BR, his spouse, and the examiner generated a series of two- to four-word functional phrases that BR was unable to produce with consistency. Some of the phrases generated appeared to be

TABLE 1
Stimulus examples used with modified
Melodic Intonation Therapy

| Automatic | Self-generated |
| --- | --- |
| I love you | Find my glasses |
| Thank you | Time for e-mail |
| Have a nice day | Grandpa is here |
| Good morning | I need my cane |

more routine or automatic phrases whereas others were intuitively more proposi-tional or individualised. It was hypothesised that these latter phrases would be more difficult for BR to generate, and therefore should be treated separately from the "automatic" phrases. Subsequently, 60 undergraduate students (two sections of the introductory communication disorders class) were asked to determine whether each of 55 phrases was an "automatic" phrase or a "self-generated" phrase, as part of an extra credit assignment. The examiner explained that an automatic phrase was a rote statement or question; the meaning of the particular phrase was based on the com-bined contribution of all the words in the phrase. In another linguistic context the individual words from the phrase would be independent and have a completely dif-ferent meaning. A self-generated phrase was identified as a statement/question that was individualised to a particular person's needs or wants; each word was independ-ent relative to contributing to the meaning of the utterance.

Only phrases that were considered automatic or self-generated by at least 95% of the students were identified as treatment stimuli for implementing MIT with BR. Analysis of the student ratings resulted in 40 phrases that met this criterion: 15 phrases were identified as automatic ("I love you"); 25 phrases were personal/self-generated ("find my glasses"). Of the latter set, 15 were randomly chosen as treat-ment stimuli and 10 as generalisation probes that were not treated, resulting in two sets of 15 treatment stimuli (30 stimuli, 10 probes). Examples of automatic and self-generated stimuli are presented in Table 1.

A multiple baseline design across the automatic and self-generated treatment stimuli was implemented. Three baselines were obtained on all treatment and probe (untreated) stimulus phrases. A criterion of 75% accuracy over two consec-utive sessions was established for both sets of treatment stimuli. Treatment was implemented on the automatic phrases while baseline measurements were continued on the self-generated phrases. When criterion was met for the automatic phrases, treatment was initiated for the self-generated stimuli. The generalisation probe (untreated) stimuli were presented to BR at the last weekly session of each week of treatment. For both baseline and untreated probe stimuli, each phrase was read aloud by the examiner with typical melodic contour and intonation. BR was required to repeat the phrase. If BR, had difficulty, the phrase was repeated using *Sprechgesang* and BR was required to repeat the production. Phrases were considered correct if each word of the phrase was uttered and each word was produced accurately and intelligibly. Intra- and inter-judge reliability for response accuracy were analysed and are presented below. Follow-up probing with all stimuli occurred at 2 and 4 weeks post-treatment. BR attended three weekly treat-ment sessions, which were approximately 1 hour in length, for 8 weeks using the modified MIT protocol.

Using the specified stimuli, MIT programming was begun with BR at the ECU Speech, Language, and Hearing Clinic, administered by the primary author. MIT was implemented without the tapping component for stages 1 and 2, using the traditional approach. Thus, in stage 1, the examiner introduced humming of intoned phrases, producing each phrase three times. During presentation of each phrase BR was primarily required to listen to each production. He could tap or nod his head in a rhythmic manner if chosen. In stage 2 BR was required to repeat the hummed phrases simultaneously with the examiner; he could tap the rhythm if chosen but this was not required, nor did he choose to do this behaviour. Tapping along with phrase production was used by the clinician for cuing only to re-focus BR when productions were inaccurate or to enhance precision of individual words. Additionally, the Eight-Step Continuum (Rosenbek, 1985; Rosenbek, Lemme, Ahern, Harris, & Wertz, 1973) was utilised to increase awareness of speech precision relative to the rhythmic components of MIT. Specifically, if BR encountered difficulty with speech production of a particular word, the Continuum was utilised with or without *Sprechgesang*. Relative to actual implementation of the Continuum, steps were utilised sequentially based on what cues BR required to establish accuracy for certain words in a phrase. Steps 1 to 5 of the Eight-Step Continuum were implemented as needed. However, primarily only steps 1 and 2 of the Continuum were needed to enhance accuracy of production. Overall, for an average session with the automatic phrases, the continuum was implemented approximately 6 times per session; for the self-generated phrases, the Continuum was implemented approximately 10 times per session. The Eight-Step Continuum is similar in nature to Auditory-Motor Feedback Training (Norton et al., 2009), which recently has been used to complement the effectiveness of MIT. This latter protocol was developed to restore volitional and purposeful communication in adults with marked to severe AOS and moderate aphasia, through use of both visual and auditory modalities as well as simultaneous and sequential production strategies. A treatment trial included all stimulation directed towards each individual treatment phrase in that particular phase of treatment. All phrases within each phrase type for that phase of treatment were typically treated at each treatment session, thus yielding approximately 15 trials per session.

MIT treatment began with the automatic phrases. Measurement of baseline data was continued on the self-generated phrases until the criterion of 75% accuracy over two consecutive sessions was achieved on the automatic phrases. Once this was attained, treatment was implemented on the self-generated phrases, with maintenance probing on automatic phrases. Accuracy of phrase production was the dependent variable; phrases were considered accurate if each word in the phrase was produced and understandable, regardless of whether BR utilised *Sprechgesang* during the particular production. Self-corrections that were correct responses were judged as accurate. Intra-judge reliability for response accuracy was determined via percentage of agreement of 10% of each session's productions; these responses were reviewed at least 2 weeks after the particular session, yielding a 98.5% agreement. For inter-judge reliability, a graduate student familiar with MIT judged response accuracy of 10% of each session's productions; percentage of agreement was 96%. All responses were audio tape-recorded using a Marantz PMD201 portable cassette recorder attached to a Shure SM58 vocal microphone.

The following tests were administered pre- and post-treatment: (1) *Western Aphasia Battery-Revised (WAB-R)* (Kertesz, 2006), Aphasia Quotient (AQ), Cortical Quotient (CQ); (2) *American Speech-Language Hearing Association Functional Assessment of Communication Skills (ASHA FACS)* (Frattali, Thompson, Holland,

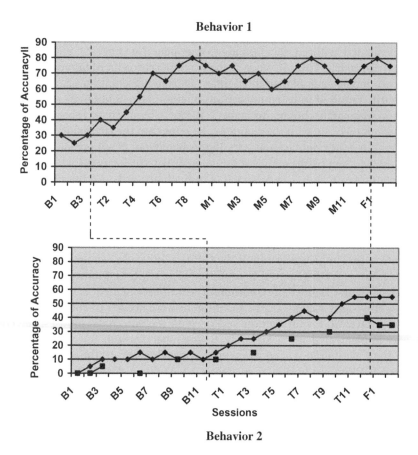

**Figure 1.** Accuracy percentage for automatic and self-generated phrases, including untreated probes, using modified Melodic Intonation Therapy protocol for 8 weeks. Behaviour 1: Automatic phrases. Behaviour 2: Self-generated phrases and Probe (untreated) phrases (untreated stimulus probes presented at end of each week of treatment). B: Baseline; T: Therapy Sessions; M: Maintenance; F: Follow-up Sessions.

Wohl, & Ferketic, 1995); (3) *American Speech-Language Hearing Association Quality of Communication Life Scale (ASHA QCL)* (Paul et al., 2003); and (4) *Communicative Effectiveness Index (CETI)* (Lomas et al., 1989).

## RESULTS

BR's performance on the automatic and self-generated phrases using MIT without tapping relative to percent accuracy is displayed in Figure 1. As can be observed, BR reached the established criterion of 75% on the automatic phrases at approximately 4 weeks (nine treatment sessions) into the MIT treatment programme. This level of accuracy was generally retained throughout the maintenance phase and was apparent at both follow-up sessions several weeks after the entire treatment programme was completed.

Treatment on the self-generated phrases was initiated once BR reached criterion on the automatic phrases. At 8 weeks post-baseline, BR's performance accuracy on the self-generated phrases was 55%. Although he had not achieved the established 75% accuracy criterion, BR made noticeable improvement from baseline, which was never higher than 13%, as seen in Figure 1. Furthermore, he maintained a 55% accuracy level at the follow-up sessions, 2 and 4 weeks post-treatment.

To determine if the effect of treatment with MIT was significant for either set of stimuli, separate Welch two sample $t$-tests were used to analyse the automatic and self-generated phrase data, respectively. This particular test was used due to the skewed nature of the data and the potential for serial dependence of data points. In addition, the Durbin-Watson statistic was applied to these data sets to determine the influence of autocorrelation or serial dependence of the data points. For the automatic phrase data, baseline performance was compared with maintenance plus follow-up performance data. The results revealed a significant difference between baseline and post-treatment data ($t = 18.7314$; $df = 6.456$; $p < .00001$). With these findings, the 95% confidence interval for improvement is 37.5% to 48.5%t. Based on these observations the Durbin-Watson statistic for autocorrelation was not significant (DW = 1.6322; $p = .1002$). For the self-generated phrase data, baseline performance was compared with follow-up performance data. The results revealed a significant difference between baseline and post-treatment data ($t = 33.3729$; $df = 10$; $p < .00001$). With these findings, the 95% confidence interval for improvement is 42% to 48%. Based on these observations the Durbin-Watson statistic for autocorrelation was not significant (DW = 2.5887; $p = .718$). In both analyses the alternative hypothesis is that the true autocorrelation must be greater than 0, thus justifying the use of this analysis as a means controlling for autocorrelation in these sets of data. Furthermore, the size of the effects as indicated by the confidence intervals strongly suggests real clinically significant effects as observed in Figure 1.

Some generalisation to untreated self-generated probe phrases was observed. Findings displayed on Figure 1 indicate that BR performed at 0% accuracy at baseline. However, with implementation of MIT, he exhibited increases in performance up to 40% accuracy at 8 weeks post-baseline and 35% accuracy at the follow-up maintenance sessions. Pre- and post-treatment scores on the *Western Aphasia Battery-Revised* (WAB-R) (Kertesz, 2006) AQ and CQ are presented in Table 2. As may be observed, these results revealed increases post-treatment in language structure skills, particularly in auditory comprehension, naming, spontaneous speech, and reading and writing skills. Pre/post-treatment ratings on the *ASHA FACS* are presented in Table 3. Improved performance was noted on all communicative independence scales, with greatest increases for two scales: reading, writing, and number concepts and daily planning.

Pre/post-treatment and difference scores on the *ASHA QCL* are presented in Table 4. These findings suggest increased participant perception of communicative effectiveness and independence. Specifically, BR showed an overall difference score of +25 across all stimuli with increases on 16 of 18 items. Most notable increase was identified for "I get out of the house and do things". Pre/post-treatment and difference scores for the CETI are presented in Table 5. The results indicated increased caregiver perception of communicative effectiveness and independence relative to BR. Results based on the ratings by BR's spouse, revealed an overall difference score of +28.2 across all stimuli, with increases on 13 of 16 items. Stimulus items with highest increases included, "Getting somebody's attention", "Getting involved in group conversations that are about him/her", "Giving yes and no answers appropriately", and "Indicating that he/she understands what is being said to him/her". For all three rating scales (ASHA FACS, ASHA QCL, CETI), the rater did not have access to pre-treatment scores when conducting post-treatment ratings.

TABLE 2
Pre- and post-treatment test scores on the Western
Aphasia Battery-Revised

| Tasks | Pre | Post |
|---|---|---|
| *Spontaneous Speech* | | |
| Information | 4 | 6 |
| Fluency | 2 | 3 |
| Total | 6 | 9 |
| *Comprehension* | | |
| Yes/No Questions | 44 | 58 |
| Word Recognition | 20 | 34 |
| Sequential Command | 18 | 30 |
| Total | 4.1 | 6.1 |
| Repetition | 2.3 | 2.6 |
| *Naming* | | |
| Object Naming | 4 | 7 |
| Word Fluency | 0 | 4 |
| Sentence Completion | 5 | 8 |
| Responsive Speech | 1 | 3 |
| Total | 1.0 | 2.2 |
| AQ | 26.8 | 39.8 |
| | | |
| *Reading and Writing* | | |
| Reading | 25 | 37 |
| Writing | 9.5 | 32.5 |
| Total | 3.45 | 6.95 |
| Praxis | 5.4 | 5.7 |
| *Construction* | | |
| Drawing | 18 | 28 |
| Block Design | 7 | 9 |
| Calculation | 18 | 20 |
| Ravens Score | 28 | 27 |
| Total | 7.1 | 8.4 |
| CQ | 33.45 | 47.05 |

TABLE 3
Pre- and post-treatment ratings on the ASHA FACS
Communication Independence Scales

| Communication Independence Scales | Pre | Post |
|---|---|---|
| Social Communication | 2.7 | 4.2 |
| Basic Needs Communication | 5.0 | 6.1 |
| Reading, Writing, Number Concepts | 3.1 | 5.7 |
| Daily Planning | 1.8 | 4.8 |
| OVERALL | 3.15 | 5.2 |

Ratings based on a 0–7 scale.

# DISCUSSION

The purpose of the current investigation was to examine the effectiveness of the techniques of a modified version of MIT as a means of enhancing verbal output in a patient with chronic Broca's aphasia of extensive duration. Overall, BR significantly increased his ability to produce short phrases using the MIT protocol without the

TABLE 4
Pre- and post-treatment testing and difference scores on the ASHA Quality
of Life Communication Scale

| Statement stimuli | Pre | Post | Diff |
|---|---|---|---|
| I like to talk to people. | 1 | 3 | +2 |
| It's easy for me to communicate. | 1 | 2 | +1 |
| My role in the family is the same. | 2 | 3 | +1 |
| I like myself. | 3 | 5 | +2 |
| I meet the communication needs of my job or school. | 1 | 1 | 0 |
| I stay in touch with family and friends. | 2 | 4 | +2 |
| People include me in conversations. | 2 | 3 | +1 |
| I follow news, sports, and stories on TV/movies. | 4 | 5 | +1 |
| I use the telephone. | 2 | 3 | +1 |
| I see the funny things in life. | 3 | 5 | +2 |
| People understand me when I talk. | 1 | 2 | +1 |
| I keep trying when people don–t understand me. | 1 | 3 | +2 |
| I make my own decisions. | 5 | 5 | 0 |
| I am confident that I can communicate. | 2 | 4 | +2 |
| I get out of the house and do things. | 2 | 5 | +3 |
| I have household responsibilities. | 2 | 4 | +2 |
| I speak for myself. | 1 | 2 | +1 |
| In general, my quality of life is good. | 4 | 5 | +1 |
| Total Difference Score | | | +25 |

Ratings based on a 5-point rating scale (1–5).

TABLE 5
Pre- and post-treatment testing and difference scores on the CETI

| Statement stimuli | Pre | Post | Diff |
|---|---|---|---|
| Getting somebody's attention | 2.8 | 7.8 | +5.0 |
| Getting involved in group conversations that are about him/her | 2 | 5 | +3.0 |
| Giving yes and no answers appropriately | 1 | 4 | +3.0 |
| Communicating his/her emotions | 1 | 3 | +2.0 |
| Indicating that he/she understands what is being said to him/her | 3.8 | 6.8 | +3.0 |
| Having coffee-time visits and conversations with friends and neighbours | 0.5 | 3.0 | +2.5 |
| Having a one-to-one conversation with you | 0.5 | 2.0 | +1.5 |
| Saying the name of someone whose face is in front of him/her | 0.5 | 1.5 | +1.0 |
| Communicating physical problems such as aches and pains | 2.0 | 3.5 | +1.5 |
| Having a spontaneous conversation | 0.5 | 0.5 | 0 |
| Responding to or communicating anything without words | 5.0 | 6.0 | +1.0 |
| Starting a conversation with people who are not close family | 0.5 | 1.7 | +1.2 |
| Understanding writing | 0.5 | 2.0 | +1.5 |
| Being part of a conversation when it is fast/ number of people involved | 2.0 | 4 | +2.0 |
| Participating in a conversation with strangers | 1.0 | 1.0 | 0 |
| Describing or discussing something in depth | 0.5 | 0.5 | 0 |
| Total Difference Score | | | +28.2 |

Ratings based on a 10 cm (point) analogue rating scale (1–10).

tapping component. Although pre-determined criterion was reached only for the automatic phrases, remarkable increases were observed for both the automatic and self-generated phrases throughout the treatment protocol. Furthermore, improved phrase production was maintained at follow-up sessions at 2 and 4 weeks post-treatment for both types of phrases. Some generalisation to the untreated phrase stimuli was observed. This increase for the self-generated probe phrases was maintained at both follow-up sessions. Increases were not as remarkable for the untreated as the treated stimuli; however, improved production was evident. Statistical analyses on the untreated stimuli were not conducted because there were too few data points.

Although tapping has been considered an integral part of MIT, this component of the technique was not used with BR, as he found this behaviour to be distracting and disruptive to his verbal output performance. Tapping in MIT or any other therapy approach (i.e., pacing board, gestural reorganisation, etc.) has been considered a form of inter-systemic reorganisation (Duffy, 2005; Rosenbek & LaPointe, 1985). In inter-systemic reorganisation a non-speech motor activity, such as tapping, is introduced to accompany production of the impaired act. Thus the impaired act is paired with internal cues generated by this more intact function (tapping). Consequently, the intact system functions as an organiser relative to enhancing verbal output. Although Schlaug et al. (2008) indicated that tapping is a critical element of MIT, it may not be essential to increase abilities in verbal output for all individuals with aphasia and/or AOS. Thus in BR's case, an additional tool such as Norton et al.'s (2009) inner rehearsal was not beneficial because of the tapping aspect of this process. Tapping may be as impaired as BR's ability to produce speech; thus attempting to use this behaviour to facilitate verbal output may be more of a hindrance than an assistive tool. Rosenbek's Eight-Step Continuum (Rosenbek, 1985; Rosenbek, et al., 1973) was utilised intermittently with BR throughout treatment, particularly during stages 1 and 2 of the MIT treatment protocol. Interestingly, it is during these stages that the tapping component of MIT is typically helpful in modulating and enhancing accuracy of production for most patients with aphasia and/or AOS. Thus it appears that BR did require some additional stimulation to increase accurate phrase production; however, he benefited from direct manipulation of his articulatory skills, rather than an inter-systemic reorganisation approach such as tapping. Thus, the successful use of the Eight-Step Continuum (Rosenbek, 1985) in conjunction with MIT with BR supports the simultaneous implementation of other similar approaches that enhance articulatory precision and volitional use of speech along with techniques addressing manipulation of the melodic and intonation components of speech (Norton et al., 2009).

Improved performance on standardised tests relative to language structure and communication skills was observed. Although some improvement was found relative to spontaneous speech and naming, most notables increases were observed for auditory comprehension and reading and writing skills. It is interesting to note that this similar pattern of improvement on standardised tests also has been observed with other chronic aphasic patients (Hough & Johnson, 2009; Hough & King, 2008; Johnson, Hough, King, Jeffs, & Vos, 2008; Steele, 2008). Furthermore, in the current investigation, improvement in perception of communicative effectiveness was reported independently by both BR and his spouse. These observations included enhanced general and functional aspects of communication as well as increased initiation of interaction with others.

There are several limitations regarding the current study that restrict the extent to which findings may be generalised to other patients with chronic Broca's aphasia and/or AOS. Although probe phrases were included in the investigation, generalisation to other spontaneous and natural contexts relative to BR's verbal output was not examined. Furthermore, maintenance data for the self-generated phrases was obtained only in follow-up sessions; unlike the data available for the automatic phrases, it is not evident whether BR maintained an improved level of accuracy for the self-generated phrases over an extended time period. However, BR showed increases in many areas of communication that were consistent with his improvements using MIT. Furthermore, his language and communication performance had been relatively stable prior to initiating this investigation; therefore it is strongly suggested that increases on self-generated phrase production were maintained.

Current results indicate that, with variations, MIT is a viable option for enhancing verbal output for some individuals with aphasia, regardless of the chronic nature or time post-stroke/injury of their aphasia (Baker, 2000; Bonakdarpour et al., 2000, 2003; Dunham & Newhoff, 1979; Goldfarb & Bader, 1979; Marshall & Holtzapple, 1976; Norton et al., 2009; Racette et al., 2006; Schlaug et al., 2008). In some individuals with aphasia there have been significant neurophysiological changes that have accompanied increases in verbal output (Carlomagno et al., 1997; Schlaug et al., 2008, 2009). Furthermore, findings with normal adults have emphasised the important combined contributions of the right hemisphere in speaking, humming, and singing (Hebert et al., 2003; Odzemir et al., 2006). Additional treatment investigations are needed to examine generalisation effects to other linguistic contexts. Efficiency issues including treatment length and intensity require further exploration relative to the efficacy and effectiveness of MIT as well as variations to the protocol that may be needed for some patients, such as BR.

Manuscript received 19 July 2009
Manuscript accepted 19 November 2009

## REFERENCES

Baker, F. A. (2000). Modifying the melodic intonation therapy program for adults with severe non-fluent aphasia. *Music Therapy Perspectives, 18*(2), 110–114.

Belin, P., Eeckhout, V., Zilbovicius, M., Remy, P., Francois, C., Guillaume, S., et al. (1996). Recovery from non-fluent aphasia after melodic intonation therapy: A PET study. *Neurology, 47*(6), 1504–1511.

Bonakdarpour, B., Eftekharzadeh, A., & Ashayeri, H. (2000). Preliminary report on the effects of melodic intonation therapy in the rehabilitation of Persian aphasic patients. *Iranian Journal of Medical Sciences, 25*, 156–160.

Bonakdarpour, B., Eftekharzadeh, A., & Ashayeri, H. (2003). Melodic intonation therapy in Persian aphasic patients. *Aphasiology, 17*(1), 75–95

Carlomagno, S., Van Eeckhout, P., Blasi, V., Belin, P., Samson, Y., & Deloche, G. (1997). The impact of functional neuroimaging methods on the development of a theory for cognitive remediation. *Neuropsychological Rehabilitation, 7*, 311–326.

Duffy, J. (2005). *Motor speech disorders* (2nd ed.). Boston: Elsevier Mosby

Dunham, M. J., & Newhoff, M. (1979). Melodic intonation therapy: Rewriting the song. In R. H. Brookshire (Ed.), *Clinical Aphasiology Conference Proceedings* (pp. 286–294*)*. Minneapolis, MN: BRK Publishers.

Frattali, C. M., Thompson, C. M., Holland, A. L., Wohl, C. B. & Ferketic, M. M. (1995). *ASHA Functional Assessment of Communication Skills (FACS)*. Rockville, MD: American Speech-Language-Hearing Association.

Gates, A., & Bradshaw, J. L. (1977). The role of the cerebral hemispheres in music. *Brain and Language, 4*, 403–431.

Goldfarb, R., & Bader, E. (1979). Espousing melodic intonation therapy in aphasia rehabilitation: A case study. *International Journal of Rehabilitation Research, 2*(3), 333–342.

Goodglass, H., & Calderon, M. (1977). Parallel processing of verbal and musical stimuli in right and left hemisphere. *Neuropsychologia, 15*, 397–407.

Hebert, S., Racette, A., Gagnon, L., & Peretz, I. (2003). Revisiting the dissociation between singing and speaking in expressive aphasia. *Brain, 126*, 1–13.

Helm-Estabrooks, N. & Albert, M. (2004). *Manual of aphasia and aphasia therapy* (2nd ed.). San Diego, CA: Singular Publishing Company.

Helm-Estabrooks, N., Nicholas, M., & Morgan, A. (1989). *MIT, melodic intonation therapy manual*. San Antonio, TX: Special Press.

Hough, M. S., & Johnson, R. K. (2009). Use of AAC to enhance linguistic communication skills in an adult with chronic severe aphasia. *Aphasiology, 23*(7), 965–974.

Hough, M. S., & King, K. A. (2008). *Enhancing word retrieval in three adults with chronic fluent aphasia*. Paper presented at the annual Clinical Aphasiology Conference, Jackson Hole, May.

Johnson, R., Hough, M. S., King, K. A., Jeffs, T., & Vos, P. (2008). Use of an augmentative system as a functional communicative device for adults with severe chronic nonfluent aphasia. *Alternative and Augmentative Communication, 24*(4), 1–12.

Kertesz, A. (2006). *Western Aphasia Battery-Revised*. New York: Grune & Stratton.

Lomas, J., Pickard, L., Bester, S., Elbard, H., Finlayson, A., & Zoghaib, C. (1989). The Communicative Effectiveness Index: Development and psychometric evaluation of a functional communication measure for adult aphasia. *Journal of Speech and Hearing Disorders, 54*, 113–124.

Marshall, N., & Holtzapple, P. (1976). Melodic intonation therapy: Variations on a theme. In R. H. Brookshire (Ed.), *Clinical Aphasiology Conference Proceedings* (pp. 115–141). Minneapolis, MN: BRK Publishers.

Naeser, M. A., & Helm-Estabrooks, N. (1985). CT scan lesion localization and response to melodic intonation therapy with nonfluent aphasia cases. *Cortex, 21*(2), 203–223.

Norton, A., Zipse, L., Marchina, S., & Schlaug, G. (2009). Melodic Intonation Therapy: Shared insights on how it is done and why it might help. *Annals of the New York Academy of Sciences, 1169*, 431–436.

Ozdemir, E., Norton, A., & Schlaug, G. (2006). Shared and distinct neural correlates of singing and speaking. *Neuroimage, 33*, 628–635.

Paul, D. R., Frattali, C. M., Holland, A. L., Thompson, C. K., Caperton, C. J., & Slater, S. C. (2003). *ASHA Quality of Communication Life Scale (QCL)*. Rockville, MD: American Speech-Language-Hearing Association.

Racette, A., Bard, C., & Peretz, I. (2006). Making non-fluent aphasics speak: Sing along! *Brain, 129*(10), 2571–2584.

Rosenbek, J. C. (1985). Treating apraxia of speech. In D. F. Johns (Ed.), *Clinical management of neurogenic communicative disorders* (2nd ed.) (pp. 267–312). Boston: Little, Brown & Company.

Rosenbek, J. C., & LaPointe, L. L. (1985). The dysarthrias: Description, diagnosis and treatment. In D. F. Johns (Ed.), *Clinical management of neurogenic communicative disorders* (2nd ed., pp. 151–210). Boston: Little, Brown & Company.

Rosenbek, J. C., Lemme, M. L., Ahern, M. B., Harris, E. H., & Wertz, R. T. (1973). A treatment for apraxia of speech in adults. *Journal of Speech and Hearing Disorders, 38*, 462–472.

Schlaug, G., Marchina, S., & Norton, A. (2008). From singing to speaking: Why singing may lead to recovery of expressive language function in patients with Broca's aphasia. *Music Perception, 25*(4), 315–323.

Schlaug, G., Marchina, S., & Norton, A. (2009). Evidence for plasticity in white-matter tracts of patients with chronic Broca's aphasia undergoing intense intonation-based speech therapy. *Annals of the New York Academy of Sciences, 1169*, 385–394.

Sparks, R. W., & Deck, J. W. (1994). Melodic intonation therapy. In R. Chapey (Ed.), *Language intervention strategies in adult aphasia* (3rd ed.) (pp. 368–379). Baltimore: Williams & Wilkins.

Sparks, R. W., Helm, N., & Albert, M. (1973). Melodic intonation therapy for aphasia. *Archives of Neurology, 29*, 130–131.

Sparks, R. W., Helm, N., & Albert, M. (1974). Aphasia rehabilitation resulting from melodic intonation therapy. *Cortex, 10*, 303–316.

Sparks R. W., & Holland A. (1976). Method: Melodic intonation therapy for aphasia. *Journal of Speech and Hearing Disorders, 41*, 287–297.

Steele, R. (2008). *Changes in chronic global aphasia at impairment and functional communication levels following SGD practice and use*. Paper presented at the annual Clinical Augmentative and Alternative Communication conference, Charlottesville, September.

Ventry, I. M., & Weinstein, B. E. (1983). Identification of elderly people with hearing problems. *American Speech-Language-Hearing Association, 25*(7), 37–42.

Ventry, I., & Weinstein, B. (1992). Considerations in screening adults/older persons for handicapping hearing impairments. *American Speech-Language-Hearing Association, 34*, 81–87.

APHASIOLOGY, 2010, 24 (6–8), 787–801

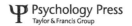

# Predicting outcomes for linguistically specific sentence treatment protocols

Michael Walsh Dickey and Hyunsoo Yoo

*University of Pittsburgh and VA Pittsburgh Healthcare System,
Pittsburgh, PA, USA*

*Background*: Linguistically motivated treatment protocols like the Treatment of Underlying Forms (TUF: Thompson & Shapiro, 2005) have shown significant success in remediating aphasic individuals' sentence production deficits. However, adults with aphasia are not uniform in their response to TUF: not all individuals trained with TUF successfully acquire the sentence types they are trained on or generalise to untrained sentence types. More research is therefore needed to determine which individuals are most likely to benefit from TUF treatment.
*Aims*: The current study analysed existing TUF treatment studies in an effort to determine what measures may be predictive of TUF outcomes for different aphasic individuals. Three different measures were tested: aphasia severity, auditory comprehension ability, and complex sentence comprehension ability.
*Methods & Procedures*: A meta-analysis was conducted based on existing TUF treatment studies drawn from the aphasiological literature. These studies included individual demographic, language-testing, and treatment data from 30 aphasic individuals. Regression analyses were conducted comparing these individuals' improvements on production of treated and untreated sentence types (treatment and generalisation effects) with the three predictor measures (severity, auditory comprehension, and complex sentence comprehension scores).
*Outcomes & Results*: Only one of the measures tested, general auditory comprehension, was predictive of the size of individuals' gains on treated sentence types. None of the measures tested was predictive of these individuals' generalisation to untrained structures.
*Conclusions*: The current results suggest that general auditory comprehension appears to be related to improved sentence production following TUF treatment. In contrast, neither overall aphasia severity nor performance with complex sentence stimuli is a strong predictor of TUF treatment outcomes. Interestingly, there were no strong relationships between any of the measures and the generalisation effect scores. These findings suggest that clinicians should consider a patient's general auditory comprehension when deciding whether TUF would be appropriate. They also suggest that partially different cognitive mechanisms may underlie treatment and generalisation effects following treatment, at least for TUF protocols.

Address correspondence to: Michael Walsh Dickey, 4033 Forbes Tower, Communication Science & Disorders, University of Pittsburgh, PA 15260, USA. E-mail: mdickey@pitt.edu

The authors are grateful to two anonymous reviewers, to Yasmeen Faroqi-Shah, Will Hula, Swathi Kiran, Laura Murray, Lew Shapiro, and Cindy Thompson, to colleagues at VA Pittsburgh Healthcare System and the University of Pittsburgh, and to audiences at the Clinical Aphasiology Conference (Keystone, CO) and the Academy of Aphasia (Boston) for very useful comments and discussion. This work was partially supported by University of Pittsburgh CRDF grant # 37769 to M. W. Dickey and by the Geriatric Research Education and Clinical Center of the VA Pittsburgh Healthcare System.

http://www.psypress.com/aphasiology      DOI: 10.1080/02687030903515354

*Keywords:* Aphasia; Treatment; Sentence production; Syntax; Outcomes.

Recent research focused on treatment of sentence-production deficits in aphasia has shown increasingly positive results. In particular, linguistically motivated treatment protocols such as the Treatment of Underlying Forms (TUF: Thompson & Shapiro, 2005) have shown significant evidence of efficacy for aphasic individuals with agrammatic language profiles. TUF trains the production of complex sentences by explicitly modelling the abstract syntactic structure of those sentences. The comprehension and production of these types of sentences, which involve non-canonical ordering of arguments resulting from syntactic movement operations, is often impaired among aphasic individuals. This impairment appears most dramatically among individuals with agrammatic language profiles (Goodglass, 1976), but it has also been found among fluent aphasic individuals (see Edwards, 2005; Murray, Ballard, & Karcher, 2004).

In TUF, participants are taught to re-order the constituents of complex sentences such as passives (which involve NP movement) or object wh-questions and object relatives (which involve wh-movement) in a metalinguistic card-manipulation task. Primary sentence constituents (such as the subject NP, object NP, and verb) are written on cards that are paired with picture stimuli depicting actions, and participants are taught re-order the constituents of simple active sentences to form more complex sentences. The steps of the re-ordering mirror the steps of the syntactic transformations involved in deriving the complex sentences that are impaired among aphasic individuals. See Thompson (2001) and Thompson and Shapiro (2005) for more detailed descriptions of the TUF treatment protocol.

In a number of studies with English-speaking agrammatic aphasic adults, TUF has been shown to result in successful acquisition of the complex sentences that are the target of training. These individuals have improved in their production of trained object wh-questions in both simple and embedded contexts (e.g., Ballard & Thompson, 1999), as well as object clefts and object relative clauses (e.g., Thompson, Shapiro, Kiran, & Sobecks, 2003). Importantly, these individuals have been shown not only to acquire trained sentence types but also to generalise to grammatically related but untrained sentence types. For example, in a study of four agrammatic individuals trained on production of wh-movement sentences (Thompson et al., 2003), two of the individuals trained to produce object relative clauses also improved on their production of untrained wh-questions and object clefts. However, these same individuals did not improve in their production of grammatically unrelated passive sentences, which involve NP rather than wh-movement (see also Thompson et al., 1997). The finding of generalisation to untrained structures in response to TUF has been replicated in a number of studies (e.g., Ballard & Thompson, 1999; Thompson, Shapiro & Roberts, 1993; Thompson, Shapiro, Tait, Jacobs & Schneider, 1996; Thompson et al., 1997). Generalisation to untrained structures is a particular strength of TUF: other sentence-treatment protocols such as Mapping Therapy (Rochon, Laird, Bose & Scofield, 2005) or HELPSS (Doyle, Goldstein & Bourgeois, 1987) have shown much more limited evidence of generalisation to untrained stimuli.

Treatment protocols inspired by TUF have also been successfully used to treat sentence production deficits among German-speaking agrammatic aphasic individuals (Stadie et al., 2008) as well as some fluent aphasic individuals with sentence-production deficits (Murray et al., 2004). There is also some evidence that TUF-like treatment protocols may be used to improve the sentence production of children with SLI (Levy & Friedmann, 2009). Furthermore, in a recent meta-analysis of existing aphasia treatment studies, TUF was shown to have the largest effect sizes of existing sentence-production treatment protocols (Beeson & Robey, 2008). In light of these findings, TUF merits special attention as a potentially clinically useful therapeutic intervention for sentence production deficits, among aphasic individuals of varying language backgrounds and profiles.

Despite TUF treatment's record of success, patients are not uniform in their response to it. This variability appears for both acquisition of trained structures and generalisation to untrained structures. For example, in a single-participant study of four aphasic individuals of varying profiles (Murray et al., 2004), only two of four individuals showed clear evidence of acquiring the sentence structures on which they were trained using TUF, object- and subject-extracted embedded questions. Similarly, in a single-participant multiple-baselines study of five agrammatic aphasic adults (Ballard & Thompson, 1999), only three of the five adults trained to produce object clefts generalised to untrained related sentences, object wh-questions. (There are also important effects of the order in which structures are trained, which will be explored in the Discussion below; see Thompson, Ballard, & Shapiro, 1998; Thompson et al., 2003). There is thus significant variability in how successfully aphasic individuals treated using TUF acquire the sentences on which they are trained, and in whether they will generalise to related but untrained forms.

Given that there is variability in individual patients' outcomes following TUF treatment, and the fact that TUF treatment has shown significant evidence of efficacy across clinical populations and studies, it is clinically and theoretically important to explore what factors determine how well aphasic individuals will respond to TUF. As a first step in this process, the current study analysed existing treatment studies using TUF to examine what measures may be predictive of TUF treatment outcomes. Three different measures were tested: aphasia severity, auditory comprehension ability, and complex sentence comprehension ability. These three measures were chosen for both theoretical and practical reasons. From a practical perspective, these variables are useful because they have been consistently reported for individual participants in existing TUF treatment studies. Other demographic variables (such as age at testing and time post-onset) have not: often only mean ages or ranges are provided as part of the participant descriptions in these studies. From a theoretical perspective, these variables have each been argued to have special significance, either for recovery or treatment outcomes, or for performance with complex sentence stimuli that are the target of TUF treatment.

Relative aphasia severity has been argued to be predictive of general potential for recovery (Porch & Callaghan, 1981). In particular, individuals with relatively mild impairments (or high peak performance on standardised measures of language abilities such as the PICA) have been argued to show better recovery in large-scale surveys of aphasic individuals' spontaneous recovery (e.g., Porch & Callaghan, 1981). These individuals are assumed to have more preserved access to pre-morbid language abilities. They are therefore expected to show better performance as they recover towards pre-morbid levels of language function. Relating this finding to TUF treatment outcomes specifically, relatively more mildly impaired aphasic individuals would be expected to show better treatment outcomes, since they have better access to pre-morbid sentence production abilities. This prediction is consistent with the general profile of individuals who have been treated using TUF in the existing literature: these individuals tend to have language-impairment scores on standardised batteries like the Western Aphasia Battery (WAB: Kertesz, 1982) which put them in the mildly to moderately impaired range (see Murray et al., 2004, for discussion).

Auditory comprehension ability has been argued to be predictive of TUF outcomes specifically: Murray et al. (2004) report that patients with better auditory comprehension abilities in their study showed larger treatment and generalisation effects. Auditory comprehension in these studies is measured by assessment of individuals' ability to identify single words, answer yes–no questions, and follow simple commands, on standardised measures such as the Western Aphasia Battery (Kertesz, 1982). Murray and colleagues also suggest that across existing TUF treatment studies, participants with better auditory comprehension abilities exhibit better TUF treatment outcomes, in particular faster and larger generalisation effects (Murray et al., 2004, p. 805). However, they do not present specific data in favour of this claim. Furthermore, this prediction is consistent with Schuell's (1960) more general observation that good auditory comprehension is crucial for successful outcomes in aphasia treatment. A number of other studies examining recovery from stroke have also pointed to the importance of auditory comprehension: for example, Mazzoni et al. (1992) found that auditory comprehension was also a leading indicator of improvement in language performance during spontaneous recovery.

Complex sentence comprehension ability may also be especially relevant for TUF performance. Sentence production and comprehension are broadly assumed to tap the same mental representations (Bock & Levelt, 1994). Relatively good comprehension performance for complex sentences indicates that aphasic individuals are still sensitive to the syntactic structure associated with the complex sentence stimuli trained in TUF, even if this sensitivity does not appear in their syntactically reduced production. Thus, good comprehension performance for complex sentence stimuli may be indicative of relatively preserved access to the abstract structure explicitly trained in TUF. It may therefore also be indicative of good potential for recovery of access to those representations in production, particularly in response to treatment protocols (like TUF) which explicitly stimulate/train those abstract syntactic representations (Thompson & Shapiro, 1995, 2005).

The current study therefore examined which of these variables (if any) was predictive of either the relative success of aphasic individuals in acquiring the complex sentence structures on which they are trained, or the likelihood of their generalising to untrained sentence structures. It did so by conducting a small-scale meta-analysis of existing TUF treatment studies, comparing the magnitude of participants' treatment gains and generalised improvement to untrained structures to their performance on the three predictor measures given above.

## METHOD

### Literature surveyed

The ANCDS Aphasia Treatment Evidence Tables (ANCDS, 2008) were surveyed to locate all treatment studies published through 2007 involving TUF, a total of 12 studies. Two additional case studies were also located in the literature (Dickey & Thompson, 2007; Murray, Timberlake, & Eberle, 2007), for a total of 14 studies. All studies involved single-participant, multiple-baseline or single-participant case studies. These studies were then reviewed to determine whether they: (a) reported individual participant data that had not been reported elsewhere, (b) reported individual data for treatment effects and generalisation to untrained stimuli, and (c) reported individual participant data for variables relevant to the analysis below (severity, general auditory comprehension, and complex sentence comprehension). The studies collected for the analysis and inclusion/exclusion information are provided in Table 1.

The 10 selected studies included 30 aphasic individuals' treatment and generalisation data, which were then used for further analysis.

## Analysis

The magnitude of the treatment effect for each of the 30 individuals was estimated by comparing pre-treatment production accuracy for trained sentence types to post-treatment production accuracy for the same sentences. These accuracy measures were derived from baseline-session probes and follow-up session probes, respectively. The reason for the choice of follow-up probes rather than maintenance-phase probes is that not all studies surveyed (especially case studies: see e.g., Dickey & Thompson, 2007) employed a full ABA single-participant, multiple-baseline design (see Beeson & Robey, 2006; Thompson, 2006). However, most of the studies surveyed had at least one follow-up probe that could serve as an estimate of post-treatment performance with the trained structures. In the absence of a follow-up probe, the final data point from the treatment phase was used as an estimate of post-treatment performance with trained structures.

Furthermore, not all studies or participants had enough observations or sufficient variability in baseline or post-treatment measurements to permit calculation of traditional effect sizes (Beeson & Robey, 2006, 2008). For instance, many participants exhibited no variability in their performance with trained structures in the baseline phase, resulting in a standard deviation of zero for pre-treatment scores. Since Cohen's *d*, the standard measure of effect size, standardises treatment effects by dividing the pre- to post-treatment difference by the pre-treatment standard deviation, a pre-treatment standard deviation of zero makes it impossible to calculate Cohen's *d* (see Beeson & Robey, 2006, for discussion). Therefore, a *treatment effect score* was calculated instead by subtracting the pre- from the post-treatment score. The generalisation effect for each participant was estimated in a similar way, but targeting untrained structures, resulting in a *generalisation effect score*.

These treatment and generalisation effect scores were then compared to the three predictor variables chosen above. *Severity scores* were based on the overall aphasia severity score for each individual included in the analysis. This score was the WAB Aphasia Quotient (AQ) in all the studies that were selected for the analysis. The WAB AQ is based on scores from subtests of language ability in four domains (comprehension, production or naming, repetition, and fluency) and ranges from 0 to 100, with a cut-off for positive aphasia diagnosis of 93.8. Severity scores were expected to correlate positively with the treatment and generalisation scores, based on the general finding that recovery is better for aphasic individuals with better performance on standardised measures of language impairment (Porch & Callaghan,

TABLE 1
Treatment studies surveyed for meta-analysis

| Treatment study | Included in analysis? |
|---|---|
| 1  Ballard, K. J., & Thompson, C. K. (1999). Treatment and generalization of complex sentence production in agrammatism. *Journal of Speech, Language, and Hearing Research, 42*, 690–707. | Yes |
| 2  Dickey, M.W., & Thompson, C.K. (2007). The relation between syntactic and morphological recovery in agrammatic aphasia: A case study. *Aphasiology, 21*, 604–616. | Yes |
| 3  Jacobs, B. J., & Thompson, C. K. (2000). Cross-modal generalization effects of training noncanonical sentence comprehension and production in agrammatic aphasia. *Journal of Speech, Language, and Hearing Research, 43*, 5–20. | Yes |
| 4  Jacobs, B. (2001). Social validity of changes in informativeness and efficiency of aphasic discourse following linguistic specific treatment (LST). *Brain and Language, 78*, 115–127. | No – patient treatment data reported elsewhere |
| 5  Murray, L. L., Ballard, K., & Karcher, L. (2004). Linguistic Specific Treatment: Just for Broca's aphasia? *Aphasiology, 18*, 785–809. | No – no measures of complex sentence comprehension |
| 6  Murray, L., Timberlake, A., & Eberle, R. (2007). Treatment of Underlying Forms in a discourse context. *Aphasiology, 21*, 139–163. | Yes |
| 7  Thompson, C. K., Shapiro, L. P., & Roberts, M. M. (1993). Treatment of sentence production deficits in aphasia: A linguistic-specific approach to wh-interrogative training and generalization. *Aphasiology, 7*, 111–133. | Yes |
| 8  Thompson, C. K., & Shapiro, L. P. (1994). A linguistic-specific approach to treatment of sentence production deficits in aphasia. In M. L. Lemme (Ed.), *Clinical Aphasiology: Vol. 22* (pp. 307–323). Austin, TX: Pro-Ed. | No – no individual data provided for auditory comprehension scores |
| 9  Thompson, C. K., & Shapiro, L. P. (1995). Training sentence production in agrammatism: Implications for normal and disordered language. *Brain and Language, 50*, 201–224. | No – no individual treatment data provided |
| 10  Thompson, C. K., Shapiro, L. P., Tait, M. E., Jacobs, B. J., & Schneider, S. S. (1996). Training wh-question production in agrammatic aphasia: Analysis of argument and adjunct movement. *Brain and Language, 52*, 175–228. | Yes |
| 11  Thompson, C. K., Shapiro, L. P., Ballard, K. J., Jacobs, B. B., Schneider, S. S., & Tait, M. E. (1997). Training and generalized production of wh- and NP-movement structures in agrammatic aphasia. *Journal of Speech, Language, and Hearing Research, 40*, 228–244. | Yes |
| 12  Thompson, C. K. (1998). Treating sentence production in agrammatic aphasia. In. N. Helm-Estabrooks & A. L. Holland (Eds.), *Approaches to the treatment of aphasia* (pp. 113–151). San Diego, CA: Singular Publishing Group. | Yes |
| 13  Thompson, C. K., Ballard, K. J., & Shapiro, L. P. (1998). The role of syntactic complexity in training wh-movement structures in agrammatic aphasia: optimal order for promoting generalization. *Journal of the International Neuropsychological Society, 4*, 661–674. | Yes |
| 14  Thompson, C. K., Shapiro, L. P., Kiran, S., & Sobecks, J. (2003) The role of syntactic complexity in treatment of sentence deficits in agrammatic aphasia: The complexity account of treatment efficacy (CATE). *Journal of Speech, Language, and Hearing Research, 46*, 591–607. | Yes |

1981) as well as the fact that most or all participants in existing TUF treatment studies are mildly to moderately impaired.

*Auditory comprehension scores* were based on general auditory comprehension measures, the WAB auditory comprehension subtest for all studies. This subtest measures comprehension for single words as well as simple sentences, and scores for the subtest range from 0 to 10. This choice of a general auditory comprehension measure is not ideal, as it is not independent of the general aphasia severity measure: the WAB auditory comprehension subtest is used to calculate WAB AQ. However, no other independent measure of general auditory comprehension was available for the studies included in the analysis. Auditory comprehension scores were expected to correlate positively with the treatment and generalisation scores, based on the general finding that positive treatment outcomes depend on good auditory comprehension (Schuell, 1960) and the specific suggestion that better TUF treatment outcomes are found for individuals with better auditory comprehension (Murray et al., 2004). Furthermore, if Murray and colleagues are correct in their suggestion that generalisation is faster and better for aphasic individuals with better auditory comprehension (Murray et al., 2004, p. 805), this correlation is expected to be stronger for generalisation scores.

*Complex sentence comprehension* scores were based on scores from assessments of comprehension of syntactically complex non-canonical sentences (object relative clauses, for example). In all the studies surveyed, complex sentence comprehension was tested using either the Northwestern Sentence Comprehension Test or the Philadelphia Comprehension Battery for Aphasia. Both these batteries assess sentence comprehension using a forced-choice sentence–picture matching paradigm and are scored using percentage correct, with scores ranging from 0 to 100. Complex sentence comprehension scores were expected to correlate positively with treatment and generalisation scores, based on the assumption that sentence comprehension and production access the same abstract syntactic representations (e.g., Bock & Levelt, 1994). Preserved access to these representations in the comprehension domain should therefore indicate that they are relatively intact and amenable to stimulation during production treatment, particularly for treatments like TUF that specifically target those representations.

## RESULTS

Consistent with the variable patterns of acquisition and generalisation for TUF treatment outcomes noted in the Introduction, there was significant variability in the size of the treatment and generalisation scores among the 30 participants. The mean treatment effect score was 76.9% ($SD$ = 20.7), with a range of 20–100%. The mean generalisation effect score was 57.9% ($SD$ = 27.2), with a range of 2.9–95.8%. These patterns provide numerical evidence that, while TUF does result in significant positive changes in sentence production performance for both trained and untrained sentence types, there is significant variation across participants in the magnitude of those gains.

The three predictor measures also exhibited significant variability across the 30 participants. The mean aphasia severity score was 67.8 ($SD$ = 7.7), with a range of 52.7–80.9. This pattern is consistent with the observation that most participants enrolled in TUF treatment studies are mildly to moderately impaired at most. The mean auditory comprehension score was 8.3 ($SD$ = 0.9), with a range of 6.1–10. This pattern indicates that most participants in published TUF treatment studies had relatively good auditory comprehension, although there was still some variability in the sample. The mean complex sentence comprehension score was 61.5% ($SD = 14.5$), with a range of 22–97.5%. This pattern indicates that there was considerable variability in comprehension ability for complex sentences (and by hypothesis, access/sensitivity to the associated abstract syntactic structure) among this sample of aphasic individuals. The variability for this predictor variable was thus much larger than that seen for the other two predictor variables.

These three predictor variables were entered into a pair of linear regressions examining the relationship between the predictor variables and the treatment and generalisation effect scores. In addition to the three predictor measures, treatment duration (defined as the number of treatment sessions a patient received) was entered as a separate variable into the regression analyses. The amount of time an aphasic individual spent in therapy could in principle affect the magnitude of his/her treatment gains and/or the likelihood of generalisation, creating another potential source of variability (and a potential confounding factor in interpreting the results).

Scatter-plots illustrating the relationship between the three predictor measures and the treatment effect scores are shown in Figure 1.

The $r$ values reported in the graphs represent zero-order correlations found in the regression analysis. The regression model as a whole (comprising all four independent variables) resulted in an $R$ value of .452, accounting for 20% of the observed variability ($R^2 = .204$). Of the individual predictor variables, only auditory comprehension was a significant predictor of patients' treatment effect scores, with an $r$ value of .401 ($t = 2.168, p < .05$). Severity was not a significant predictor ($r = .192; t = -.619, p > .05$), nor was complex sentence comprehension ($r = -.058; t = -.948, p > .05$). Finally, treatment duration was negatively related to treatment score ($r = -.073$) and was not a significant predictor ($t = -.580, p > .05$). The size of TUF treatment effects does not appear to be related to (or confounded by) the duration of treatment in this patient sample.

Scatter-plots illustrating the relationship between the three predictor measures and the generalisation effect scores are shown in Figure 2.

The $r$ values reported in the graphs represent zero-order correlations found in the regression analysis. The regression model as a whole (comprising all four independent variables) resulted in an $R$ value of .209, accounting for 4% of the observed variability ($R^2 = .044$). None of the individual predictor variables was a significant predictor of patients' treatment effect scores: not severity ($r = -.163; t = -.893, p > .05$), complex sentence comprehension ($r = .052; t = .438, p > .05$), or auditory comprehension ($r = -.055; t = .340, p > .05$). Finally, treatment duration was also negatively related to generalisation score ($r = -.044$) and was not a significant predictor ($t = .296, p > .05$). Parallel to the treatment effect data, the size of TUF generalisation effects does not appear to be related to (or confounded by) the duration of treatment in this patient sample.

## DISCUSSION

The Treatment of Underlying Forms syntactic treatment protocol (TUF) targets production of complex sentences and has shown significant evidence of efficacy in a number of case studies and single-participant studies. The current study examined

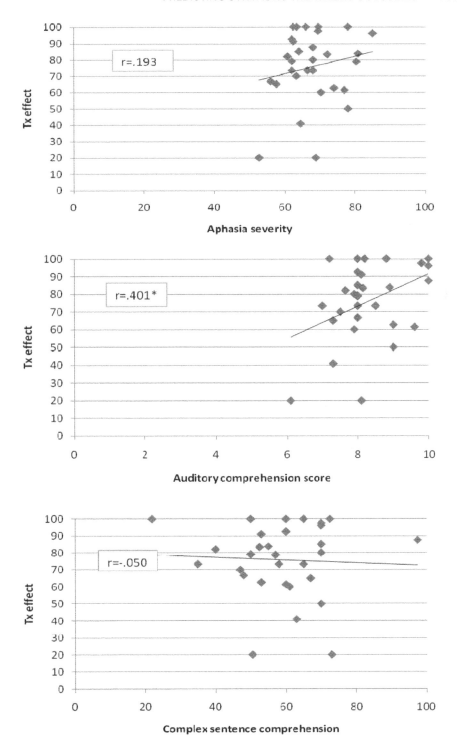

**Figure 1.** Relationship between predictor measures and treatment effects.

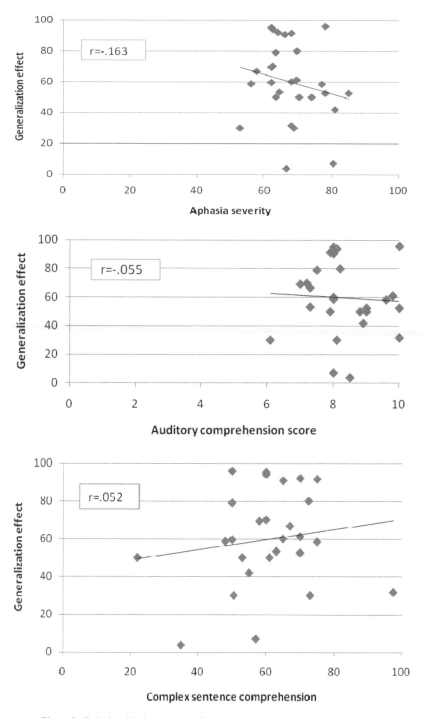

**Figure 2.** Relationship between predictor measures and generalisation effects.

the variability of individual patient outcomes among published TUF treatment studies, with the aim of identifying factors that favour positive treatment outcomes following TUF. The results suggest that only one of the factors considered is correlated with positive treatment outcomes. They also highlight important differences between treatment and generalisation effects following treatment.

Examining the treatment and generalisation effects themselves revealed that aphasic individuals do exhibit substantial gains in their sentence production ability for complex sentences in response to TUF. The mean treatment effect score was 76.9%, a figure in line with Beeson and Robey's (2008) finding that TUF treatment studies showed the largest effect sizes among the syntactic treatment studies they surveyed. The mean generalisation effect score was also high: 57.9%. This is consistent with the finding that individuals trained with TUF are likely not only to acquire the sentence forms they are trained on, but also to generalise to untrained but related sentence forms (Ballard & Thompson, 1999; Thompson et al., 1997, 1998, 2003). However, for both treatment and generalisation effect scores there was considerable variability: treatment effect scores ranged from 20% to 100%, while generalisation effect scores ranged from 2.9% to 95.8%. This variability highlights the importance of identifying factors that will predict which aphasic individuals are most likely to benefit from TUF treatment.

Examining the relationship between treatment effect scores and the three predictor measures (severity, general auditory comprehension, and complex sentence comprehension) revealed that neither overall aphasia severity nor performance with complex sentence stimuli was strongly related TUF treatment outcomes. These findings are surprising, especially if comprehension and production use the same abstract syntactic structures (Bock & Levelt, 1994), and performance for complex sentences is indicative of relatively preserved access to the grammatical structures involved. The absence of a correlation between severity and treatment outcomes is also surprising, particularly given previous evidence suggesting a relationship between severity on standardised language measures and aphasia recovery (for example, Porch & Callaghan, 1981).

The relatively weak relationship between impairment severity and treatment gains for TUF may be due in part to how severity was measured in these studies. The WAB AQ may simply be too broad a measure to be of predictive value for a linguistically specific protocol like TUF, since it samples language behaviours across many domains. It may therefore not be relevant to the specific behaviours or structures trained in TUF. The range of severity among participants in these TUF studies was also relatively limited: TUF has typically been used with patients with mild-to-moderate levels of impairment. Both these possibilities would weaken the relationship between severity and treatment outcome measures. Teasing these two possibilities apart is a question for further research.

The weak relationship between non-canonical sentence comprehension and TUF outcomes may also be due to measurement issues. The assumption behind using noncanonical sentence comprehension as a predictor variable is that it should measure preserved sensitivity to the syntactic distinctions that are specifically trained in TUF. However, sentence–picture matching (the sentence comprehension task used in all the TUF studies surveyed) may not be the best measure of aphasic adults' sensitivity to grammatical structure. Linebarger, Schwartz, and Saffran (1983) and others have argued that grammaticality judgement provides a better measure of preserved access to grammatical structure. Similarly, online measures like eye tracking (Dickey, Choy, & Thompson, 2007), auditory moving window paradigms (Caplan & Waters, 2003), or cross-modal lexical priming (Love, Swinney, Walenski, & Zurif, 2008) have revealed preserved sensitivity to grammatical structure that does not appear in sentence–picture matching tasks. Either on-line processing or grammaticality-judgement measures might therefore be better predictor measures than sentence–picture matching.

General auditory comprehension did appear to be related to improved sentence production following TUF treatment. This finding is consistent with Murray and colleagues' (2004) suggestion that aphasic individuals with better auditory comprehension show better TUF treatment outcomes, and it is also consistent with Schuell's (1960) observations regarding the importance of auditory comprehension for good clinical outcomes among aphasic individuals. Furthermore, it suggests that clinicians should consider a patient's general auditory comprehension when deciding whether TUF would be appropriate.

However, it is an open question why general auditory comprehension ability should be predictive of outcomes for a linguistically specific protocol like TUF. One possibility is that good general auditory comprehension is a necessary prerequisite for TUF training. TUF is a complex treatment protocol, involving multiple treatment steps that require successful word identification, yes/no question comprehension, and execution of simple commands. These are exactly the comprehension behaviours assessed in the general auditory comprehension measure used in the studies surveyed (WAB auditory comprehension subscore). A second (related) possibility is that good general auditory comprehension will be predictive of outcomes for any treatment protocol (cf. Schuell, 1960). Since all language treatments involve responding to spoken cues, good general auditory comprehension may be necessary for any therapy. Again, further research is required to tease these possibilities apart, perhaps comparing TUF and other therapies.

A third possibility is that good auditory comprehension is indicative of preserved domain-general cognitive abilities, such as working memory or executive function. TUF demands effortful learning and makes significant working memory and executive function demands on patients. Many researchers have suggested that working memory is important for processing of sentence-level stimuli like those trained in TUF (e.g., Sung et al., 2009). Recent work has also emphasised the role of executive function in mediating treatment outcomes (e.g., Fillingham, Sage, & Lambon-Ralph, 2006; see also Murray, 2004), and a number of studies have furthermore pointed to the importance of cognitive functions in stroke recovery (e.g., Nys et al., 2005). If auditory comprehension indirectly measures these domain-general cognitive functions, a relationship between auditory comprehension and TUF treatment outcomes is to be expected.

Interestingly, there were no strong relationships between any of the measures and the generalisation effect scores. This finding is not consistent with Murray et al.'s (2004) observation that individuals with better auditory comprehension show better and faster generalisation in response to TUF. Further research is needed to see whether auditory comprehension may be predictive of generalisation in larger samples of patients, as well as to see which other measures may be useful in predicting whether aphasic individuals are likely to generalise to untrained stimuli in response to TUF. Also of interest will be to examine whether these measures are predictive of outcomes for other sentence-level treatment protocols (such as Mapping Therapy, Rochon et al., 2005, or VNeST, Edmonds, Nadeau & Kiran, 2009). Furthermore, additional research is needed to determine whether the order in which sentence types are trained will affect the magnitude of TUF generalisation effects (cf. Thompson et al., 2003). Regardless of the answers to these additional questions, the current results do provide novel insight into the relationship between treatment outcomes and generalisation in response to TUF: the two processes appear to be subserved by partially different cognitive mechanisms. General auditory comprehension was related to the magnitude of treatment gains in response to TUF, but not the magnitude of generalisation. This distinction suggests that there may be important differences between the ability to acquire a trained form in response to explicit treatment (likely a form of explicit learning) and the ability to generalise to related but untrained forms (likely a form of implicit learning).

The current results are preliminary, in that they examined only a small number of factors that may be relevant to treatment outcomes following one specific treatment protocol. It is important to note that a number of other factors that have been shown to be prognostic of recovery and treatment outcomes—such as age, lesion site and extent, comorbid conditions, and cognitive function—were not addressed in this study. While such data were unavailable for the treatment studies surveyed here, they should be included in future prospective studies of treatment outcomes. Inclusion of these other variables will be crucial for improving the predictive power of future models of treatment gains and generalisation: the four-variable regression model used here explained only 20% of the observed variance for the treatment effect scores. However, the current results do represent a first step in determining which individuals are most likely to benefit from a linguistically specific treatment like TUF, as well as what factors are likely to underlie not only successful acquisition but generalisation in response to treatment.

Manuscript received 24 July 2009
Manuscript accepted 26 November 2009
First published online 7 May 2010

# REFERENCES

ANCDS. (2008). *The ANCDS aphasia treatment evidence tables.* Available online from: http://www.u.arizona.edu/~pelagie/ancds/index.html

Ballard, K. J., & Thompson, C. K. (1999). Treatment and generalization of complex sentence production in agrammatism. *Journal of Speech, Language, and Hearing Research, 42,* 690–707.

Beeson, P. M., & Robey R. R. (2006). Evaluating single-subject treatment research: Lessons learned from the aphasia literature. *Neuropsychological Review, 16,* 161–169.

Beeson, P. M., & Robey, R. R. (2008, May). *Meta-analyses of aphasia treatment outcomes: Examining the evidence.* Invited platform presentation at the Annual Clinical Aphasiology Conference, Jackson Hole, Wyoming.

Bock, K., & Levelt, W. (1994). Language production: Grammatical encoding. In M. A. Gernsbacher (Ed.), *Handbook of psycholinguistics.* San Diego, CA: Academic Press.

Caplan, D., & Waters, G. (2003). On-line syntactic processing in aphasia: Studies with auditory moving window presentation. *Brain and Language, 84*(2), 222–249.

Dickey, M. W., Choy, J. W. J., & Thompson, C. K. (2007). Real-time comprehension of wh- movement in aphasia: Evidence from eyetracking while listening. *Brain and Language, 100*(1), 1–22.

Dickey, M. W., & Thompson, C. K. (2007). The relation between syntactic and morphological recovery in agrammatic aphasia: A case study. *Aphasiology, 21,* 604–616.

Doyle, P. J., Goldstein, H., & Bourgeois, M. (1987). Experimental analysis of syntax training in Broca's aphasia: A generalisation and social validation study. *Journal of Speech and Hearing Disorders, 52,* 143–155.

Edmonds, L. A., Nadeau, S. E., & Kiran, S. (2009). Effect of verb network strengthening treatment (VNeST) on lexical retrieval of content words in sentences in persons with aphasia. *Aphasiology, 23*(3), 402–424.

Edwards, S. (2005). *Fluent aphasia.* Cambridge, UK: Cambridge University Press.

Fillingham, J. K., Sage, K., & Lambon Ralph, M. A. (2006). The treatment of anomia using errorless learning. *Neuropsychological Rehabilitation*, *16*, 129–154.

Goodglass, H. (1976). Agrammatism. In H. Whitaker & A. Whitaker (Eds.), *Studies in neurolinguistics* (Vol. 1). New York: Academic Press.

Jacobs, B. (2001). Social validity of changes in informativeness and efficiency of aphasic discourse following linguistic specific treatment (LST). *Brain and Language*, *78*, 115–127.

Jacobs, B. J., & Thompson, C. K. (2000). Cross-modal generalization effects of training noncanonical sentence comprehension and production in agrammatic aphasia. *Journal of Speech, Language, and Hearing Research*, 43, 5–20.

Kertesz, A. (1982). *Western Aphasia Battery*. San Antonio, TX: Psychological Corp.

Levy, H., & Friedmann, N. (2009). Treatment of syntactic movement in syntactic SLI: A case study. *First Language*, *29*, 15–50.

Linebarger, M. C., Schwartz, M. F., & Saffran, E. M. (1983). Sensitivity to grammatical structure in so-called agrammatic aphasics. *Cognition*, *13*(3), 361–392.

Love, T., Swinney, D., Walenski, M., & Zurif, E. (2008). How left inferior frontal cortex participates in syntactic processing: Evidence from aphasia. *Brain and Language*, *107*(3), 203–219.

Mazzoni, M., Vista, M., Pardossi, L., Avila, L., Bianchi, F., & Moretti, P. (1992). Spontaneous evolution of aphasia after an ischemic stroke. *Aphasiology*, 6, 387–396.

Murray, L., Timberlake, A., & Eberle, R. (2007). Treatment of Underlying Forms in a discourse context. *Aphasiology*, *21*, 139–163.

Murray, L. L. (2004) Cognitive treatments for aphasia: Should we and can we help attention and working memory problems? *Medical Journal of Speech-Language Pathology*, *12*, xxi–xxxviii.

Murray, L. L., Ballard, K., & Karcher, L. (2004). Linguistic Specific Treatment: Just for Broca's aphasia? *Aphasiology*, *18*, 785–809.

Nys, G. M., van Zandvoort, M. J., de Kort, P. L., van der Worp, H. B., Jansen, B. P., Algra, A., et al. (2005). The prognostic value of domain-specific cognitive abilities in acute first-ever stroke. *Neurology*, *64*, 821–827.

Porch, B., & Callaghan, S. (1981). Making predictions about recovery: Is there HOAP? In R. H. Brookshire (Ed.), *Clinical Aphasiology Conference Proceedings: 1981*. Minneapolis, MN: BRK Publishers.

Rochon, E., Laird, L., Bose, A., & Scofield, J. (2005). Mapping therapy for sentence production impairment in aphasia. *Neuropsychological Rehabilitation*, *15*(1), 1–36.

Schuell, H. (1960). Clinical findings in aphasia. *The Lancet*, *80*, 482–490.

Stadie, N., Schroder, A., Postler, J., Lorenz, A., Swoboda-Moll, M., Burchert, F., et al. (2008). Unambiguous generalisation effects after treatment of non-canonical sentence production in German agrammatism. *Brain and Language*, *104*(3), 211–229.

Sung, J. E., McNeil, M. R., Pratt, S. R., Dickey, M. W., Hula, W. D., Szuminsky, N. J., et al. (2009). Verbal working memory and its relationship to sentence-level reading and listening comprehension in persons with aphasia. *Aphasiology*, *23*, 1040–1052.

Thompson, C. K. (1998). Treating sentence production in agrammatic aphasia. In N. Helm-Estabrooks & A. L. Holland (Eds.), *Approaches to the treatment of aphasia* (pp. 113–151). San Diego, CA: Singular Publishing Group

Thompson, C. K. (2001). Treatment of underlying forms: A linguistic specific approach for sentence production deficits in agrammatic aphasia. In R. Chapey (Ed.), *Language intervention strategies in adult aphasia* (4th ed.). Baltimore: Williams & Wilkins.

Thompson, C. K., Ballard, K. J., & Shapiro, L. P. (1998). The role of syntactic complexity in training wh-movement structures in agrammatic aphasia: Optimal order for promoting generalization. *Journal of the International Neuropsychological Society*, *4*, 661–674.

Thompson, C. K., & Shapiro, L. P. (1994). A linguistic-specific approach to treatment of sentence production deficits in aphasia. In M. L. Lemme (Ed.), *Clinical aphasiology* (Vol. 22, pp. 307–323). Austin, TX: Pro-Ed.

Thompson, C. K. & Shapiro, L. P. (1995). Training sentence production in agrammatism: Implications for normal and disordered language. *Brain and Language*, *50*, 201–224.

Thompson, C. K., & Shapiro, L. P. (2005). Treating agrammatic aphasia within a linguistic framework: Treatment of Underlying Forms. *Aphasiology*, *19*(10–11), 1021–1036.

Thompson, C. K., Shapiro, L. P., Ballard, K. J., Jacobs, B. B., Schneider, S. S., & Tait, M. E. (1997). Training and generalized production of wh- and NP-movement structures in agrammatic aphasia. *Journal of Speech, Language, and Hearing Research*, *40*, 228–244.

Thompson, C. K., Shapiro, L. P., Kiran, S., & Sobecks, J. (2003) The role of syntactic complexity in treatment of sentence deficits in agrammatic aphasia: The complexity account of treatment efficacy (CATE). *Journal of Speech, Language, and Hearing Research, 46*, 591–607.

Thompson, C. K., Shapiro, L. P., & Roberts, M. M. (1993). Treatment of sentence production deficits in aphasia: A linguistic-specific approach to wh-interrogative training and generalization. *Aphasiology, 7*, 111–133.

APHASIOLOGY, 2010, 24 (6–8), 802–813

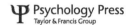

# Semantic typicality effects in acquired dyslexia: Evidence for semantic impairment in deep dyslexia

Ellyn A. Riley and Cynthia K. Thompson

*Northwestern University, Evanston, IL, USA*

*Background*: Acquired deep dyslexia is characterised by impairment in grapheme-phoneme conversion and production of semantic errors in oral reading. Several theories have attempted to explain the production of semantic errors in deep dyslexia, some proposing that they arise from impairments in both grapheme-phoneme and lexical-semantic processing, and others proposing that such errors stem from a deficit in phonological production. Whereas both views have gained some acceptance, the limited evidence available does not clearly eliminate the possibility that semantic errors arise from a lexical-semantic input-processing deficit.

*Aims*: To investigate semantic processing in deep dyslexia this study examined the typicality effect in deep dyslexic individuals, phonological dyslexic individuals, and controls using an online category verification paradigm. This task requires explicit semantic access without speech production, focusing observation on semantic processing from written or spoken input.

*Methods & Procedures*: To examine the locus of semantic impairment, the task was administered in visual and auditory modalities with reaction time as the primary dependent measure. Nine controls, six phonological dyslexic participants, and five deep dyslexic participants completed the study.

*Outcomes & Results*: Controls and phonological dyslexic participants demonstrated a typicality effect in both modalities, while deep dyslexic participants did not demonstrate a typicality effect in either modality.

*Conclusions*: These findings suggest that deep dyslexia is associated with a semantic processing deficit. Although this does not rule out the possibility of concomitant deficits in other modules of lexical-semantic processing, this finding suggests a direction for treatment of deep dyslexia focused on semantic processing.

*Keywords:* Deep dyslexia; Semantic typicality.

Caused by an acquired disease of the central nervous system such as stroke or traumatic brain injury, acquired dyslexia results from damage to the mature reading system and manifests as an impairment in the comprehension of written language (Ellis & Young, 1988). Deep dyslexia and phonological dyslexia are two subtypes of acquired dyslexia. Although the literature offers varying descriptions of deep dyslexia, patients exhibit several hallmark symptoms including: (1) severely impaired pseudoword reading, (2) semantic errors in oral reading, (3) visual errors in oral reading, (4) morphological

Address correspondence to: Ellyn Riley, Northwestern University, 2240 Campus Drive, Evanston, IL 60208, USA. E-mail: e-riley@u.northwestern.edu

http://www.psypress.com/aphasiology                                DOI: 10.1080/02687030903422486

errors in oral reading, and (5) an imageability effect in word reading with greater success in reading concrete, imageable words (Coltheart, 1980; Ellis & Young, 1988). In contrast, the hallmark of phonological dyslexia is impairment in pseudoword reading in conjunction with an absence of semantic reading errors (Beauvois & Dérouesné, 1979; Dérouesné & Beauvois, 1979; Ellis & Young, 1988). These patients may also show visual errors and imageability effects, as in deep dyslexia. However, the presence of semantic errors distinguishes between the two reading disorders (Friedman, 1996; Glosser & Friedman, 1990).

Several theories of semantic error production in deep dyslexia have been proposed, but the theories relevant to the current study include the multiple-deficit hypothesis (Morton & Patterson, 1980) and the failure of inhibition theory (Buchanan, McEwen, Westbury, & Libben, 2003). The multiple-deficit hypothesis suggests that reading deficits in deep dyslexia stem from more than one source. Referencing patient data from several case studies, Morton and Patterson (1980) suggested damage to both the non-lexical grapheme-phoneme route (to account for pseudoword reading deficits) and lexical-semantic routes (to account for semantic errors). Shallice and Warrington (1980) further proposed multiple candidates for impairment constrained to the lexical-semantic processing route: (1) impaired *access* to the semantic system, (2) impaired *processing* within the semantic system, and (3) impaired *phonological retrieval* following semantic processing. Some studies support impaired access to the semantic system, reporting differences in performance accuracy on visual and auditory tasks (Shallice & Coughlan, 1980; Shallice & Warrington, 1975). In contrast, other studies support a central semantic processing deficit, reporting individuals with deep dyslexia who show poor performance accuracy in both visual and auditory word–picture matching tasks (Newcombe & Marshall, 1980; Patterson, 1978). Still other studies support a phonological impairment, with evidence of deep dyslexic patients producing semantic errors in naming as well as reading (Marshall & Newcombe, 1966; Patterson, 1978; Saffran & Marin, 1977). Although Shallice and Warrington (1980) were able to specify possible deficit locations, they acknowledged that supporting evidence exists for all three possibilities and the problem of locating the lexical-semantic impairment still remains.

In contrast, the failure of inhibition theory (FIT) proposes that semantic errors in deep dyslexia are caused by failure to inhibit incorrect responses at the level of phonological production (Buchanan et al., 2003). Within this theoretical framework, when a word is read aloud the word's stored orthographic representation is activated, followed by activation of its semantic representation as well as spreading activation of semantically related neighbours and, in turn, these entries in the phonological lexicon are activated. In a normal reading system, incorrect responses would be inhibited, however, in deep dyslexia, FIT hypothesises that the inhibition mechanism is impaired, resulting in production of semantic errors (Buchanan et al., 2003). One critical aspect of FIT relates to how orthographic, semantic, and phonological representations are accessed, a feature of the model referred to as PEIR (Production, Explicit access, Implicit access, Representation) (Buchanan et al., 2003). PEIR proposes that production relies on explicit access, which relies on implicit access, which relies on intact representations (Buchanan et al., 2003; Colangelo & Buchanan, 2007). Authors of FIT propose that deep dyslexia is the result of a deficit in explicit access at the level of phonological production (Colangelo & Buchanan, 2007).

This hypothesis is based primarily on data from a single case of deep dyslexia, patient JO, whose responses the authors interpret as intact implicit access to semantics, intact explicit access to semantics in the absence of production, and deficient explicit access in tasks requiring production (Colangelo & Buchanan, 2005, 2007). To test implicit access, JO completed a lexical decision task and performed within accuracy ranges of controls, leading the authors to conclude that implicit semantic processing was intact (Colangelo & Buchanan, 2005). To test explicit access to semantics with a production component, performance on an oral reading task was compared in a semantically blocked condition and an unrelated condition. JO produced significantly more semantic errors in the semantically blocked condition, so the authors argued that FIT was supported in that explicit access to phonology was not achieved (Colangelo & Buchanan, 2005, 2007). In order to further specify that this explicit access related to the phonological lexicon and not semantics, JO was given a forced choice trial for multiple lists of semantically related words, requiring silent reading of the list, followed by selection of the most semantically associated word from a field of two choices (Colangelo & Buchanan, 2005, 2007). JO's accuracy on this task was within the range of control participants' performance; thus it was concluded that explicit access to the semantic system was not impaired. Although, on the surface, this evidence may appear convincing, it is to date the only piece of evidence directly addressing the explicit semantic access capabilities of deep dyslexic individuals and is only based on data from a single case study. Additionally, although the task examined semantic access, the only measure was overall accuracy of performance, which could potentially be insensitive to processing impairments that may be detected by online measures such as reaction time.

In summary, both models of deep dyslexia discussed here provide supporting evidence, but neither is able to adequately address all the evidence, especially regarding semantic error production. To investigate semantic processing in deep dyslexia, the current study examined the semantic typicality effect using a task that requires explicit semantic access without production.

## SEMANTIC TYPICALITY EFFECTS

Semantic typicality is a factor that affects the organisation of semantic categories in the mental lexicon. While the classical view of semantic categorisation considers each category to possess a set of defining features, it has been shown that not all members of a category represent these features to the same degree (Rosch, 1973, 1975). Some items in a category can be considered good or typical exemplars that possess many of the defining features of the category (e.g., *robin* in the category of *birds*), whereas others can be considered poor or atypical exemplars that possess fewer defining features of the same category (e.g., *ostrich*). Some studies have shown that typical members of a category are processed faster than atypical members, an effect known as the typicality effect (Kiran & Thompson, 2003; Rosch, 1975).

In healthy control participants the typicality effect has been found in several studies using a variety of experimental paradigms, including item ranking, lexical decision, category verification, and category naming (Casey, 1992; Hampton, 1995; Rosch, 1973, 1975). This effect also has been found for people with nonfluent Broca's, but not fluent Wernicke's aphasia. Using a category verification task Kiran and Thompson (2003) found faster reaction times (RTs) for typical as compared to atypical exemplars of category items for the nonfluent patients. However, for the fluent patients no RT differences were found for the two types of words, a finding associated with an underlying semantic deficit.

The purpose of the current study was to test for a semantic processing impairment in deep dyslexia using an online category verification paradigm identical to that used by Kiran and Thompson (2003). This task requires explicit access to the semantic system without requiring oral production. The following questions were posed: (1) Do individuals with deep dyslexia fail to show a typicality effect, which would suggest impaired semantic processing? (2) In the event that deep dyslexic readers fail to show this effect, does the impairment show up when processing both visual and auditory words? It was predicted that, in contrast to participants with deep dyslexia, both healthy control participants and phonological dyslexic participants would show a typicality effect in both visual and auditory modalities. Whereas we predicted that if a semantic impairment underlies semantic errors in deep dyslexia, the typicality effect would be absent in one or both modalities. A deficit in visual, but not auditory, processing would suggest a deficit in accessing semantic representations from the written form of lexical items; whereas deficient processing in both modalities would indicate an amodal central semantic deficit.

## METHOD

### Participants

Nine individuals served as adult control participants (six females; age 22 to 29, $M = 24.5$; years of education 16 to 20, $M = 17.4$) and eleven individuals with acquired dyslexia participated in this study (four females; age 47 to 69, $M = 58.2$; years of education 12 to 19, $M = 15.5$). All were monolingual English speakers, had normal or corrected-to-normal vision, and normal hearing. None reported a history of psychiatric, developmental speech-language, or neurological disorders, other than stroke in the patient participants. All patient participants demonstrated behavioural characteristics consistent with acquired dyslexia subsequent to left hemisphere cerebrovascular accident (CVA); time elapsed after CVA ranged from 2.5 to 17.5 years ($M = 6.9$ years). Control participants were recruited from Northwestern University and the surrounding community, and acquired dyslexia participants were recruited from the Northwestern University Aphasia and Neurolinguistics Laboratory and the Northwestern University Speech and Language Clinic. All participants gave informed consent in accordance with Northwestern University's Institutional Review Board.

Six individuals showed patterns consistent with a diagnosis of phonological dyslexia and five showed "deep dyslexia" patterns. Participants in the deep dyslexia group were not significantly different from those in the phonological dyslexia group for age, years of education, or years post-CVA—age, $t(9) = -0.053$, $p = .61$; years education, $t(9) = -1.46$, $p = 0.18$; years post-CVA, $t(9) = -0.87$, $p = .41$. Participants with acquired dyslexia were not significantly different from controls in years of education, $t(18) = 1.97$, $p = .07$, but control participants were significantly younger, $t(18) = -14.67$, $p < .05$.

To determine a diagnosis of acquired dyslexia, participants were administered the *Western Aphasia Battery-Revised* (*WAB-R*) (Kertesz, 2007), a subtest from the *Woodcock Johnson-III Diagnostic Reading Battery* (*WJDRB-III*) (Woodcock, Mather, & Schrank, 2004), and selected subtests from the *Psycholinguistic Assessment of Language Processing in Aphasia* (*PALPA*) (Kay, Lesser, & Coltheart, 1992). Although a diagnosis of aphasia was not a criterion for participant inclusion, all acquired dyslexic participants presented with aphasia as measured by the *WAB-R*, with Aphasia Quotients ranging from 51.4 to 87.6. All dyslexic participants also demonstrated deficits in pseudoword reading on the *WJDRB-III* and on the *Nonword Reading* subtest of the *PALPA* (see Table 1). To ensure integrity of the written version of the experimental task, all dyslexic participants were required to demonstrate the ability to match single written words to pictures on the *Written Word-Picture Matching* subtest of the *PALPA*.

To distinguish between the phonological and deep dyslexia patient groups, additional subtests of the *PALPA* were administered, including the *Imageability and Frequency Reading* subtest (*PALPA* 31) and *Regularity Reading* subtest (*PALPA* 35). Individuals included in the deep dyslexia group produced semantic errors in single-word oral reading, whereas individuals in the phonological dyslexia group did not. Additionally, although participants in both the deep and phonological dyslexia groups showed effects of imageability— deep dyslexia, $t(4) = 5.404$, $p < .01$; phonological dyslexia, $t(5) = 5.809$, $p < .05$—in single-word oral reading as demonstrated by the *Imageability and Frequency Reading* subtest of the *PALPA*, individuals in the deep dyslexia group demonstrated imageability effects of a significantly greater magnitude, $t(9) = -4.804$, $p < .01$) (see Table 1).

## Materials

The stimuli used in this study were based on those used by Kiran and Thompson (2003) in their online category verification task. Three animate superordinate categories were used (birds, vegetables, and fish), with each category containing 15 typical and 15 atypical items for a total of 90 items. The typicality norms for each category were obtained from Kiran (2001), derived by asking groups of healthy young and elderly individuals to rate items on a 7-point scale based on category typicality. Within this scale a low rank (e.g., 1) indicated items judged as good members of a category, and a high rank (e.g., 7) indicated items judged as poor members of a category. The items for each category were then rank ordered using $z$-scores. Because low ranks represented "typical" items and high ranks represented "atypical" items, $z$-score calculations resulted in a range of $z$-scores from $-1.2$ on the extreme end of "typical" items to 1.3 on the extreme end of "atypical" items. For each category, typical exemplars were selected based on the 15 items with the lowest $z$-scores (range: $-1.2$ to $-0.45$) and atypical exemplars were selected based on the 15 items with the highest $z$-scores (range: 0.01 to 1.3). An additional 90 items belonging to different superordinate categories served as non-member exemplars (Kiran & Thompson, 2003). For the online category verification task each item was paired with a superordinate category label (i.e., bird, vegetable, fish), resulting in 180 word pairs. The order of stimulus presentation was randomised during the experimental task. For each superordinate category, 30 items matched the category ("yes" response) and 30 items did not match the category ("no" response).

The same 180 word pairs were used for both the visual and auditory online category verification tasks. For the visual task stimulus words were presented in 48-point Arial Black font. For the auditory task stimuli were recorded in a soundproof booth using a female voice and presented through external speakers adjusted to each participant's sound comfort level. A Mac Book computer with Superlab 4.0 was used to present stimuli and collect accuracy and reaction time data. In the visual online category verification task the superordinate prime word was presented for 750 ms, followed by a 200-ms Inter-Stimulus Interval (ISI) and then the target word, which remained on the screen until the participant responded. This sequence was followed by a 1500-ms

TABLE 1
Language testing data for acquired dyslexic participants

| | P1 | P2 | P3 | P4 | P5 | P6 | group mean | D1 | D2 | D3 | D4 | D5 | group mean |
|---|---|---|---|---|---|---|---|---|---|---|---|---|---|
| *Western Aphasia Battery-Revised* | | | | | | | | | | | | | |
| Aphasia Quotient | 87.6 | 78.2 | 78.1 | 72.6 | 68.1 | 66.8 | 75.2 | 51.4 | 81.8 | 85 | 54.3 | 59.6 | 66.4 |
| Reading Score | 19.8 | 12.8 | 17.4 | 15 | 12.2 | 18.2 | 15.9 | 13.8 | 17.8 | 18.2 | 11.2 | 10.2 | 14.2 |
| *Psycholinguistic Assessment of Language Processing in Aphasia* | | | | | | | | | | | | | |
| Nonword reading | 33% | 0% | 0% | 33% | 6% | 22% | 16% | 6% | 22% | 17% | 0% | 6% | 10% |
| Written word picture matching | 100% | 98% | 100% | 100% | 100% | 100% | 100% | 100% | 100% | 93% | 88% | 85% | 93% |
| Imageability & Frequency Reading | | | | | | | | | | | | | |
| high imageability | 93% | 95% | 98% | 93% | 65% | 100% | 91% | 75% | 98% | 98% | 45% | 35% | 70% |
| low imageability | 90% | 90% | 90% | 88% | 55% | 95% | 85% | 25% | 68% | 77% | 0% | 15% | 37% |
| Regularity Reading | | | | | | | | | | | | | |
| regular | 90% | 76% | 87% | 87% | 33% | 87% | 77% | 70% | 100% | 93% | 13% | 40% | 63% |
| exception | 87% | 83% | 93% | 80% | 50% | 77% | 78% | 63% | 97% | 87% | 16% | 43% | 61% |
| *Woodcock Johnson-III* | | | | | | | | | | | | | |
| Nonword reading | 28% | 9% | 19% | 25% | 9% | 28% | 20% | 0% | 37% | 34% | 9% | 13% | 19% |
| % semantic errors in total number of single words read | 0% | 0% | 0.01% | 0.01% | 0.01% | 0.01% | 0.01% | 5% | 4% | 5% | 34% | 6% | 11% |

P1 through P6 represent phonological dyslexic participants and D1 through D5 represent deep dyslexic participants.

inter-trial interval (ITI). For the auditory online category verification task the super-ordinate prime word was presented for the duration of the audio file (500–700 ms), followed by a 200-ms ISI and the audio presentation of the target word. A 1500-ms ITI followed each participant response and the next superordinate prime was presented. For both task modalities, the participant's response time was recorded from the onset of the target word.

All participants completed both the visual and auditory versions of the task, which were presented in two separate sessions on different days, with at least 5 days between the two. The order of modality presentation was counterbalanced across participants. For both modalities, participants were seated in front of the computer screen with one hand resting on a button response box. Participants were instructed to either read or listen to (depending on modality) each word pair presented and decide if the target word belonged to the preceding category. If the word was judged to be a member of the category, the participant was instructed to press the green "yes" response button on the button box. If the word was judged not to be a member of the preceding category, the participant was instructed to press the red "no" response button on the button box.

After receiving the task instructions, a 10-item training session was completed to allow practice with items similar to those used in the actual experiment and feedback on the accuracy of the participant's response was provided by Superlab 4.0. Participants were instructed to respond as quickly and as accurately as possible for all items. After the training session was completed, the experimental task was begun. To avoid effects of fatigue, during the experiment, participants were given an opportunity for two breaks, the first when a third of the items were completed and the second when two-thirds of the items were completed.

## Data analysis

Accuracy and response times for each participant were recorded by Superlab 4.0. For each participant and participant group the mean and median proportions of accurate responses and response times were calculated for each independent variable. Only the response times of correct responses were included in the final statistical analysis. Due to the small number of participants in each group as well as the uneven number of participants representing each group, nonparametric statistics were used to analyse the data. For between-participants comparisons of group accuracy, Kruskal-Wallis tests were performed. For within-participants comparisons of reaction time across typicality, Friedman tests were performed to assess overall differences within participant groups and Wilcoxon Signed Rank tests were performed for pairwise comparisons of typical and atypical RTs within each participant group. To reduce the possibility of Type I statistical error, only comparisons critical to answering the research questions were conducted, resulting in a single pairwise typicality comparison (typical versus atypical) within each participant group.

## RESULTS

### Accuracy

Analysis of the response accuracy data showed that, in the visual task, no significant differences were found for any level of typicality—$H(2) = 0.40$, *ns*, typical; $H(2) = 1.24$, *ns*, atypical; $H(2) = 4.15$, *ns*, non-member. In the auditory task no significant differences were found for any level of typicality—$H(2) = 4.08$, *ns*, typical; $H(2) = 2.32$, *ns*, atypical—except for non-member items, $H(2) = 8.90$, $p < .05$. Although a significant difference was found for non-member items in the auditory task, because this was not one of the critical questions of this study no post-hoc tests were conducted for this analysis.

## Reaction time

*Visual condition analysis.* Analysis of the reaction time data resulted in a significant difference between typical and atypical items for the control group, $\chi^2(2) = 8.667$, $p < .05$, and the phonological dyslexic group, $\chi^2(2) = 9.00$, $p < .05$, but not for the deep dyslexic group, $\chi^2(2) = 2.8$, *ns*. To address the research questions and identify the specific level of difference within each group, a single comparison between typical and atypical items was completed. This analysis revealed that, for the control group and phonological dyslexic group, typical responses were significantly faster than atypical responses ($T = 2.00$, $p < .05$, controls; $T = 0.00$, $p < .05$, phonological dyslexic participants). However, for deep dyslexic participants this analysis revealed no significant difference between the two ($T = 3.00$, *ns*) (see Figure 1).

*Auditory condition analysis.* Analysis of the reaction time data resulted in a significant difference between typical and atypical items for the control group, $\chi^2(2) = 16.22$, $p < .05$, phonological dyslexic group, $\chi^2(2) = 5.33$, $p < .05$, and deep dyslexic group, $\chi^2(2) = 7.6$, $p < .05$. To address the research questions and identify the specific level of difference within each group, a single comparison between typical and atypical items was completed. This analysis revealed that, for the control group and phonological dyslexic group, typical responses were significantly faster than atypical responses ($T = 0.00$, $p < .05$, controls; $T = 0.00$, $p < .05$, phonological dyslexic participants). However, for deep dyslexic participants this analysis revealed no significant difference between the two ($T = 0.00$, *ns*) (see Figure 1).

## DISCUSSION

The purpose of the current study was to identify and locate the potential semantic impairment in deep dyslexia using a task that would specifically require explicit semantic access from both visual and auditory input without requiring an oral response, thus avoiding a confound of speech production. Results indicated that healthy control and phonological dyslexic participant groups demonstrated a typicality effect in both visual and auditory modalities, but deep dyslexic participants did not demonstrate this effect in either modality. These results will be discussed in relation to each of the two research questions posed in the current study. Taking this new evidence into account, a modified theory of deep dyslexia is proposed.

The first question concerned whether or not a semantic impairment exists in deep dyslexia. The failure of inhibition theory (FIT) suggests that semantic reading errors result from failure to inhibit incorrect responses at the level of the phonological output lexicon, with all prior levels of processing intact (Buchanan et al., 2003). The evidence used to support this theory was that performance accuracy levels similar to normal controls were found for their patient, for a task requiring implicit access to semantics and a task requiring explicit access to semantics without oral production.

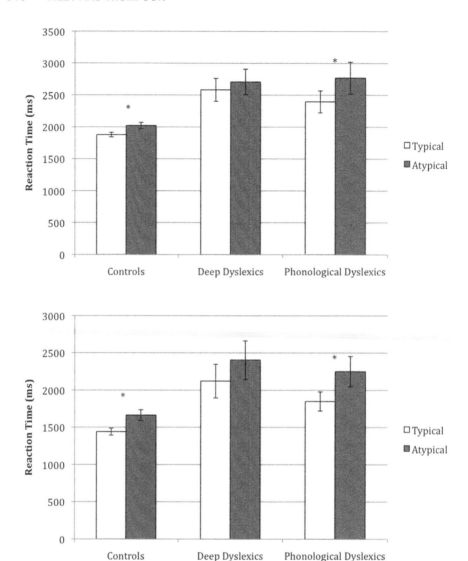

**Figure 1.** Mean response times for correct responses to typical and atypical in the visual task (top) and auditory task (bottom).

Although accuracy measures for this single case study did not differ from control participants, no other more sensitive measures were collected to explore the possibility of semantic processing differences. The current study examined explicit access to semantics without requiring oral production by testing a well-documented lexical-semantic processing effect (semantic typicality) using reaction time as a primary dependent measure.

It was predicted that in the visual task, if deep dyslexic participants showed a typicality effect similar to control participants, then this would suggest intact semantic processing. Conversely, differing typicality effects between the two groups would suggest impaired semantic processing. Results showed that whereas control participants demonstrated a typicality effect, deep dyslexic participants did not. These findings suggest that in a task requiring semantic processing of written lexical items, deep dyslexic participants process semantic information differently from control participants, thus indicating a semantic impairment.

While the evidence presented here supports a semantic impairment in deep dyslexia, it does not directly test the presence or absence of a deficit at the level of the phonological output lexicon or the claim that semantic errors result from failure of inhibition. It is entirely possible, even likely, that the mechanism for semantic errors is an inability to inhibit incorrect responses. However, the current study now calls into question the level of processing at which this inhibition mechanism fails. Perhaps it is a failure to inhibit at both the semantic and phonological output lexicon levels, which is subtle at the level of semantics and only obviously detectable at the level of production.

The second question addressed the locus of the semantic impairment along the lexical-semantic reading route. Most models of lexical processing represent the semantic system as a single processing system accessed by all modalities. In order to test whether or not the semantic processing impairment in deep dyslexia affects general semantic processing or semantic access from written input, the current study examined category verification in both the visual and auditory modalities. Whereas control participants (and phonological dyslexic participants) demonstrated a typicality effect in both the visual and auditory modalities, deep dyslexic participants did not demonstrate a typicality effect in either modality. This pattern suggests that deep dyslexic participants demonstrate impairment in semantic processing. The multiple-deficit hypothesis (Morton & Patterson, 1980) conceptualises deep dyslexia as a disorder involving two separate impairments: a lexical-semantic impairment and grapheme-phoneme conversion impairment. Whereas the current study did not address grapheme-phoneme conversion, it directly addressed the locus of impairment along the lexical-semantic reading route, with the results supporting the existence of a semantic impairment in deep dyslexia. The design of the experimental task allowed a direct comparison of semantic system processing and access, with deep dyslexic participants showing impairment in semantic processing.

## Toward a modified theory of deep dyslexia

Although the current study has provided additional evidence supporting and opposing various parts of the previously discussed theories, it appears that neither of these theories accounts for all the evidence. Therefore we propose a modified version of FIT. In deep dyslexia, as FIT proposes, selection inhibition is impaired. However, the lack of a semantic typicality effect in deep dyslexia may indicate an inability to efficiently select a correct lexical-semantic representation, suggesting that selection inhibition becomes impaired beginning at the level of semantics.

## Summary

FIT provides a comprehensive view of deep dyslexia that compliments other theories by proposing a mechanism for semantic error production. Proponents of FIT suggest that semantic processing is intact in deep dyslexia; however, the current study suggests that deep dyslexics demonstrate semantic processing impairments. These data suggest a modification to the FIT model, conceptualising failure of inhibition beginning at the level of semantic processing.

Manuscript received 23 July 2009
Manuscript accepted 19 October 2009
First published online 3 February 2010

## REFERENCES

Beauvois, M. F., & Dérouesné, J. (1979). Phonological alexia: Three dissociations. *Journal of Neurology Neurosurgery Psychiatry, 42*(12), 1115–1124.

Buchanan, L., McEwen, S., Westbury, C., & Libben, G. (2003). Semantics and semantic errors: Implicit access to semantic information from words and nonwords in deep dyslexia. *Brain and Language, 84*, 65–83.

Casey, P. J. (1992). A re-examination of the roles of typicality and category dominance in verifying category membership. *Journal of Experimental Psychology: Learning, Memory and Cognition, 12*(2), 237–267.

Colangelo, A., & Buchanan, L. (2005). Semantic ambiguity and the failure of inhibition hypothesis as an explanation for reading errors in deep dyslexia. *Brain and Cognition, 57*(1), 39–42.

Colangelo, A., & Buchanan, L. (2007). Localizing damage in the functional architecture: The distinction between implicit and explicit processing in deep dyslexia. *Journal of Neurolinguistics, 20*(2), 111–144.

Coltheart, M. (1980). Deep dyslexia: A review of the syndrome. In M. Coltheart, K. Patterson, & J. Marshall (Eds.), *Deep dyslexia*. London: Routledge & Kegan Paul.

Dérouesné, J., & Beauvois, M. F. (1979). Phonological processing in reading: Data from alexia. *Journal of Neurology, Neurosurgery, and Psychiatry, 42*(12), 1125–1132.

Ellis, A. W., & Young, A. W. (1988). *Human cognitive neuropsychology*. Hove, UK: Lawrence Erlbaum Associates Ltd.

Friedman, R. B. (1996). Recovery from deep alexia to phonological alexia: Points on a continuum. *Brain and Language, 52*, 114–128.

Glosser, G., & Friedman, R. B. (1990). The continuum of deep/phonological alexia. *Cortex, 26*(3), 343–359.

Hampton, J. A. (1995). Testing the prototype theory of concepts. *Journal of Memory and Language, 34*, 686–708.

Kay, J., Lesser, R., & Coltheart, M. (1992). *The Psycholinguistic Assessment of Language Processing in Aphasia (PALPA)*. Hove, UK: Lawrence Erlbaum Associates Ltd.

Kertesz, A. (2007). *Western Aphasia Battery-Revised*. San Antonio, TX: PsychCorp.

Kiran, S. (2001). *Effects of exemplar typicality on naming deficits in fluent aphasia*. Dissertation, Northwestern University, Evanston, IL.

Kiran, S., & Thompson, C. K. (2003). Effect of typicality on online category verification of animate category exemplars in aphasia. *Brain & Language, 85*(3), 441–450.

Marshall, J. C., & Newcombe, F. (1966). Syntactic and semantic errors in paralexia. *Neuropsychologia, 4*, 169–176.

Morton, J., & Patterson, K. (1980). A new attempt at an interpretation, or, an attempt at a new interpretation. In M. Coltheart, K. Patterson, & J. Marshall (Eds.), *Deep dyslexia*. London: Routledge & Kegan Paul.

Newcombe, F., & Marshall, J. (1980). Response monitoring and response blocking in deep dyslexia. In M. Coltheart, K. Patterson, & J. Marshall (Eds.), *Deep dyslexia*. London: Routledge & Kegan Paul.

Patterson, K. (1978). Phonemic dyslexia: Errors of meaning and the meaning of errors. *The Quarterly Journal of Experimental Psychology, 30*, 587–601.

Rosch, E. (1973). On the internal structure of perceptual and semantic categories. In T. E. Moore (Ed.), *Cognitive development and the acquisition of language*. New York: Academic Press.

Rosch, E. (1975). Cognitive representations of semantic categories. *Journal of Experimental Psychology: General, 104*(3), 192–233.

Saffran, E., & Marin, O. (1977). Reading without phonology: Evidence from aphasia. *The Quarterly Journal of Experimental Psychology, 29*(3), 515–525.

Shallice, T., & Coughlan, A. K. (1980). Modality specific word comprehension deficits in deep dyslexia. *British Medical Journal, 43*(10), 866.

Shallice, T., & Warrington, E. (1975). Word recognition in a phonemic dyslexic patient. *Quarterly Journal of Experimental Psychology*, *27*, 187–199.

Shallice, T., & Warrington, E. (1980). Single and multiple component central dyslexic syndromes. In M. Coltheart, K. Patterson, & J. Marshall (Eds.), *Deep dyslexia*. London: Routledge & Kegan Paul.

Woodcock, R. W., Mather, N., & Schrank, F. A. (2004). *The Woodcock-Johnson III Diagnostic Reading Battery*. Rolling Meadows, IL: Riverside Publishing.

APHASIOLOGY, 2010, 24 (6–8), 814–825

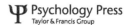

# Sound Production Treatment:
# Application with severe apraxia of speech

Julie L. Wambaugh

*VA Salt Lake City Healthcare System and University of Utah, Salt Lake City,
UT, USA*

Shannon C. Mauszycki

*VA Salt Lake City Healthcare System, Salt Lake City, UT, USA*

*Background*: Acquired apraxia of speech (AOS) has been shown to be responsive to behavioural intervention. Although numerous treatments for AOS have been developed, most have received limited study. Specifically, the AOS treatment evidence base is compromised by a lack of replication of treatment effects. Sound Production Treatment (SPT; Wambaugh, Kalinyak-Fliszar, West, & Doyle, 1998) has undergone more systematic examination than other AOS treatments and has been documented to result in predictable improvements in consonant production. However, SPT has not been studied with persons with severe AOS and perseverative speech behaviours.
*Aims*: The purpose of this investigation was to examine the acquisition, response generalisation, and maintenance effects of SPT with a speaker with severe AOS, significant nonfluent aphasia, and verbal perseverations.
*Methods & Procedures*: A single-participant, multiple baseline design across behaviours was employed to examine the effects of treatment on production of six consonants in monosyllabic words. Treatment was applied sequentially to two sets of items, with three consonants targeted in each set. A third phase of treatment entailed training of all target sounds. Follow-up probing was conducted at 10 and 15 weeks post-treatment.
*Outcomes & Results*: Improved productions were observed for all trained items and response generalisation to untrained exemplars of trained items was positive. Across-sound generalisation was not evident. Maintenance effects were strong at 10 weeks post-treatment, but diminished considerably for most of the sounds by 15 weeks.
*Conclusions*: Results for this speaker with severe AOS and verbal perseverations were similar to those previously reported for SPT. The decrease in performance from 10 weeks to 15 weeks indicated that changes in behaviour had not been sufficiently instantiated. Furthermore, these findings suggested that maintenance probing may need to be conducted over a considerably longer period of time than has previously been reported in the literature.

*Keywords:* Apraxia of speech; Aphasia; Treatment.

Address correspondence to: Julie L. Wambaugh, 151A, 500 Foothill Blvd., Salt Lake City, UT, USA 84148. E-mail: julie.wambaugh@health.utah.edu

This research was supported by the Department of Veterans Affairs, Rehabilitation Research and Development.

http://www.psypress.com/aphasiology          DOI: 10.1080/02687030903422494

Acquired apraxia of speech (AOS) is a neurologic speech disorder that is characterised by slowed rate of speech, difficulties in sound production, and disrupted prosody (McNeil, Robin, & Schmidt, 2009). A critical review of the AOS treatment literature by the Academy of Neurologic Communication Disorders and Sciences (ANCDS) AOS guidelines committee indicated that although the evidence base for AOS treatment was relatively sparse and lacking in many respects, there was sufficient support for the statement that "individuals with AOS can be expected to make improvements in speech production as a result of treatment, even when AOS is chronic" (Wambaugh, Duffy, McNeil, Robin, & Rogers, 2006, p. lxiii).

Various treatments for AOS may result in improved speech production, but there is a limited understanding of the effects of specific techniques or treatment factors that contribute to positive changes (Wambaugh et al., 2006). In fact, in order to provide qualitative ratings of the AOS treatment evidence, the ANCDS AOS guidelines committee grouped treatment investigations by "general approach" because there was insufficient evidence for any one treatment/technique (Wambaugh et al., 2006).

Of the general approaches to AOS treatment, articulatory-kinematic approaches have received the most study (Wambaugh et al., 2006). Such approaches are designed to increase the accuracy of the speaker's production of sounds through improvements in the movement and/or positioning of the articulators. Techniques that are considered to be articulatory-kinematic in nature include integral stimulation (i.e., "watch me, listen to me, say it with me"), modelling-repetition, articulatory placement instructions, repeated practice, feedback concerning articulation (e.g., verbal feedback, biofeedback), contrastive practice, shaping, and tactile-kinaesthetic cueing.

Sound Production Treatment (SPT) is an articulatory-kinematic treatment for AOS that combines modelling-repetition, minimal contrast practice, integral stimulation, articulatory placement cueing, repeated practice, and verbal feedback (Wambaugh et al., 1998). Additionally, it incorporates aspects of principles of motor learning (Maas et al., 2008) such as blocked and random practice and a reduced feedback schedule. SPT has received more extensive and systematic study than any other specific treatment for AOS (Duffy, 2005; Wambaugh, 2002). Although much remains to be specified concerning SPT and its application, its acquisition, response generalisation, and maintenance effects have been demonstrated to be robust and relatively predictable. SPT has been shown to improve articulatory accuracy of consonant production in words, phrases, and sentences for trained and untrained items (Wambaugh, 2004; Wambaugh & Nessler, 2004). To date, the effects of SPT have not been studied with persons with severe AOS who have extremely limited sound repertoires. Furthermore, it has not been studied in speakers with significant verbal motor perseveration.

It was considered that aspects of SPT such as integral stimulation and articulatory placement cueing should promote differentiated consonant production with AOS speakers with limited sound production capabilities. Given that perseveration may result from reduced speech/language processing efficiency (Moses, Nickels, & Sheard, 2007), it was further speculated that treatment focused on facilitating speech production would be appropriate even in the presence of significant perseveration. Furthermore, aspects of the treatment such as minimal contrast practice and random practice of multiple sounds was thought to have potential benefit if competing activation was a source of perseverative behaviour.

As indicated in the ANCDS AOS guidelines report, one of the biggest liabilities of the AOS treatment evidence base is a lack of replications of treatment effects (Wambaugh et al., 2006). The purpose of this investigation was to conduct a systematic replication of the effects of SPT with a speaker with more severe deficits than previously studied participants. Specifically, the investigation was designed to examine the acquisition, response generalisation, and maintenance effects of SPT in an individual with severe AOS, verbal motor perseverations, and stereotypic productions.

# METHOD

## Participant

The participant was a 55-year-old Caucasian male who was 2 years post-onset of a left CVA. Radiological reports indicated a large cortical lesion involving the entire distribution of the middle cerebral artery. The participant was a native-English speaker, passed a pure-tone hearing screening at 40dB for each ear, and had hemiparesis of the right leg and arm. He was a retired wood-worker with 14 years of formal education. Additional demographic data are shown in Table 1.

Pre-treatment assessment findings are presented in Table 2. The participant attained a *Porch Index of Communicative Abilities* (PICA; Porch, 2001) overall percentile score of 19 and a *Western Aphasia Battery* aphasia quotient (WAB AQ; Kertesz, 1982) of 14.8 Performance on the WAB was consistent with a classification of Broca's aphasia.

The participant presented with severe AOS, with speech behaviours that were consistent with diagnostic criteria described by McNeil et al. (2009): (1) sound errors that were predominantly distortions, (2) errors that were consistent in terms of location and type, (3) slow rate of speech production, and (4) disrupted prosody. His spontaneous, verbal productions were extremely limited and reflected a very restricted sound repertoire, consisting primarily of /w, h, d, ʌ, aɪ, ɝ n, h, o, j, ɪ/. He combined these sounds in various ways with some combinations being stereotypic in nature (e.g., /wʌhaɪə/). He often perseverated on these stereotypic productions.

An evaluation of the participant's consonant production in monosyllabic words (five exemplars of all English consonants in word-initial and word-final positions) revealed that only word-initial /w/ and /n/ were produced accurately on a consistent basis (i.e., >50% accuracy). Examples of the participant's errors in response to the monosyllabic word repetition task are provided in Appendix A.

TABLE 1
Participant demographic information

| Characteristic | Participant |
|---|---|
| Gender | Male |
| Age | 55 |
| Months post-onset CVA | 24 |
| Area of infarct | Left cortex – entire middle cerebral artery distribution |
| Years of education | 14 |
| Premorbid handedness | Right |
| Marital status | Married |
| Residence | Own home |
| Former profession | Wood-worker |

TABLE 2
Assessment results

| Measure | Performance |
| --- | --- |
| Porch Index of Communicative Ability (Porch, 2001) | |
|     Overall Percentile | 19th |
|     Verbal Percentile | 11th |
|     Auditory Percentile | 21st |
| Western Aphasia Battery (Kertesz, 1982) | |
|     Aphasia Quotient | 14.8 |
|     Aphasia Classification | Broca's Aphasia |
| Raven's Coloured Progressive Matrices (Raven, Raven, & Court, 2003) | 26/36 |
| Assessment of Intelligibility of Dysarthric Speech (Yorkston & Beukelman, 1981) | |
|     Word Intelligibility (multiple choice) | 0% |
| AOS Behaviours | |
|     Sound errors | Predominately distortions |
|     Consistent location and type of errors | Yes |
|     Slow rate of production | Yes |
|     Disrupted prosody | Yes |

The participant was originally recruited to participate in a rate control treatment study, but was unable to demonstrate the minimal repetition skills necessary for inclusion in that investigation. He did not participate in any other speech/language therapy at the time of the investigation. According to his family, one of his early speech/language experiences involved working exclusively on the phrase, "I want water." His errors and stereotypic productions appeared to be closely related to this phrase (see Appendix A).

## Experimental stimuli

Six sounds were selected for treatment and were grouped into two sets of three sounds each: Set 1 = /b, s, l/, and Set 2 = / m, d, f/. Manner and place of production were considered in the selection and grouping of experimental sounds. The targeted sounds were elicited in the context of monosyllabic, real words with either CV or CVC shapes. A total of 13 words were selected for each sound; 8 words were used for treatment and 5 words were untreated in order to assess response generalisation (see Appendix B).

The experimental words were also selected so that minimal pair items could be devised to be used during treatment. Because the participant most often produced a variant of "water" for all items, the minimal pair items were all word-initial /w/ words (e.g., target item = buy, minimal pair item = why; target item = say, minimal pair item = way).

## Experimental design

A multiple baseline design across behaviours was used to examine the acquisition and response generalisation effects of treatment. Production of the six consonants in the context of monosyllabic words was measured repeatedly in baseline probes.

Treatment was then applied to three of the six sounds, while the other three sounds remained untreated. Following 25 treatment sessions, treatment was withdrawn from the first three sounds and extended to the remaining three sounds. After the second phase of treatment, treatment was applied to all six sounds simultaneously.

*Baseline phase.* Five probes were conducted during the initial baseline phase for all six sounds of interest. A minimum of five probes was selected a priori to allow adequate evaluation of variability. An additional criterion of non-rising trends for all groups of sounds (trained and generalisation items) was employed to determine baseline length.

Each set of items representing three target sounds was presented as a group. The 39 items (8 treatment and 5 generalisation items for each of the 3 sounds) were randomised and presented verbally, one at a time. The investigator instructed the participant to produce each word as well as he could A single repetition of the item by the examiner was provided upon request of the participant. The order of presentation of the two sets of items was randomised for each probe session.

*Treatment phase.* During the first two treatment phases, the set of items receiving treatment was probed every session, while the set not receiving treatment was probed after every five treatment sessions. During the final treatment phase, probes were conducted after every two treatment sessions for all sounds. This change in probing schedule was due to the treatment time (per session) being slightly extended because all six sounds were receiving treatment. Probes were always conducted prior to treatment. During probes (baseline and treatment phases), no feedback regarding accuracy of articulation was provided. General encouragers (e.g., "you're trying hard") were given.

*Follow-up phase.* Follow-up probes were conducted at 10 and 15 weeks after the cessation of all treatment. Probes had originally been planned for 2 and 6 weeks post-treatment, but health issues prohibited this (described further in Discussion).

## Dependent variable

Accuracy of articulation of the target sounds produced in the experimental words during probes served as the dependent variable. In cases where the participant self-corrected, the self-correction was scored. The participant's productions were scored for accuracy of consonant production using binary (+/–) scoring. That is, only the target consonant was required to be produced accurately to receive a score of "correct". Productions were scored online, with audio recordings used to verify scoring. Percentage of correct productions was calculated for each of the sounds, with separate percentages calculated for treatment and for generalisation items.

## Reliability

A total of 10% of all probes were rescored by the investigator who did not conduct and perform the original scoring of the probe. Point-to-point agreement for scoring of each item was calculated and ranged from 92% to 100%, with an average of 96%.

## Treatment

Treatment was applied in the form of a response contingent hierarchy. Specifically, the steps of the hierarchy were applied only as needed (i.e., in the event of a preceding incorrect response). The treatment hierarchy is shown in Appendix C and includes the following techniques: modelling-repetition, minimal contrast practice, graphemic cueing, integral stimulation, articulatory placement cueing, repeated practice, and verbal feedback. In the first two treatment phases (treatment of Sets 1 and 2 separately), application of the treatment hierarchy to each of the 24 treatment words constituted one treatment trial. Three to four treatment trials were completed in each treatment session when three sounds were under treatment. In the final phase of treatment, when all six sounds received treatment, a trial consisted of application of treatment to each of the 48 treatment words and two trials were completed each session.

Treatment was administered by an ASHA certified speech/language pathologist (i.e., the authors) three times per week. Sessions were approximately 45 to 60 minutes in length, including the probe, during the first two treatment phases. Sessions were approximately 60 minutes in length during the third treatment phase. Therapy was conducted in the research lab or the participant's home, at the preference of the participant and his family.

## RESULTS

Probe data, reflecting acquisition and generalisation effects of treatment, are shown in Figure 1. Across the five baseline probes, accuracy of production ranged from 0% to 25% correct with *average* percentages of accuracy as follows: /b/ 3%, /s/ 0%, /l/ 5%, /m/ 10%, /d/ 0%, /f/ 0%.

Following application of treatment to the first group of sounds (/b, s, l/), increases in accuracy of production of /b/ and /l/ were observed. These increases were seen for both trained and untrained items. Changes in accuracy of /s/ production were not observed until the last two probe sessions. During training of the first group of sounds, no changes were observed for the untrained sounds /d/ and /f/. Slight but unstable increases were seen for untrained /m/ during this period.

As seen in Figure 1, when treatment was applied to the second group of sounds (/m, d, f/), increases in accuracy of production were seen for all three sounds for trained and untrained items. Maintenance of the previously trained set of sounds was measured after every fifth treatment session during training of the second set. Production of trained and untrained /b/ remained at high levels as did production of /l/ for most of the second treatment phase. However, accuracy levels of /l/ appeared to be declining by the end of the phase. Productions of /s/ remained at low accuracy levels during training of the second set of sounds.

When treatment was applied to all six sounds simultaneously, high levels of accuracy were achieved for /b/, /s/, /d/, and /f/. Some decreases in correct productions were observed for /m/ and /l/ during this training period.

Follow-up probes conducted at 10 weeks post-treatment revealed the following levels of accuracy: /b/ 100%, /s/ 75%, /l/ 100%, /m/ 50%, /d/ 38%, and /f/ 88% Probes at 15 weeks post-treatment revealed the following accuracy levels: /b/ 37%, /s/ 13%, /l/ 75%, /m/ 0%, /d/ 25%, and /f/ 88%.

Effect sizes were calculated for all sounds; baseline performance was compared to performance during the last phase of treatment.The *d* Index statistics (Bloom,

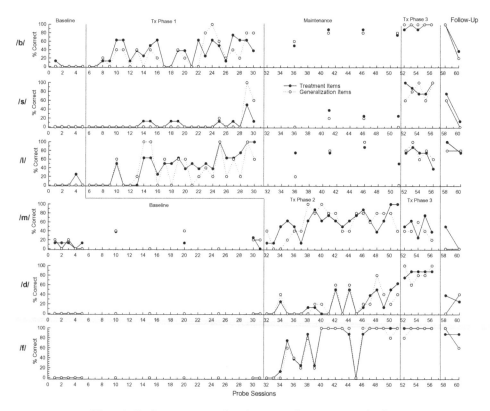

**Figure 1.** Performance on probes: Accuracy of consonant production.

Fischer, & Orme, 2003) were as follows: b = 14.1; s = 9.89; l = 4.1; m = 2.7; d = 22.29; f >30.9. Additionally, the conservative dual-criteria (CDC; Fisher, Kelley, & Lomas, 2003) method was used as an aid to visual inspection to make a determination of treatment effects. The CDC method has been found to optimally control Type 1 error rates even in the presence of high degrees of autocorrelation (Fisher et al.) The CDC procedure entailed creating two criterion lines using the baseline data: a trend line based on the binomial test and a mean line. These criterion lines were both raised by .25 standard deviations and were superimposed on the treatment phases. Interpretation of reliable treatment effects using the CDC method is dependent on a pre-specified number of data points falling above both lines (i.e., 15 of 25 data points, Phase 1; 14 of 20 data points, Phase 2). According to the CDC method, a reliable treatment effect was found for /b/, /l/, /m/, and /f/ during the first application of treatment (Phase 3 was not analysed due to an insufficient number of data points).

## DISCUSSION

Findings were consistent with previous investigations of SPT that involved speakers with less severe AOS and minimal verbal motor perseveration. That is, treatment resulted in improved production of trained sounds in treated words with similar improvements seen for sound production in untreated words. Generalisation to untrained sounds was limited, which is also consistent with previous findings. Probable interference of training sounds with similar place of production was observed during the last phase of training. Specifically, decreasing accuracy of production of /m/ and /l/ were due largely to overgeneralisation of /b/ and /d/, respectively. Similar overgeneralisation has been reported previously with SPT (Wambaugh, Martinez, McNeil, & Rogers, 1999).

It was somewhat surprising to observe overgeneralisation in the third phase of training when all six sounds were being trained and practised in a random presentation context. Furthermore, all target sounds were practised in varied phonetic contexts. As discussed by Maas et al. (2008), both variable motoric practice and random practice are likely to result in generalisation and maintenance of learned behaviours. Furthermore, contrastive practice is consistent with models of speech production/learning that stress the importance of refining target regions through contrastive somatosensory feedback (Guenther, 2006). Currently there are no data concerning the relative merits of variable versus constant practice in the treatment of AOS and limited (albeit promising) data suggesting that random practice is superior to blocked practice (Knock, Ballard, Robin, & Schmidt, 2000).

In a previous investigation of SPT involving overgeneralisation, "booster treatment" involving training of all sounds simultaneously (as in this investigation) resulted in differentiated sound production that was maintained (Wambaugh et al., 1999). Perhaps the participant in the current investigation was unable to fully utilise somatosensory and auditory feedback from contrastive and random practice to develop clearly differentiated speech sound target regions. Feedback from the clinician focused on differentiating sounds with similar place of production might have been beneficial.

Guenther and colleagues' neural model of speech production, "directions into velocities of articulators" (DIVA; Guenther, 2006), indicates that the feedforward commands for speech sounds become tuned by the feedback subsystem in repeated production attempts. Early in the learning process, production relies heavily on the feedback system, but "eventually the feedforward command by itself is sufficient to produce the sound in normal circumstances" (p. 353). The decrease in sound production accuracy observed at 15 weeks post-treatment indicates that the participant's feedforward commands were insufficiently tuned or instantiated. It is likely that the improved accuracy observed in earlier phases of the study reflected improvements in the feedback control subsystem and that the lengthy period without treatment resulted in a deterioration in that subsystem. Given the presence of overgeneralisation in the last phase of treatment, it may be the case that the somatosensory and/or auditory target regions were not adequately tuned, which theoretically should result in inadequate tuning of the feedforward commands.

Perhaps treatment should have included specific training to recognise and self-monitor various somatosensory and auditory cues. That is, although feedback was provided concerning accuracy of production and instructions for improving production, this information was completely clinician generated. After the final follow-up probe, informal probes were conducted to assess the participant's skill in judging accuracy of production. The participant was very accurate in judging correct and incorrect productions made by the therapist, but demonstrated that he had great difficulty in determining if his own productions were accurate or inaccurate. It may be prudent to assess such skills prior to developing a therapy programme. In the case of very poor self-monitoring skills, therapy may need to be modified to include training and application of self-monitoring of auditory and somatosensory feedback.

As the data clearly show, the participant was able to utilise feedback to modify his productions, but increasing focus or conscious awareness of critical auditory and somatosensory features may have assisted in solidifying feedforward commands for speech sound production. It is possible that additional practice with the same treatment may have been sufficient to promote lasting maintenance of gains. As noted by Ludlow and colleagues (2008, p. S243) in discussing principles of experience-dependent neural plasticity (Kleim & Jones, 2008), "changes in neural substrates will occur only as a result of extensive and prolonged practice and that neural changes may not become consolidated until later in the training process".

Maintenance of AOS treatment gains has typically not been measured for periods as extended as in the current investigation. Follow-up probes were originally scheduled for 2 and 6 weeks post-treatment. Unfortunately, the participant was hospitalised prior to the first scheduled probe and underwent surgery (not neurological in nature) several weeks later. Although the participant had been provided with "homework" and a practice log, he did not complete any practice during the period from the last treatment session to the 15-week probe. Given the lack of practice and the medical issues, his excellent performance at 10 weeks post-treatment was unexpected. Weather prohibited scheduling another probe for more than a month, which resulted in the 15-week probe. Had these complications not arisen, the decrease in performance at 15 weeks would likely not have been detected. It is suggested that future AOS treatment studies include extended follow-up probes when possible.

Another health issue was present during the second phase of treatment. The participant developed mononucleosis, which persisted throughout the second phase of treatment. This did not appear to have an impact on his performance in comparison to the first treatment phase. Despite health issues and the presence of severe AOS, severe aphasia, and verbal perseveration, this participant made impressive gains in consonant production. Unfortunately, verbal motor perseverations and stereotypic productions were not tracked quantitatively. Anecdotally, such behaviours appeared to decrease across the course of treatment. Following completion of this investigation, booster treatment and "homework" have resulted in regaining accuracy levels of production of all sounds and the participant is currently practising production in the context of sentence completion.

Maintenance effects of SPT and other AOS treatments may not be as stable as previously assumed. Modifications to the SPT protocol may be needed to solidify treatment gains. In particular, testing of self-monitoring or and/or awareness of errors and subsequent modifications in SPT may be warranted in future investigations of this treatment. However, the severe nature of this participant's speech and language deficits may have been the primary factor contributing to less than optimal maintenance. Further replications are obviously warranted.

Manuscript received 24 July 2009
Manuscript accepted 19 October 2009
First published online 23 March 2010

## REFERENCES

Bloom, M., Fischer, J., & Orme, J. G. (2003). *Evaluating practice – Guidelines for the accountable professional* (4th ed.). Boston: Allyn & Bacon, Pearson Education, Inc.

Duffy, J. R. (2005). *Motor speech disorders. Substrates, differential diagnosis, and management* (2nd ed.). St. Louis, MO: Elsevier Mosby.

Fisher, W. W., Kelley, M. E., & Lomas, J. E. (2003). Visual aids and structured criteria for improving visual inspection and interpretation of single-case designs. *Journal of Applied Behaviour Analysis, 36*, 387–406.

Guenther, F. H. (2006). Cortical interactions underlying the production of speech sounds. *Journal of Communication Disorders, 39*, 350–365.

Kertesz, A. (1982). *The Western Aphasia Battery*. New York: Grune & Stratton.

Kleim, J., & Jones, T. (2008) Principles of experience-dependent neural plasticity: Implications for rehabilitation after brain-injury. *Journal of Speech and Hearing Research, 51*, S225–S239.

Knock, T., Ballard, K. J., Robin, D. A., & Schmidt, R. A. (2000). Influence of order of stimulus presentation on speech motor learning: A principled approach to treatment for apraxia of speech. *Aphasiology, 14*, 653–668.

Ludlow, C. L., Hoit, J., Kent, R., Ramig, L., Shrivastav, R., Smith, A., et al. (2008). Translating principles of neural plasticity into research on speech motor control recovery and rehabilitation. *Journal of Speech, Language and Hearing Research, 51*, S240–S258.

Maas, E., Robin, D. A., Austermann Hula, S. N., Wulf, G., Ballard, K. J., & Schmidt, R. A. (2008). Principles of motor learning in treatment of motor speech disorders. *American Journal of Speech Language Pathology, 17*, 277–298.

McNeil, M. R., Robin, D. A., & Schmidt, R. A. (2009). Apraxia of speech: Definition, differentiation, and treatment. In M. R. McNeil (Ed.), *Clinical management of sensorimotor speech disorders* (2nd ed., pp. 249–268). New York: Thieme.

Moses, M. S., Nickels, L. A., & Sheard, C. (2007). Chips, cheeks and carols: A review of recurrent perseveration in speech production. *Aphasiology, 21*(10/11), 960–974.

Porch, B. (2001). *Porch Index of Communicative Ability: Vol. 2. Administration, scoring and interpretation* (4th ed.). Albuquerque, NM: PICA Programs

Raven, J., Raven, J. C., & Court, J. H. (2003). *Manual for Raven's Progressive Matrices and Vocabulary Scales. Section 1: General Overview*. San Antonio, TX: Harcourt Assessment.

Wambaugh, J. L. (2002). A summary of treatments for apraxia of speech and review of replicated approaches. *Seminars in Speech and Language, 23*(4), 293–308.

Wambaugh, J. L. (2004). Stimulus generalisation effects of sound production treatment for apraxia of speech. *Journal of Medical Speech Language Pathology, 12*(2), 77–97.

Wambaugh, J. L., Duffy, J. R., McNeil, M. R., Robin, D. A., & Rogers, M. (2006). Treatment guidelines for acquired apraxia of speech: Treatment descriptions and recommendations. *Journal of Medical Speech Language Pathology, 14*(2), xxxv–ixvii.

Wambaugh, J. L., Kalinyak-Fliszar, M. M., West, J. E., & Doyle, P. J. (1998). Effects of treatment for sound errors in apraxia of speech. *Journal of Speech, Language, and Hearing Research, 41*, 725–743.

Wambaugh, J. L., Martinez, A. L., McNeil, M. R., & Rogers, M. (1999). Sound production treatment for apraxia of speech: Overgeneralisation and maintenance effects. *Aphasiology, 9–11*, 821–837.

Wambaugh, J. L., & Nessler, C. (2004). Modification of Sound Production Treatment for aphasia: Generalisation effects. *Aphasiology, 18*(5//6/7), 407–427.

Yorkston, K. M., & Beukelman, D. R. (1981). *Assessment of intelligibility of dysarthric speech*. Austin, TX: Pro-Ed.

# APPENDIX A

## Examples of errors on the word repetition task

mom → mɑd
den → waɪdɪlwaɪ
beep → maɪə
my → maɪ
sigh → wɔdɚ
sam → o jɛs
mow → waɪə
bill → bəiɑ
bore → jɛə
four → wɔdɚ

day → wɔdɚ
fur → ohɔɪə
food → wɔdɚ
due → wɔdɚ
fay → aɪə
sue → əheɪə
duck → wɔdɚ
mike → wɔdɚ

# APPENDIX B

## Experimental stimuli

*Set 1 Items*

/b/

Treatment items: buy, bee, bite, bay, bore, beep, ben, bill
Minimal pair items: why, we, white, way, war, weep, when, will
Generalisation items: boo, bar, bib, bait, bean

/s/

Treatment items: say, sill, sit, sue, Sam, seal, sew, see
Minimal pair items: way, will, wit, woo, wham, wheel, whoa, we
Generalisation items: sigh, sail, sip, saw, sat

/l/

Treatment items: lie, low, lit, lee, lay, lick, line, late
Minimal pair items: why, who, wit, we, way, wick, wine, wait
Generalisation items: Lou, law, lane, lead, lip

*Set 2 Items*

/m/

Treatment items: may, mow, me, Mike, mat, mom, mail, men
Minimal pair items: way, whoa, we, wick, what, womb, whale, when
Generalisation items: my, moo, more, main, mill

/d/

Treatment items: day, due, dog, dear, date, dome, den, dye
Minimal pair items: way, woo, wag, we're, wait, womb, when, why
Generalisation items: doll, done, duck, door, dough

/f/

Treatment items: fee, four, fun, foam, fill, fat, food, fay
Minimal pair items: we, war, one, womb, will, what, wood, way
Generalisation items: few, phone, fur, foe, fit

# APPENDIX C

## Sound Production Treatment hierarchy

1. Therapist says word and requests repetition.
   (a) If correct, request additional repetitions (5 times*) and go to next item.
   (b) If incorrect, give feedback and say, "Now let's try a different word" and produce minimal pair word and request a repetition.

- If correct, give feedback and say, "Now let's go back to the other word" and go to #2 with the target word.
- If incorrect, give feedback, attempt with integral stimulation up to 3 times, then go to #2 with the target word.

2. Therapist shows the printed letter of the target sound, says word, and requests repetition.
   (a) If correct, request addition repetitions (5 times) and go to the next item.
   (b) If incorrect, go to #3.

3. Therapist uses integral stimulation: "Watch me, listen to me, say it with me" up to three times.
   (a) If correct, request addition repetitions (5 times) and go to the next item.
   (b) If incorrect, go to #4.

4. Therapist provides verbal articulatory placement cues appropriate to error. Therapist elicits production using integral stimulation.
   (a) If correct, request addition repetitions (5 times) and go to the next item.
   (b) If incorrect, go to next item.

*Provide feedback for accuracy for approximately 3 of the 5 productions

*Note: the hierarchy is response-contingent (subsequent steps are used only upon incorrect production) and does not reverse directions.*

APHASIOLOGY, 2010, 24 (6–8), 826–837

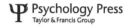

# Treating apraxia of speech (AOS) with EMA-supplied visual augmented feedback

William F. Katz

*The University of Texas at Dallas, Dallas, TX, USA*

Malcolm R. McNeil

*Pittsburgh Veterans Administration Medical Center, PA, USA*

Diane M. Garst

*The University of Texas at Dallas, Dallas, TX, USA*

*Background*: Previous studies have suggested that visual augmented feedback provided by electromagnetic articulography (EMA) helps persons with apraxia of speech (AOS) recover speech motor control following stroke (e.g., Katz et al., 2007). However, the data are few, both in terms of the variety of participants and the speech motor targets investigated.

*Aims*: This study was designed to determine whether EMA supplied feedback improves articulatory accuracy in an adult with acquired AOS. We also examined whether reduced feedback frequency results in (1) decreased performance during acquisition and (2) enhanced maintenance and generalisation of the targeted behaviours.

*Methods & Procedures*: A multiple-baseline across-behaviours design was used to assess the efficacy of this treatment for an individual with AOS. Over a 27-week period, the participant received visual feedback provided by an EMA system for treatment of three groups of speech motor targets (SMTs): /j/, /θ/, and /tʃ/ with various following VCs. The consonant clusters /br/ and /sw/ served as untreated controls. Frequency of feedback scheduling was 100% for /j/ and /tʃ/, and 50% for /θ/.

*Outcomes & Results*: For the first group of SMTs treated, /j/, there was acquisition for 4/5 trained words. These were maintained post-treatment and at the long-term probe. Improved performance and maintenance were also noted for 5/8 untreated stimuli, with maintenance shown for most of these words by 1 month post-treatment. The next treated SMT, /θ/, showed acquisition for all five treated items. Two of these five targets were maintained one month post-treatment. All three untreated /θ/ probes showed generalisation, with two of these showing maintenance post-treatment. The third treated group of SMTs, /tʃ/, showed improved performance for all of the five treated words. However, these gains could only be attributed to /tʃ/ treatment for three of the five words. Two treated items appeared well maintained at 1 month post-treatment. Generalisation and maintenance were also noted for all six untreated /tʃ/ words. However, generalisation from previously

Address correspondence to: William F. Katz PhD, The University of Texas at Dallas, Callier Center for Communication Disorders, 1966 Inwood Rd., Dallas, TX 75235, USA. E-mail: wkatz@utdallas.edu

This research was supported by the Department of Veterans Affairs, Veterans Health Administration, Rehabilitation Research and Development Service (award #B3670R to Malcolm R. McNeil). The authors thank the participant and her family for their help in this study. We also appreciate the assistance of clinicians at the Callier Center for Communication Disorders for help in contacting potential research participants.

http://www.psypress.com/aphasiology                DOI: 10.1080/02687030903518176

treated /j/ and /tʃ/ targets was involved in their improved performance. The untrained (control) word data suggested that the gains noted for treated items did not result from across-the-board improvement or unassisted recovery. There were no consistent differences corresponding with low- versus high-frequency feedback conditions.

*Conclusions*: Augmented kinematic feedback provided by an EMA system improved production for some, but not all, treated targets. Generalisation to untreated probes was also evident. Predictions concerning the effects of feedback frequency on the acquisition, maintenance, and transfer of trained behaviours were not supported.

*Keywords:* Apraxia of speech; Treatment; Electromagnetic articulography; Speech motor control; Feedback.

Apraxia of speech (AOS) is a speech motor deficit thought to involve motor planning (Van der Merwe, 1997) or planning / programming impairments (McNeil, Robin, & Schmidt, 1997). Although AOS has traditionally been considered difficult to treat, the application of motor learning principles to its treatment may provide new optimism for clinicians (see reviews by Ballard, Granier, & Robin, 2000; McNeil, Doyle, & Wambaugh, 2000).

A treatment method currently being explored involves providing augmented feedback of articulatory movements by means of an electromagnetic articulography (EMA) system. EMA is a non-invasive method for tracking speech movement (including the tongue) using low-strength magnetic fields. In this specialised clinical application, EMA is used to show a participant the position of the articulators during intended movements. The aim is to use visual feedback to clarify movement aspects of speech as a restitutive treatment for AOS and related disorders.

Two single-participant studies conducted in our laboratory have suggested that EMA can be used to treat speech motor deficits in individuals with Broca's aphasia and AOS. Katz, Bharadwaj, and Carstens (1999) explored EMA as a means of remediating fricative articulation deficits in the speech of a 63-year-old woman with Broca's aphasia and moderate-to-severe AOS. Over a 1-month period the participant was provided with (1) EMA visual feedback for tongue tip position during fricative production, and (2) foil treatment in which a computer program delivered voicing-contrast stimuli for simple repetition. The results suggested lasting improvement from the visually guided feedback, while the phonetic contrast treated in the foil condition showed only slight improvement, with a return to baseline 10 weeks later.

Katz, Bharadwaj, Gabbert, and Stettler (2002) investigated EMA therapy for a 67-year-old male talker with anomia and mild-to-moderate AOS. A similar experimental design was employed, with two error-prone groups of speech motor targets (SMTs) assigned to EMA treatment (/θ/, /tʃ/) and two assigned to a foil treatment condition. Treatment was provided bi-weekly for a 1-month period. The results of a perceptual assessment indicated that groups of SMTs treated with EMA were notably improved over baseline levels, while the groups of SMTs treated in the foil condition showed no evidence of improvement. The group of /θ/ SMTs was maintained 6 weeks post-training, while the group of /tʃ/ targets declined near baseline levels. Taken together, the data of these two studies suggest superior performance under EMA training for the small sets of SMTs investigated.

The theoretical underpinnings of EMA treatment derive from studies conducted in the framework of *schema theory*, an influential view of motor control and learning (Schmidt, 1975, 1976). Schema theory assumes that when individuals practise a particular class of movements they acquire a set of rules (or schema) that are used to determine the parameter values necessary to produce different versions of the action. Two key concepts in schema theory are *generalised motor programs (GMPs)* and *parameters*. GMPs contain invariant, abstract information about relative timing, structure, and force that allow an individual to produce different versions of a movement. Parameters are the values assigned to the GMP that allow individuals to adjust a movement pattern to meet specific environmental demands.

Schema theory makes an important distinction between the initial acquisition of a skill and its maintenance or transfer. A number of studies (e.g., Shea & Morgan, 1979; Wright, Black, Immink, Brueckner, & Magnuson, 2004; Wulf & Schmidt, 1989) have shown that facilitatory effects noted during treatment sessions are not necessarily predictive of post-treatment retention of skills (i.e., learning). Rather, a number of variables interact to affect motor learning in a complex fashion. These variables include (1) type of feedback, (2) the amount of repetitive practice, (3) the schedule under which the practice trials are performed, and (4) the supporting cognitive mechanisms for learning shown by the participant, including attention, memory, and motivation.

The primary goal of the current study was to determine whether EMA-derived visual feedback improved speech production accuracy in an adult with acquired AOS and concomitant aphasia. It was hypothesised that SMTs treated with EMA would demonstrate robust acquisition, maintenance, and generalisation (i.e., improved performance with untrained items) in comparison with unrelated control SMTs.

A secondary question addressed the schedule under which EMA feedback information was provided. Studies of limb motor movement have suggested that reducing the frequency of feedback presentation (e.g., from 100% to 50%) may decrease the rate of acquisition but enhance retention and generalisation to similar (untreated) behaviours (Bruechert, Lai, & Shea, 2003; Wulf, Schmidt, & Deubel, 1993). Similar patterns have been noted in recent studies of speech production, including articulation (Adams & Page, 2000; Austermann et al., 2008; Clark & Robin, 1998) and voice (Steinhauer & Grayhack, 2000).

Austermann and colleagues (2008) examined frequency feedback effects in the speech treatment of four individuals with AOS. Treatment involved producing nonword syllables or syllable sequences. Transfer was tested to untreated stimuli of similar complexity and to more complex real words related to the treated behaviours. Feedback was given on 60% of productions in the low-frequency feedback condition, and on 100% of the productions in the high-frequency feedback condition. It was found that one participant showed enhanced performance during acquisition under the high-frequency feedback condition and two participants showed enhanced maintenance and transfer during the low-frequency feedback condition. These findings were interpreted as qualified support for reduction of feedback in the structured intervention of AOS.

Feedback frequency research has mostly focused on a type of feedback known as *knowledge of results* (KR), which describes the outcome of a motor act. However, it has generally been assumed that the principles discovered for KR would be applicable when feedback is about movement quality, known as *knowledge of performance* (KP) (Schmidt & Lee, 1999, p. 325; Weeks & Kordus, 1998). In the current research a combined form of KR and KP visual feedback is provided to treat tongue-tip positioning after stroke, with feedback frequency manipulated to investigate this particular prediction of schema theory. We further predict that low-frequency feedback would result in reduced acquisition but enhanced generalisation and maintenance of treated behaviours (in comparison to high-frequency feedback).

# METHOD

## Participant

The participant was a 50-year-old female monolingual speaker of American English who sustained a left-hemisphere middle cerebral artery CVA 9 months before treatment. She is a homemaker with 12 years of education. Prior to enrolling in this study she had received individual and group therapy for approximately 7 months on an outpatient basis. Table 1 shows initial cognitive, linguistic, and speech assessment data. The participant was diagnosed with a moderate Broca's aphasia, based on clinical examination and results of the Short Form Boston Diagnostic Aphasia Exam BDAE-3; (Goodglass, Kaplan, & Barresi, 2001).

An oral mechanism examination revealed no oral apraxia. Participant behaviours were consistent with the unique pattern of speech characteristics of AOS as defined by McNeil et al. (1997), including overall slow rate, extended segment (consonants and vowels) and inter-segmental durations (with occasional schwa insertion), phoneme distortions, and prosodic impairment. For instance, when attempting the word "flashlight" she produced [flæ#tʃəlaɪt].

## Experimental stimuli

Treated SMTs, (/j/, /θ/, and /tʃ/) in varying CVC contexts, and two untreated controls (/br/ and /sw/) were selected based on frequency and consistency of errors produced on a 200-item list of phonetically balanced single words. For the treated SMTs, the majority of errors were incorrect place of articulation. The control SMTs also included some schwa-intrusion errors. Treated groups of SMTs were assigned (in counterbalanced fashion) to frequent and infrequent feedback conditions, with /j/ and /tʃ/ SMTs receiving 100% feedback and /θ/ SMTs receiving 50% feedback. As part of a larger study investigating SMTs in different syllable positions, and based on this participant's unique error pattern, the SMTs containing /j/ and /tʃ/ for this participant were assigned to initial position, and those containing /θ/ were assigned to the medial position.

TABLE 1
Participant speech, language, and cognitive characteristics

| Assessment measure | Score |
| --- | --- |
| Boston Diagnostic Aphasia Exam (BDAE) Articulatory agility (Goodglass et al., 2001) | 3/7 |
| BDAE Phrase length | 4/7 |
| BDAE Grammatical form | 3/7 |
| BDAE Melodic line | 2/7 |
| BDAE Word finding relative to fluency | 5/7 |
| BDAE Auditory comprehension | 30% |
| Story Retell Procedure (SRP)(McNeil et al., 2007) | Mean % IU: 12 * |
| Immediate and Delayed Story Retell Subtests (Arizona Battery for Communication Disorders of Dementia) (Bayles & Tomoeda, 1993) | Ratio: 100 ** |
| Assessment of Intelligibility of Dysarthric Speech (Single Words) (Yorkston & Beukelman, 1984) | Intelligibility: 46% |
| Word intelligibility task(Kent, Weismer, Kent, & Rosenbek, 1989) | Intelligibility: 38% |

*Percentage of available information units produced by the participant.

**Ratio of the delayed retell compared to the initial retell (the delayed recall/immediate recall × 100) on the *Story Retelling Test* of the *Arizona Battery for Communication Disorders of Dementia*.

Five repetitions of a probe list containing five words for each treated SMT group, between three to eight words[1] for the untreated SMTs (to determine response generalisation), and between 17 to 26 control SMTs (assigned by a Latin square method) were audio-recorded at the beginning of each session. To avoid potential confounds of EMA sensor interference, experimental probe items were elicited without EMA sensors. The words in the experimental probe lists contained a variety of vowels and consonants (but were not closely matched on phonetic structure). All treated and untreated stimuli were probed before each treatment session and thus reflect any maintenance of performance accuracy resulting from the previous treatment session(s).

## Experimental design

The design was multiple baseline across behaviours with frequent and infrequent feedback conditions. The participant's baseline performance was measured during the first four sessions. Treatment was then applied sequentially to the five words representing the selected SMT (one SMT at a time) until the average of treated targets for three consecutive probes reached 80% correct or higher, or a total of 20 training sessions had elapsed. Long-term maintenance was determined in two sessions conducted one month post-treatment.

An important difference between the current intervention and more conventional approaches is that it is assumed each target item is potentially a distinct SMT, for which the participant is separately baselined and trained with a unique constellation of visual kinematic feedback patterns. Thus mastery of one /j/-containing word is not automatically assumed to be linked to other phonetic combinations containing /j/. For instance, the visuo-motor feedback patterns for the phonetic combination /jut/ of *Utah* are quite different from those of /jɔɹ/ in *yourself*.

## Treatment sessions and procedure

The participant was instructed that she would receive visual feedback information regarding the position and movement of her tongue during speech, and that she should attempt to "hit the targets" with her tongue during treatment. Aside from a customary 5-minute warm-up period (to allow patients to accommodate to having an EMA sensor in the mouth), no other instructions or practice trials were given. During baseline testing, productions were elicited from a spoken and written stimulus provided by the investigator. Treatment was then applied sequentially to the /j/-containing word targets, followed by the /θ/-containing word targets, then the /tʃ/-containing word targets. During the /j/ sessions, one word was practised until 40 correct responses were elicited, then the next /j/-containing target word was practised, and so on, for a minimum of 200 accurate trials per session (5 targets × 40 responses). After reaching criteria over several sessions, the participant was switched to /θ/-containing words, then /tʃ/-containing words. Thus the words within each session were in blocked order, with order randomised over sessions. Treatment sessions lasted approximately 45 min and were held three times a week. Blocked stimulus presentation was used in

---

[1]A completely balanced design would have included five treated and untreated SMTs. However, it was difficult to obtain sufficient /θ/-containing words that had not already been used in the assessment. To provide a roughly similar number of treated and untreated items, extra SMTs were added to the /j/ and /tʃ/ groups.

each session both for practical reasons (difficulty resetting spatial targets for different groups of SMTs in real time) and to compare results with previous studies that have presented data in blocked fashion (Katz et al., 1999, 2002).

During treatment, EMA feedback was delivered with a Carstens AG100 Articulograph equipped with real-time feedback display software. The participant was seated in a sound-treated room wearing the articulograph helmet with one sensor attached 1 cm posterior to the tongue tip (for the /θ/ and /tʃ/ SMTs), or one attached to the tongue dorsum for the /j/ SMTs. She faced a monitor displaying an image of her current tongue position. Using a mouse drawing tool, investigators designated a "target zone" of fixed dimensions, corresponding to the participant's accurate placement of the tongue tip for the selected SMT. This information was used by the participant to guide her tongue towards the correct place of articulation. Target words were repeated following a spoken and written example provided by the investigator. During treatment the investigator was positioned out of view so that no visual cues were available during the spoken model. Spatially accurate movement patterns (i.e., reaching the target) were followed by a tone, and a rising balloon image moved on the display. Feedback was given one trace at a time, with the screen cleared after each attempt. In the 50% feedback condition (for the /θ/ SMTs) the video monitor was programmed to randomly blank out for half the trials. During this time, the participant could not view her tongue tip position. Additional details on the EMA feedback procedure are given in Katz et al. (1999).

## Scoring procedure and reliability

Productions from each audio-recorded probe list were played to a trained examiner (DG). A production was scored as "correct" if both the targeted consonant and subsequent vowel were judged to be produced accurately and intelligibly. An analysis of inter-rater reliability using a second judge on 5% of the data indicated 88% agreement.

## RESULTS

Because of considerable individual SMT variability, and because canonical phonemes are not assumed to represent a response class, the typical method of displaying results as a staggered graph of pooled phoneme acquisition (e.g., /j/, followed by the next phoneme, and so forth) was not used. Instead, the data are displayed separately by individual SMT (Figures 1 to 4). In all cases, treatment outcome was first determined by visual inspection, then by consideration of Cohen's $d$ effect sizes for true baseline vs treatment, baseline vs post-treatment, and baseline vs long-term maintenance comparisons (Beeson & Robey, 2006). Effect sizes were calculated based on all data points in each experimental phase, and not on a certain number of points within each phase. Visual inspection was conducted by two expert judges who were unfamiliar with this participant. Judgements of generalisation (i.e., determining if treatment influenced untreated behaviours during a given treatment phase) were made by these same judges, with 94% inter-rater reliability. Visual inspection judgements were based on changes in trial-to-trial variability, and the magnitude and slope of change from the baseline and across preceding phases.

For the first group of SMTs (initial /j/), acquisition was judged to occur for 4/5 trained words, with $d$ values ranging from 1.1 to 7.74 (x = 4.24). These SMTs were maintained post-treatment ($d$ = 1.47 to 7.83; x = 4.61) and at the 1-month long-term probe ($d$ = 1.41 to 6.09; x = 3.64). Improved performance and short-term maintenance were

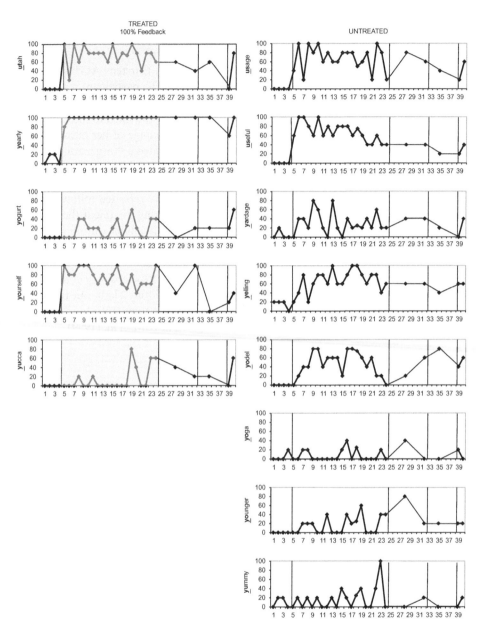

**Figure 1.** Baseline, acquisition, maintenance, and follow-up data for /j/, the first treated group of SMTs. For the treated words (left column) the treatment sessions are shaded. The untreated words (right column) probed response generalisation. Accuracy is percent correct out of five repetitions per session per word. A check indicates positive outcome for acquisition, maintenance, or long-term maintenance.

also judged for five of the eight untreated stimuli included as "near" target probes for response generalisation (*usage, useful, yardage, yelling, yodel*), with *d* values ranging from 1.89 to 5.20 (generalisation; x = 3.22), and 2.75 to 4.74 (post-treatment maintenance; x = 3.75). With one exception, production was also maintained in these words at 1 month post-treatment. There was little evidence of generalisation during /j/-containing probe items from the treatment of the subsequent /θ/- and /tʃ/-containing SMTs.

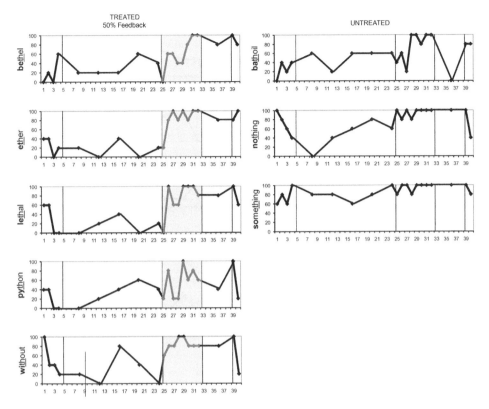

**Figure 2.** Baseline, acquisition, maintenance, and follow-up data for /θ/, the second treated group of SMTs. For the treated words (left column) the treatment sessions are shaded. The untreated words (right column) probed response generalisation. Accuracy is percent correct out of five repetitions per session per word. A check indicates positive outcome for acquisition, maintenance, or long-term maintenance.

The next treated SMT, medial /θ/, was produced with higher baseline accuracy than the /j/ SMTs, and with considerably more variability. All five treated items were judged as showing acquisition ($d$ = 1.26 to 3.61; x = 1.95). Two of these five SMTs (*bethel* and *without*) were maintained at 1 month post-treatment ($d$ = 2.83 to 4.05). All three untreated probes showed improved performance ($d$ = 1.26 to 3.61; x = 1.31), with two of these showing maintenance at 1 month post-treatment ($d$ = 0.78 and 4.05).

The third treated group of SMTs, initial /tʃ/, was judged as showing improved performance for all of the five treated SMTs. However, these gains could only be specifically attributed to /tʃ/ treatment for three of the five targets ($d$ = 2.05 to 3.06), because of generalisation from prior treated /j/- and /tʃ/-containing targets. Two of the treated items appeared well maintained (relative to baseline) at 1 month post-treatment ($d$ = 2.09 to 2.57). Improved performance and maintenance ($d$ = 0.81 to 2.31; x = 1.26) were also judged for all six untreated targets. However, generalisation from previously treated targets was clearly involved in the improvement of these items.

The majority of the untreated (control) words showed increased variability during the training phases for the three treated targets. However, there was little improvement by 1 month post-treatment, and there were many instances of no change during the course of the experiment. In summary, there were sufficient stable baselines to suggest that the gains noted for treated items did not result from across-the-board improvement

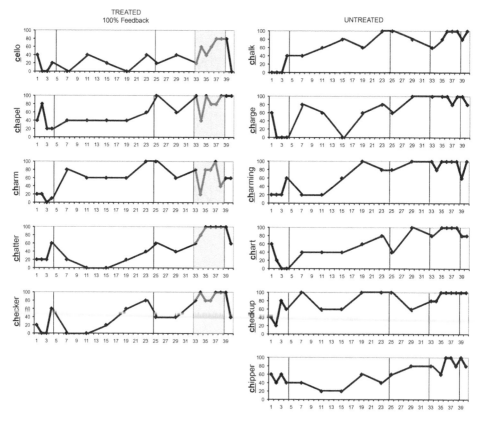

**Figure 3.** Baseline, acquisition, maintenance, and follow-up data for /tʃ/, the third treated group of SMTs. For the treated words (left column) the treatment sessions are shaded. The untreated words (right column) probed response generalisation. Accuracy is percent correct out of five repetitions per session per word. A check indicates positive outcome for acquisition, maintenance, or long-term maintenance.

or unassisted recovery. Contrary to predictions, treatment of /θ/-containing SMTs with 50% feedback corresponded with relatively rapid acquisition and poor overall maintenance, compared to the targets treated with 100% feedback.

## DISCUSSION

The main finding of this study is that augmented kinematic feedback improved production for a majority of treated targets for an individual with AOS. For the first treated SMT, organised around the /j/ gesture, most of the targets probed showed acquisition, post-treatment maintenance, and long-term maintenance. Adequate controls (i.e., unrelated probe items obtained over the course of treatment) suggested that the cases of the /j/ SMT acquisition could be attributed to the treatment. Similar patterns were noted for the next treated group of SMTs, /θ/, with most items acquired and maintained, both immediately post-treatment and at 1 month post-treatment. The third treated group of SMTs, /tʃ/, presented a greater challenge for interpretation: Improved performance and maintenance were noted for all treated and some untreated SMTs, although generalisation from previously treated targets (i.e., /j/ and /θ/ groups of SMTs) occurred for some items.

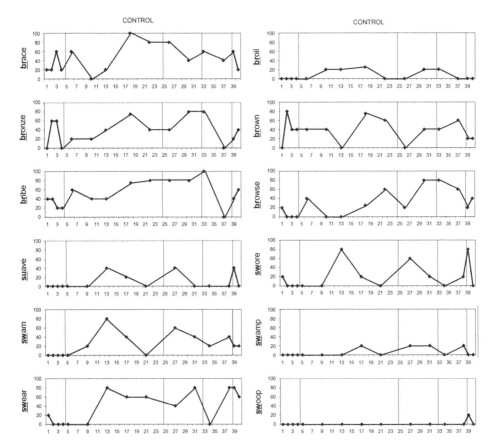

**Figure 4.** Accuracy for producing the untrained (control) sounds /br/ and /sw/ during the baseline, acquisition, maintenance, and follow-up phases of the experiment. Accuracy is percent correct out of five repetitions per session per word. A check indicates positive outcome for acquisition, maintenance, or long-term maintenance.

Considered in the framework of schema theory, the general outcome of the intervention may be attributed to strengthening of the GMP, parameters, or both. At a more detailed level, the patterns of SMT generalisation observed are puzzling: Within a given set of SMTs there was item-specific variability among the treated (e.g., *Utah* vs *yucca*) and untreated (e.g., *usage* vs *yummy*) items. At a minimum, this suggests that EMA feedback treatment does not operate uniformly at the level of a canonical phoneme. However, these differences do not seem to be attributable to phonetic context effects at the level of the syllable, since there were also cases in which a treated item generalised to an untreated item sharing the same CV context (e.g., *yogurt*, *yodel*), but did not generalise to other untreated items in the same SMT category (e.g., *yoga*). In addition, there were untreated CV combinations acquired (e.g., *yardage*, *yelling*) that were not treated. There are a number of possible explanations for these patterns, including lexical-level issues or motoric/planning demands for segments larger than the CV syllable. Although the details are not yet clear, an explanation in terms of underlying motoric complexity is suspected to provide the best understanding of these and related data.

A secondary finding is that treatment of /θ/ SMTs with 50% feedback corresponded with relatively rapid acquisition and a low degree of overall maintenance, compared to the targets treated with 100% feedback. This finding does not agree with some of the patterns noted in studies of limb (e.g., Bruechert et al., 2003) and speech (e.g., Austermann et al., 2008; Clark & Robin, 1998) motor learning. However, the present data must be considered with caution, as a small number of stimuli were involved and the stimuli were not balanced across frequency conditions.

The effect sizes for Cohen's $d$ ranged from 0.86 to 7.74, with averages for the /j/ SMTs falling in the high 3 to 4 range, the /θ/ SMTs averaging approximately 1.5, and the /tʃ/ SMTs averaging in the 1.5 to 3 range. Although there are no motor-based treatment data from which to derive comparable benchmarks, Robey, Schultz, Crawford, and Sinner (1999) reported values drawn from a number of interventions for various language functions and used in the interpretation of data in several recent studies (2.6, 3.9, and 5.8, corresponding to small-, medium-, and large-sized effects). If these comparisons were relevant, the current findings would represent relatively small effect sizes. However, this would not be particularly surprising as the current data represent a limited, experimental intervention rather than a full-fledged therapy programme. While the eventual goal is to incorporate this type of technology into a hierarchical therapy model, the current participant received only brief motor practice guided by the machine display.

One last point deserves mention: Whereas the participant received visual feedback for consonant place of articulation, her productions were scored using more stringent criteria, i.e., perceptually correct production of CV portions of the word (across place, manner, and voicing). Thus the current data likely underestimate actual training effects because the place of articulation for target SMTs probably improved at a better rate than whole-syllable performance.

In summary, the findings of this study provide qualified evidence that kinematic feedback improved the speech of this individual with AOS. Systematic replication of this technique on additional individuals with varying factors known to affect motor and verbal learning will determine the conditions under which this technique is efficacious and effective.

Manuscript received 24 July 2009
Manuscript accepted 29 November 2009

## REFERENCES

Adams, S., & Page, A. (2000). Effects of selected practice and feedback variables on speech motor learning. *Journal of Medical Speech-Language Pathology, 8*, 215–220.

Austermann, S., Hula, W., Robin, D., Maas, E., Ballard, K., & Schmidt, R. (2008). Effects of feedback frequency and timing on acquisition, retention, and transfer of speech skills in acquired apraxia of speech. *Journal of Speech, Language, and Hearing Research, 51*, 1088–1113.

Ballard, K. J., Granier, J. P., & Robin, D. A. (2000). Understanding the nature of apraxia of speech: Theory, analysis, and treatment. *Aphasiology, 14*, 969–995.

Bayles, K. A., & Tomoeda, C. K. (1993). *Arizona Battery for Communication Disorders of Dementia.* Tucson, AZ: Canyonlands.

Beeson, P. M., & Robey, R. R. (2006). Evaluating single-subject treatment research: Lessons learned from the aphasia literature. *Neuropsychology Review, 16*, 161–169.

Bruechert, L., Lai, Q., & Shea, C. (2003). Reduced knowledge of results frequency enhances error detection. *Research Quarterly for Exercise and Sport, 74*, 467–472.

Clark, H., & Robin, D. (1998). Generalised motor programme and parameterization accuracy in apraxia of speech and conduction aphasia. *Aphasiology, 12*, 699–713.

Goodglass, H., Kaplan, E., & Barresi, B. (2001). *The assessment of aphasia and related disorders* (3rd ed.). Philadelphia, PA: Lippincott, Williams & Wilkins.

Katz, W., Bharadwaj, S., & Carstens, B. (1999). Electromagnetic articulography treatment for an adult with Broca's aphasia and apraxia of speech. *Journal of Speech, Language, and Hearing Research, 42,* 1355–1366.

Katz, W., Bharadwaj, S., Gabbert, G., & Stettler, M. (2002). Visual augmented knowledge of performance: Treating place-of-articulation errors in apraxia of speech using EMA. *Brain and Language, 83,* 187–189.

Katz, W., Garst, D., Carter, G., McNeil, M., Fossett, T., Doyle, P., et al. (2007). Treatment of an individual with aphasia and apraxia of speech using EMA visually augmented feedback. *Brain and Language, 103,* 213–214.

Kent, R. D., Weismer, G., Kent, J. F., & Rosenbek, J.C. (1989). Toward phonetic intelligibility testing in dysarthria. *Journal of Speech and Hearing Disorders, 54,* 482–499.

McNeil, M., Doyle, P. J., & Wambaugh, J. (2000). Apraxia of speech: A treatable disorder of motor planning & programming. In S. E. Nadeau, L. J. Gonzales Rothi, & B. Crosson (Eds.), *Aphasia and language: Theory to practice* (pp. 221–266). New York, USA: Guilford Press.

McNeil, M., Robin, D., & Schmidt, R. (1997). Apraxia of speech: Definition, differentiation and treatment. In M. R. McNeil (Ed.), *Clinical management of sensorimotor speech disorders* (pp. 311–344). New York, USA: Thieme Medical Publishers.

McNeil, M. R., Sung, J. E., Yang, D., Pratt, S. R., Fossett, T. R., Pavelko, S., et al. (2007). Comparing connected language elicitation procedures in person with aphasia: Concurrent validation of the Story Retell Procedure. *Aphasiology, 21,* 775–790.

Robey, R., Schultz, M, Crawford, A., & Sinner, C. (1999). Single-subject clinical-outcome research: Designs, data, effect sizes, and analyses. *Aphasiology, 13,* 445–473.

Schmidt, R. A. (1975). A schema theory of discrete motor skill learning. *Psychological Review, 82,* 225–260.

Schmidt, R. A. (1976). The schema as a solution to some persistent problems in motor learning theory. In G. E. Stelmach (Ed.), *Motor control: Issues and trends* (pp. 41–64). New York: Academic Press.

Schmidt, R. A., & Lee, T. D. (1999) *Motor control and learning: A behavioral emphasis* (3rd ed.) Champaign, IL: Human Kinetics.

Shea, J. B., & Morgan, R. L. (1979). Contextual interference effects on the acquisition, retention, and transfer of a motor skill. *Journal of Experimental Psychology: Human Learning and Memory, 5,* 179–187.

Steinhauer, K., & Grayhack, J. (2000). The role of knowledge of results in performance and learning of a voice motor task. *Journal of Voice, 14,* 137–145.

Van der Merwe, A. (1997). A theoretical framework for the characterization of pathological speech sensorimotor control. In M. R. McNeil (Ed.), *Clinical management of sensorimotor speech disorders* (pp. 1–25). New York, USA: Thieme Medical Publishers.

Weeks, D. L., & Kordus, R. N. (1998). Relative frequency of knowledge of performance and motor skill learning. *Research Quarterly for Exercise and Sport, 69,* 224–230.

Wright, D. L., Black, C. B., Immink, M. A., Brueckner, S., & Magnuson, C. (2004). Long-term motor programming improvements occur via concatenating movement sequences during random but not blocked practice. *Journal of Motor Behavior, 36,* 39–50.

Wulf, G., & Schmidt, R. (1989). The learning of generalised motor programs: Reducing the relative frequency of knowledge of results enhances memory. *Journal of Experimental Psychology: Learning, Memory and Cognition, 15,* 748–757.

Wulf, G., Schmidt, R., & Deubel, H. (1993). Reduced feedback frequency enhances generalised motor program learning but not parameterization learning. *Journal of Experimental Psychology: Learning, Memory, and Cognition, 19,* 1134–1150.

Yorkston, K. M., & Beukelman, D. R. (1984). *Assessment of intelligibility of dysarthric speech.* Austin, TX: Pro-Ed.

APHASIOLOGY, 2010, 24 (6–8), 838–855

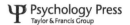

# Variability in apraxia of speech: Perceptual analysis of monosyllabic word productions across repeated sampling times

Shannon C. Mauszycki, Julie L. Wambaugh, and Rosalea M. Cameron

*VA Salt Lake City Healthcare System, University of Utah, Salt Lake City, UT, USA*

*Background*: Variability in speech sound errors has been regarded as a primary characteristic of apraxia of speech (AOS). Early research deemed errors extremely unpredictable, resulting in a number of different error types on repeated productions of the same stimuli. However, recent research has suggested that errors may not be variable, but there are limited data regarding variability over time (i.e., beyond a single sampling occasion). Furthermore, the influence of conditions of stimulus presentation (i.e., blocked vs random) on sound errors remains unclear.
*Aims*: The purpose of this investigation was to examine variability of sound errors in 11 individuals with AOS and aphasia. Of particular interest were the effects of repeated sampling and method of speech elicitation on the variability of error types as evaluated with narrow phonetic transcription.
*Methods & Procedures*: A total of 28 monosyllabic words served as experimental stimuli. There were four exemplars for each of the seven initial target phonemes (i.e., /h, f, m, d, s, r, n/). Stimuli were elicited on three sampling occasions over a 7-day period with each sampling occasion separated by 2 days. At each sampling time productions were elicited under two conditions: blocked presentation (blocked by sound) and randomised presentation. Speech productions were analysed perceptually utilising narrow phonetic transcription.
*Outcomes & Results*: Findings revealed a similar overall mean percentage of errors for the group in both conditions of stimulus presentation across the three sampling times. The target phoneme with the least number of errors was /h/. The target phoneme with the greatest number of errors was /s/. The predominant error type across target phonemes was distortions. However, the predominant error type varied across target phonemes and appeared to be influenced by number of errors.
*Conclusions*: Repeated sampling or method of speech elicitation did not influence errors, with a similar overall mean percentage of errors for the group in both conditions of stimulus presentation across the three sampling times. Distortions were found to be the predominant error type for the majority of target sounds. A comparison of the number of error types produced by the group in each condition across the three sampling times found no obvious pattern of responding by the group in either condition for individual phonemes. That is, condition of elicitation did not appear to influence the variability of error type for any given sound.

*Keywords:* Apraxia of speech; Aphasia; Perceptual analysis; Variability; Error analysis.

Address correspondence to: Shannon C. Mauszycki, Aphasia/Apraxia Research Lab, 151-A, Building 2, 500 Foothill Blvd, Salt Lake City, UT 84148, USA. E-mail: Passbrat@aol.com

This research was supported in part by Rehabilitation Research and Development, Department of Veterans Affairs.

http://www.psypress.com/aphasiology      DOI: 10.1080/02687030903438516

Acquired apraxia of speech (AOS) is a sensorimotor speech disorder that is linked to damage in the dominant language hemisphere of the brain (McNeil, Robin, & Schmidt, 2008). The primary identifying features of AOS are phoneme distortions, distorted sound substitutions, and prosodic abnormalities, as well as reduced rate of speech associated with lengthened sound segments and intersegment durations (McNeil et al., 2008). Other symptoms that frequently co-occur with AOS are articulatory groping, perseverative errors, increasing errors as word length increases, and speech initiation difficulties, but these symptoms are non-discriminatory in terms of differential diagnosis (McNeil et al., 2008; Wambaugh, Duffy, McNeil, Robin, & Rogers, 2006).

The characteristics that define AOS have continued to evolve since its initial description and remain controversial with regard to a number of speech behaviours. In particular, the variability or predictability of speech sound errors in AOS has not been resolved (Croot, 2002). Variability in speech sound errors was long considered a primary characteristic of AOS (Deal & Darley, 1972; Johns & Darley, 1970; Wertz, LaPointe, & Rosenbek, 1984). Speakers with AOS were considered to be unpredictable with regard to the location of errors (i.e., error location within a word) (Johns & Darley, 1970; LaPointe & Johns, 1975) and the type of error produced (Johns & Darley, 1970; LaPointe & Horner, 1976) on repeated productions of the same words. The early investigation by Johns and Darley (1970) claiming a high degree of variability offers less than compelling evidence for this early descriptor, but is frequently cited as evidence of variability of errors in speakers with AOS. The study examined the articulatory accuracy of 10 speakers with AOS on monosyllabic words in different conditions of stimulus presentation (i.e., random and blocked by word, one model to one response, and one model to three responses), but this had no influence on errors. Also, no data were presented regarding consistency of error location or error types across repeated productions. Only anecdotal evidence was provided by these authors concerning the variability of performance in speakers with AOS. Subsequent research with "pure" AOS speakers and speakers with AOS and aphasia has suggested that errors may not be variable (Skenes & Trullinger, 1988; Mauszycki, Dromey, & Wambaugh, 2007; McNeil, Odell, Miller, & Hunter, 1995; Odell, McNeil, Rosenbek, & Hunter, 1990; Shuster & Wambaugh, 2003; Wambaugh, Nessler, Bennett, & Mauszycki, 2004).

A study by LaPointe and Horner (1976) investigated group and individual performance of AOS speakers on repeated productions of five monosyllabic and five multisyllabic words. The authors examined two different conditions of stimulus presentation (i.e., 1 model to 1 response versus 1 model to 10 responses) with seven participants with AOS and aphasia. Results revealed that conditions of stimulus presentation had no influence on number of errors for the group or individuals. However, LaPointe and Horner also examined variability across repeated productions by calculating how frequently a subsequent production of a word differed from a previous production. Variability ranged from 23% to 50% across participants. They found no differences in the number of errors when comparing the first five productions to the last five productions for the group.

The reported variability across participants in early AOS research may be the consequence of participant selection criteria resulting in the inclusion of speakers with phonemic paraphasia (McNeil et al., 2008). Therefore it is possible that the nature of some sound errors reflect linguistic (phonologic) rather than motoric impairment. The bulk of AOS research has been conducted with participants with co-occurring aphasia rather than participants with pure AOS, due to the infrequent occurrence of pure AOS (Duffy, 2005).

McNeil and colleagues (1995) utilised narrow phonetic transcription to examine the consistency of error location and variability of error type on repeated productions with four speakers with relatively pure AOS. Ten mono-, bi-, and trisyllabic words served as stimuli and three consecutive productions were elicited from participants. The types of errors that occurred on the consecutive productions of stimuli only differed on average by 13% (range of 0% to 16%). Errors occurred in the same location of words 90% of the time (range 86% to 94%). Findings revealed a high degree of predictability for errors in these speakers with pure AOS.

More recent research found that error types may vary by sounds for speakers with AOS (Mauszycki et al., 2007; Wambaugh et al., 2004). Wambaugh and colleagues examined repeated productions of monosyllabic words with initial stop consonants from a speaker with AOS and aphasia. Stimuli were elicited on three occasions via blocked (by sound) and randomised presentation. Variability in error types ranged from 0% (i.e., the same type of error was produced for a sound) to 58%. The most predictable errors were voiced sounds in the blocked condition with variability ranging from 0% to 33%. The sounds more frequently in error were produced with fewer error types indicating some predictability for sounds errors based on the severity of the disruption for a particular sound.

Another study by Mauszycki et al. (2007) examined monosyllabic words comprising initial stop consonants in a speaker with AOS and aphasia. Stimuli were elicited randomly on three sampling occasions. Results revealed a small number of errors (0–7%) for target sounds at each sampling time. The same type of error tended to occur for a sound at each sampling time (0–25% range of variability) and across sampling occasions suggesting some degree of predictability in errors for certain sounds. Both investigations (Mauszycki et al., 2007; Wambaugh et al., 2004) examined variability of speech sound errors over time with individual speakers with AOS and aphasia, hence limiting external validity. However, these two studies display the likelihood that AOS speakers may exhibit patterns of responding associated with different sounds that may subsequently be influenced by conditions of stimulus presentation.

Certainly, variability has implications in terms of planning treatment. If speech sound errors were consistent across time (i.e., same error type produced for a sound on repeated sampling occasions), then therapy would be aimed at treating the specific sounds. However, if sound errors were inconsistent across time, then a non-sound specific treatment approach would be warranted.

A theoretical characterisation of AOS by McNeil et al. (2008) suggests that impairment involves disturbed "translation of a well-formed and filled phonologic frame to previously learned kinematic parameters assembled for carrying out the intended movement" (p. 264). This definition involves concepts of motor programs and parameterisation proposed by the schema theory (Schmidt, 1975) suggesting that the deficits in AOS are related to the accessing or retrieving previously realised motor programs. Examination of the consistency or variability of speech sound errors in speakers with AOS may offer information about whether access or retrieval of particular motor programs may be specific or general in nature. If an apraxic speaker demonstrates both consistency and variability in a session it may be possible that the speaker is exhibiting a pattern that could be transient in nature. Neural connections may be associated with this particular pattern, especially the weight of those connections. However, if an apraxic speaker exhibits consistency in a session this may be the consequence of a specific or general retrieval/access problem. A consistent pattern of performance over time may suggest the loss of a motor program or deficits due to retrieval or access, but a more simplistic explanation would be a specific access problem over time rather than a general access problem.

Perceptual analyses have primarily been used to study speakers with AOS providing descriptions of speech behaviours for diagnosis and treatment, including variability. Broad phonetic transcription has been more frequently employed to examine speech production, which can make classification of speech sound errors challenging. Narrow phonetic transcription has the ability to capture more detailed and subtle articulatory information regarding speech production that could not be obtained had broad phonetic transcription been employed. However, only a limited number of studies have utilised narrow phonetic transcription in AOS (McNeil et al., 1995; Odell et al., 1990, 1991; Shuster & Wambaugh, 2000). Findings from these investigations revealed more distortion errors that deviated from traditional AOS findings (i.e., using broad phonetic transcription) where substitutions were the prevalent error type.

Based on the recent findings examining variability with carefully selected apraxic speakers (Mauszycki et al., 2007; McNeil et al., 1995; Wambaugh et al., 2004), it was theorised that the speech sound errors produced by speakers would be invariable (i.e., fewer error types) within and across sampling times based on findings that patterns of errors were related to different phonemes (Mauszycki et al.; Shuster & Wambaugh, 2000, 2003). Additionally, it was hypothesised that conditions of stimulus presentation (i.e., blocked and random) would further influence errors with more predictable patterns of speech errors including fewer types of errors produced (i.e., less variable) in the blocked condition (Wambaugh et al., 2004).

The purpose of this investigation was to further examine variability of speech production in individuals with AOS and aphasia. Of particular interest were the effects of repeated sampling and method of speech elicitation (i.e., random and blocked by sound) on the variability of error types as evaluated by narrow phonetic transcription.

## METHOD

### Participants

A total of 11 individuals with AOS and aphasia participated in this investigation. The five males and six females ranged in age from 25 to 63 years ($M = 49$ years, $SD = 12$ years). All participants were non-hospitalised and at least 3 months post onset of brain injury. The time post onset ranged from 4 months to 15 years, 7 months ($M = 4$ years, $SD = 4$ years 9 months). Although some participants were currently receiving speech/language therapy, their treatment was suspended during the period of data collection. All participants were native English speakers and passed a pure tone air conduction hearing screening at 35 dB at 500, 1000, and 2000 Hz in at least one ear.

Brain-imaging information was collected, but was not used for participant selection. Nine participants suffered an embolic cerebral vascular accident, one participant suffered a haemorrhagic cerebral vascular accident, and another suffered a traumatic brain injury (i.e., penetrating skull fracture). All participants had negative histories for mental illness, alcohol/substance abuse, and neurological problems other than the presence of AOS and aphasia (see Table 1 for a summary of participant characteristics).

The diagnosis of AOS was judged perceptually by a certified speech language pathologist (SLP) and a confirmatory diagnosis of AOS was made independently by another certified SLP who is an internationally recognised expert in AOS. The presence of AOS was judged perceptually by both clinicians via live and/or audio-recorded samples. The diagnosis of AOS was based on the performance on Subtest 1 from the *Apraxia Battery for Adults-2*, alternating and sequential motion rates (i.e., AMRs and SMRs), and Subtest 2, words of increasing length (Dabul, 2000), as well as connected speech samples via discourse tasks from Nicholas and Brookshire (1993). The following criteria by McNeil et al. (2008) were utilised to make the diagnosis of AOS: speech production characterised by difficulty producing speech sounds, consistently reduced rate of speech, segregated syllable production, and disturbed prosody. The above symptoms may have been accompanied by the following behaviours, but these behaviours were not utilised to make the diagnosis of AOS: articulatory groping, repeated production attempts, and awareness of errors. See Table 2 for a summary of assessment results.

## Experimental design

This study involved a single-group, repeated-measures design. The investigation was designed to examine the number and types of speech sound errors produced over three sampling times in two different conditions of stimulus presentation. Stimuli were elicited at three different sampling times over a 7-day period with each participant. Each sampling time was separated by 2 days (e.g., Tuesday, Friday, and Monday) with each administration occurring at the same time of day on each sampling occasion.

At each sampling time, stimuli were elicited under two conditions: blocked and randomised presentation. The blocked condition consisted of all exemplars of a sound presented sequentially (e.g., all initial /m/ words). The word order within the block was randomised, as was the order of the blocks. In the blocked condition participants were presented with a word and produced that word five times with a model prior to each production. In the random condition each target word was randomly presented five times among all exemplars.

In each condition (i.e., blocked, random) each exemplar (168 words) was elicited five times. Thus there were 840 productions per condition, with a total of 1680 productions at each sampling time. Over the three sampling times, 5040 tokens were elicited from each speaker. However, only a subset of words are presented in this report (i.e., 28 monosyllabic words). The order of the conditions was pseudo-randomised across and within each sampling time. Each data collection session was no longer than 3 hours in length with a rest break between sampling conditions.

## Instrumentation

Participants were seated in a quiet room for the experiment. A high-quality head-mounted microphone (AKG Acoustics C420) and a digital recorder (M-Audio Microtrak 24/96) were utilised to capture the speech signals for perceptual analyses. A microphone-to-mouth distance of approximately 7 cm was maintained within and across participants to ensure uniform recording conditions.

TABLE 1
Participant characteristics

| Characteristic | P-1 | P-2 | P-3 | P-4 | P-5 | P-6 | P-7 | P-8 | P-9 | P-10 | P-11 |
|---|---|---|---|---|---|---|---|---|---|---|---|
| Age | 35 | 56 | 46 | 47 | 56 | 25 | 41 | 62 | 63 | 58 | 52 |
| Gender | Male | Female | Female | Male | Female | Female | Male | Female | Female | Male | Male |
| Years of education | 18 | 14 | 12 | 13 | 10 | 12 | 14 | 15 | 13 | 20 | 11 |
| Aetiology | CVA | CVA | CVA | CVA | CVA | CVA | TBI | CVA | CVA | CVA | CVA |
| Yrs/Mos | 1 yr | 2 yrs | 1 yr | 15 yrs | | | 6 yrs | | 9 yrs | 4 yrs | |
| Post-onset | 9 mos | 9 mos | 2 mos | 7 mos | 9 mos | 9 mos | 1 mos | 4 mos | 4 mos | 10 mos | 8 mos |

TABLE 2
Assessment results

| Assessment Tool | P-1 | P-2 | P-3 | P-4 | P-5 | P-6 | P-7 | P-8 | P-9 | P-10 | P-11 |
|---|---|---|---|---|---|---|---|---|---|---|---|
| *Apraxia Battery for Adults-2* (Dabul, 2000) | | | | | | | | | | | |
| Level of Impairment | Mild AOS | Mild-Mod AOS | Mod-Severe AOS | Mod-Severe AOS | Mod-Severe AOS | Severe AOS | Mod-Severe AOS | Mild AOS | Mild AOS | Mod-Severe AOS | Severe AOS |
| *Western Aphasia Battery* (Kertesz, 1982) | | | | | | | | | | | |
| Aphasia Quotient | 94.0 | 71.2 | 45.1 | 83.6 | 76.7 | 42.7 | 36.9 | 92.5 | 97.3 | 47.0 | 52.6 |
| Classifi-cation | Anomic | Broca's | Broca's | Broca's | Broca's | Broca's | Broca's | Anomic | Anomic | Broca's | Broca's |
| *Assessment of Intelligibility of Dysarthric Speech* (Yorkston & Beukelman, 1981) | | | | | | | | | | | |
| Word Level | 92% | 94% | 98% | 84% | 78% | 82% | 90% | 98% | 100% | 92% | 90% |
| *Raven's Coloured Progressive Matrices* (Raven, Raven, & Court, 1998) (36 possible) | | | | | | | | | | | |
| Score | 33 | 30 | 28 | 30 | 30 | 35 | 32 | 33 | 31 | 36 | 28 |

## Data collection

An ASHA-certified SLP conducted the sampling. The SLP provided a verbal model for each stimulus item at a normal rate of production and asked the participant to repeat the model. No feedback was provided regarding the accuracy of productions.

## Experimental stimuli

A total of 28 monosyllabic words served as experimental stimuli. There were four exemplars for each of seven initial target phonemes (/h, f, m, d, s, r, n/). Selection of experimental stimuli was guided by findings from research concerning phoneme frequency research in adult speech (Mines, Hanson, & Shoup, 1978). Mines et al. (1978) examined the occurrence of phonemes in initial, medial, and final position of words in casual conversation (i.e., interview) with 26 speakers of American English. For the present investigation, phoneme selection was based on frequency of occurrence with the seven initial phonemes selected across the frequency continuum (e.g., /h/ = 92%, /f/ = 63%, /d/ = 25%, /n/ = 12%).

Monosyllabic words were of consonant-vowel-consonant (CVC) structure and were constrained by position of target phoneme (i.e., initial). Four vowels /æ, i, o, u/ were also utilised to select monosyllabic exemplars for each target phoneme. In selecting exemplars, attempts were made to limit affricates and fricatives in non-target positions in order to maintain the same level of difficulty across exemplars for each target phoneme. Also, words with repeated consonants or vowel-consonants (i.e., final position of words; sap, soap, soup) were avoided and phonetic context varied among the four exemplars of a target phoneme. Although word frequency was not controlled, all exemplars were nouns. The following words served as experimental stimuli: ham, heat, hope, hoot, fat, feed, phone, fool, map, meat, mole, moon, sack, seed soap, suit, rack, reed, rope, room, nap, need, note, and noose.

## Data analyses

Audio-recordings were utilised to perceptually analyse all speech samples via narrow phonetic transcription (Shriberg & Kent, 2003). Both consonant and vowel segments were transcribed; however, only the target phonemes are reported for the purpose of this study. On occasion, when speakers audibly groped to find an articulatory position or sound in the initial position of words, these attempts were noted but were not phonetically transcribed. Only the participant's first complete production of each stimulus item was analysed, although participants frequently attempted additional productions due to inaccurate production of a stimulus item.

Analysis of each transcribed target phoneme segment involved coding segments as either correct or incorrect. Productions were considered correct if they were perceived as correct, based on transcriptions from the *Cambridge English Pronouncing Dictionary* (Jones, 2003). Then each target phoneme segment considered in error was coded according to type.

Errors on target phonemes were coded according to predetermined categories and included substitutions, distortions, distorted substitutions, and omissions (Odell et al., 1990, 1991). A substitution was considered a phonetically accurate production of a non-target English phoneme. A distortion was considered an attempt at the target phoneme that did not cross the phoneme boundary but was produced with perceptible place, timing, manner, or voice deviation(s) from the accurate production. A distorted substitution was a production that not only crossed phoneme boundaries of the target phoneme but was also distortion of the substitution (e.g., dome > (d o͜s). An omission was a deleted phoneme.

*Statistical analyses.* The Friedman test was utilised to examine the effects of the independent variable (i.e., conditions of stimulus presentation) on the number of errors produced in each condition across the three sampling times for each target phoneme (i.e., a test for the blocked condition; time 1, 2, 3, then the random condition; time 1, 2, 3 for each phoneme). This non-parametric test for related samples was utilised (with alpha set at 0.05) due to concerns of violating normality assumptions associated with the repeated measures ANOVA. Post hoc comparisons were conducted using the Wilcoxon Signed Ranks test if significant differences were revealed (via the Friedman test) utilising the Holms step-down procedure to adjust for Type I error with alpha set at 0.05 for each set of comparisons (i.e., three comparisons for each stimulus condition). Subsequent statistical analyses involved comparing the number of errors produced in each condition of stimulus presentation by time in order to examine the effects of stimulus presentation for each target phoneme (i.e., Time 1: Blocked vs Random for each phoneme). The non-parametric Wilcoxon Signed Ranks test was utilised due to concerns with violating assumptions associated with the parametric test. Again, the Holms step-down procedure was utilised to adjust for Type I error with alpha set at 0.05.

## Dependent measures

Dependent measures included mean percentage of errors by sound and predominant error type by sound, and were conducted for each participant in both conditions of stimulus presentation at each sampling time.

*Mean percentage of errors by sound.* The mean percentage of errors by sound was calculated by determining the mean number of times the phoneme was in error for the group and dividing by the total number of occasions the phoneme occurred. This resulted in a percentage that allowed comparison among target sounds for the same participant and/or across participants. The measurement was computed overall and for each target phoneme in both conditions of stimulus presentation at each sampling time for each speaker in order to determine if there was any pattern of performance over time and/or by condition.

*Predominant error type by sound.* The predominant error type used on erred productions for each target sound was examined *within* and *across* sampling times. A percentage was computed by determining the number of productions that were produced with a predominant error type and dividing by the total number of erred productions.

## Reliability

A total of 15% of the productions for each participant at each sampling time were randomly selected for reanalysis of narrow phonetic transcription as well as error classification, for the purpose of determining intra- and inter-judge reliability. Inter-judge reliability was completed by an experienced certified speech-language pathologist familiar with neurogenic speech and language disorders but not involved in the investigation. Overall item-to-item agreement for narrow phonetic transcription for target phonemes was calculated at 83% including transcription differences considered functionally equivalent (i.e., /d/; partially devoiced /d̥/ vs. /t/; partially voiced /t̬/ = functionally equivalent), which is deemed acceptable for narrow phonetic transcription (Shriberg, Kwiatkowski, & Hoffman, 1984). Overall item-to-item agreement for error classification on inaccurate target phonemes was 90%.

For intra-judge reliability, the original transcriber re-transcribed 15% of productions for each participant at each time within four to six weeks of the initial transcription. Overall item-to-item agreement for narrow phonetic transcription for target phonemes was calculated at 91% including transcription differences considered functionally equivalent. Overall item-to-item agreement for error classification on inaccurate target phonemes was 95%.

## RESULTS

### Mean percentage of errors by sound

The mean percentage of errors and standard deviation for all target phonemes for the group in each condition across sampling times is displayed in Figure 1. The mean percentage of errors ranged from 37% to 43% for the group.

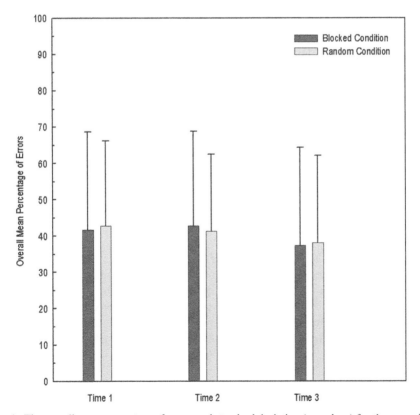

**Figure 1.** The overall mean percentage of errors and standard deviation (error bars) for the group in the blocked and random conditions across the three sampling times.

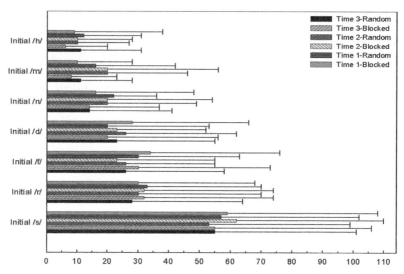

**Figure 2.** The mean percentage of errors and standard deviation (error bars) for the group for each target phoneme in both stimulus presentation conditions at each sampling time.

The mean percentage of errors was calculated for the group for each target phoneme in both conditions across the three sampling times. The mean percentage of errors for target phonemes from least number of errors to the greatest number of errors was as follows: /h, m, n, d, f, r, s/. Figure 2 depicts the mean percentage of errors and standard deviation for each target phoneme in both conditions across the three sampling times.

*Statistical analyses by condition across sampling times.* The Friedman test was utilised to examine the effects of condition of stimulus presentation on the number of errors produced in each condition across the three sampling times for each target phoneme. Statistically significant differences were found only in the random condition for /m/, $\chi^2$ (2, $N = 11$) = 7.913, $p = .019$, in the median values. Post hoc comparisons via Wilcoxon Signed Ranks test identified significant differences between time 2 and time 3, $z = -2.264$, $p = .024$ adjusting for Type I error via the Holms step-down procedure. The results indicated a greater number of errors at sampling time 2 for words with initial /m/ in the random condition.

*Statistical analyses between random and blocked conditions.* The Wilcoxon Signed Ranks test was utilised to compare conditions of stimulus presentation on the number of errors produced for each sampling time for each target phoneme (e.g., blocked time 1 vs random time 1) again utilising the Holms step-down procedure. Results from these analyses did not identify statistically significant differences among target phonemes between the blocked and random conditions at sampling time 1, 2, or 3.

## Predominant error type by sound

The percentage of different error types on erred productions for all target phonemes in the blocked and random conditions are displayed in Figure 3. The predominant error

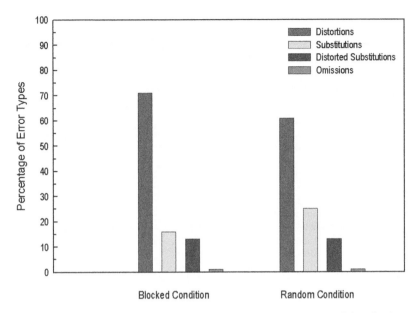

**Figure 3.** The overall percentage of error types in the blocked and random conditions for the group.

type across all sounds was distortions, followed by substitutions, distorted substitutions, and omission errors in both conditions of stimulus presentation. There was a higher percentage of distortions in the blocked condition and substitution errors in the random condition. The percentage of difference for distortions and substitution errors between conditions was 10% and 9% respectively. The percentage of errors for distorted substitutions and omission errors was identical in both conditions of stimulus presentation. Although distortions were the overall dominant error type across conditions, the dominant error type varied across sampling times and/or conditions for individual sounds. Table 3 provides a summary of number of errors and error types (percentage) for each phoneme at the three sampling times in the blocked and random conditions.

The dominant error type for the target phonemes /m/, /f/, /r/, /s/ was distortions within and across sampling times in both conditions. The predominant error type for /h/ varied between substitution and distorted substitution errors across sampling times in the blocked and random conditions. Distortion errors tended to be the dominant error type for /d/, except at sample time 3 in the random condition, where there were a comparable number of distortion and substitution errors. For /n/, substitution errors tended to be the predominant error type. However, at sampling time 2 there were a similar number of distortion and substitution errors in both conditions for this phoneme.

## DISCUSSION

This investigation was designed to examine speech production in 11 individuals with AOS and aphasia, specifically the effects of repeated sampling and method of speech elicitation (blocked and random) on the number of errors and predominant error type for seven target phonemes.

TABLE 3
Errors and error types

| Phoneme & sampling time | Condition | Number of errors | Distortion | Substitution | Distorted substitution | Omission |
|---|---|---|---|---|---|---|
| /h/ | | | | | | |
| Time 1 | Blocked | 20 | 10% | **45%** | 40% | 5% |
| | Random | 27 | 22% | 30% | **33%** | 15% |
| Time 2 | Blocked | 22 | 9% | **59%** | 32% | NA |
| | Random | 21 | 14% | 34% | **52%** | NA |
| Time 3 | Blocked | 14 | NA | 29% | **71%** | NA |
| | Random | 25 | 16% | **48%** | 36% | NA |
| /m/ | | | | | | |
| Time 1 | Blocked | 21 | **62%** | 14% | 24% | NA |
| | Random | 36 | **50%** | 39% | 11% | NA |
| Time 2 | Blocked | 45 | **69%** | 20% | 11% | NA |
| | Random | 45 | **60%** | 31% | 7% | 2% |
| Time 3 | Blocked | 18 | **39%** | 28% | 33% | NA |
| | Random | 25 | **48%** | 40% | 12% | NA |
| /n/ | | | | | | |
| Time 1 | Blocked | 36 | 14% | **50%** | 36% | NA |
| | Random | 49 | 31% | **45%** | 18% | 6% |
| Time 2 | Blocked | 45 | **40%** | 38% | 20% | 2% |
| | Random | 43 | **35%** | **35%** | 25% | 5% |
| Time 3 | Blocked | 30 | 10% | **47%** | 43% | NA |
| | Random | 31 | 23% | **42%** | 32% | 3% |
| /d/ | | | | | | |
| Time 1 | Blocked | 61 | **55%** | 16% | 29% | NA |
| | Random | 43 | **49%** | 30% | 21% | NA |
| Time 2 | Blocked | 51 | **53%** | 31% | 16% | NA |
| | Random | 57 | **53%** | 28% | 14% | 5% |
| Time 3 | Blocked | 45 | **47%** | 33% | 20% | NA |
| | Random | 51 | 41% | **45%** | 14% | NA |
| /f/ | | | | | | |
| Time 1 | Blocked | 75 | **86%** | 11% | 3% | NA |
| | Random | 67 | **64%** | 22% | 14% | NA |
| Time 2 | Blocked | 51 | **98%** | NA | 2% | NA |
| | Random | 57 | **63%** | 26% | 11% | NA |
| Time 3 | Blocked | 66 | **91%** | 6% | 3% | NA |
| | Random | 58 | **59%** | 29% | 12% | NA |
| /r/ | | | | | | |
| Time 1 | Blocked | 65 | **88%** | 6% | 6% | NA |
| | Random | 72 | **73%** | 17% | 10% | NA |
| Time 2 | Blocked | 70 | **89%** | 10% | 1% | NA |
| | Random | 65 | **74%** | 20% | 6% | NA |
| Time 3 | Blocked | 71 | **89%** | 11% | NA | NA |
| | Random | 62 | **76%** | 19% | 5% | NA |
| /s/ | | | | | | |
| Time 1 | Blocked | 130 | **85%** | 5% | 10% | NA |
| | Random | 125 | **76%** | 14% | 10% | NA |
| Time 2 | Blocked | 136 | **86%** | 4% | 10% | NA |
| | Random | 117 | **81%** | 12% | 7% | NA |
| Time 3 | Blocked | 122 | **80%** | 11% | 9% | NA |
| | Random | 122 | **82%** | 10% | 8% | NA |

Number of errors and error types (Percentage) for each target phoneme at each sampling time in both stimulus presentation conditions with predominant error type in bold. NA = No errors.

## Mean percentage of errors

Repeated sampling was found not to have influenced the mean percentage of errors produced by the group. The overall mean percentage of errors and the standard deviation was similar in both conditions of stimulus presentation across the three sampling times. The stability of errors over time has seldom been addressed in the study of AOS; however the present findings are similar to those of Haley and colleagues who found speech intelligibility measures for a group of AOS speakers to be relatively consistent across repeated sampling sessions carried out on the same day (Haley & Gottardy, 2007; Haley, Wertz, & Ohde, 1998).

Recent research suggested that the number of errors produced by individual speakers with AOS and aphasia may vary across repeated sampling occasions and may reflect specific sound difficulties as well as sound location within syllables (Mauszycki & Wambaugh, 2006; Wambaugh et al., 2004). In this investigation, sampling time had no effect for most sounds for the group of AOS speakers. There was only one occasion in which significant differences were revealed among the seven experimental sounds and three sampling time comparisons (of a possible 21 differences). However, in this study, the number of errors by sound was not examined for individual speakers across sampling times. Perhaps the performance of individual speakers in the group may have been comparable to speakers in previous investigations than what was uncovered by group performance. Certainly, additional analyses are warranted to examine the performance of individual speakers as well as the influence that syllable frequency may have on sound errors based on the research by Aichert and Ziegler (2004). These authors identified a greater number of errors on words with a lower syllable frequency, suggesting that motor programs comprising syllables and errors reflect damage to specific motor program rather than impaired access to those motor programs.

Repeated practice of stimuli in a short span of time (7 days) had the potential to promote motor learning, which could have resulted in a decline in errors on later sampling occasions. In contrast, repeated practice of incorrect productions could have served to increase the number of errors at subsequent sampling times (i.e., lack of feedback may serve as reinforcement for erred productions). Also, motivation could have diminished over the course of the three sampling times resulting in more errors. Nevertheless, it appears repeated practice did not positively or negatively influence the number of errors produced by this group of speakers with AOS and aphasia.

## Blocked versus randomised conditions of stimuli presentation

Conditions of stimulus presentation (i.e., blocked by sound vs random) did not exhibit any effect on the percentage of errors produced by the group for the 28 monosyllabic words comprising seven initial target phonemes. These findings are consistent with previous research that found conditions of stimulus presentation had no influence on repeated productions of monosyllabic words in terms of number of errors for groups of AOS speakers (Johns & Darley, 1970; LaPointe & Horner, 1976). The present findings are not consistent with recent research by Wambaugh and colleagues (2004), who found a pattern of performance on monosyllabic word productions of certain initial stop consonants in the blocked condition of stimulus presentation across three sampling occasions for a speaker with moderate AOS and aphasia.

There is evidence in the motor-learning literature that random practice in the training of novel limb movements in unimpaired individuals produces greater retention of a skill rather than blocked practice (Schmidt & Lee, 1999). Blocked practice has been found to increase the rate of acquisition of a new skill, but does not serve to enhance retention and transfer of the novel skill (Schmidt & Lee, 1999). Only one investigation has applied these motor-learning principles to the treatment of speakers with AOS. Knock and colleagues (Knock, Ballard, Robin, & Schmidt, 2000) conducted a single-participant alternating-treatment study utilising blocked and random practice with two speakers with severe AOS. Findings revealed increased accuracy in the production of treatment stimuli in the random condition post treatment for both speakers, but with no generalisation to untrained items. This is one of the first investigations to systematically examine the influence of principles of motor learning, and findings suggest these principles may have value in the treatment of speakers with AOS. The present investigation did not involve treatment on experimental stimuli, but speakers produced stimulus items under blocked and random conditions at each of the three sampling times over a short span of time (a week). However, it appears random practice of this nature did not facilitate performance in terms of speech production accuracy for the individuals in this investigation.

## Predominant error type by sound

Distortions were found to be the predominant error type for the majority of target sounds. This finding is consistent with previous research by Odell and colleagues (1990) with speakers with pure AOS. Although the participants in this investigation presented with AOS and aphasia, a large portion (61–71%) of their speech sound errors in both conditions of stimulus presentation appeared to be motoric in nature. It is hypothesised that distortions reflect problems in motor planning involving deficits in recalling or adapting movement as well as monitoring or maintaining parameters of movements in speakers with AOS based on schema theory as it is applied to AOS (Ballard, Grainer, & Robin, 2000) as well as a model of speech production proposed by Van der Merwe (2008). Distortion errors are therefore considered to be the result of disrupted spatial and temporal parameters for the intended target phoneme in speakers with AOS. A comparison of the number of error types produced by the group in both conditions across the three sampling times found no apparent pattern of responding by the group in either condition for target phonemes. That is, condition of elicitation did not appear to influence the variability of error type for any given sound.

Findings revealed that speakers tended to exhibit a dominant error type for phonemes more frequently in error. When a low number of errors were produced for a phoneme, no predominant error type emerged among speakers. However, as the percentage of errors increased across target phonemes, a greater number of speakers tended to produce a dominant error type across conditions and sampling times. These findings uncovered a fewer number of different error types were produced for a phoneme more frequently in error as hypothesised, and are comparable to findings by Wambaugh et al. (2004). Findings by Wambaugh and colleagues also revealed a pattern of responding in the blocked condition, with a limited number of error types produced for a speaker with AOS and aphasia. However, contrary to hypothesised results, the present investigation did not reveal any pattern of performance due to conditions of stimulus presentation.

The findings from this investigation revealed greater consistency in speech sound errors for the group regardless of conditions of stimulus presentation or sampling time. It appears there was a predictable pattern of sounds errors uncovered for the group based on target phonemes. The majority of errors were motoric in nature, although speakers presented with concomitant aphasia. Findings are similar to research by McNeil et al. (1995) with "pure" AOS speakers, which uncovered errors that were invariable in type across consecutive word productions as well as predictable pattern of errors associated with different phonemes in speakers with AOS and aphasia across repeated sampling times (Mauszycki et al., 2007; Shuster & Wambaugh, 2000; Wambaugh et al., 2004). One possible explanation for differing results between more recent research findings and early AOS research examining sound errors is methods of analysis (i.e., narrow vs broad transcription). Without the use of narrow phonetics in the current investigation, the bulk of sound errors (i.e., primarily distortions) would have been missed and the results could have resembled early AOS findings (i.e., greater variability in speech sound errors). From a clinical perspective, blocked and random conditions did not facilitate a pattern of performance for sound errors for these individuals with AOS. However, narrow transcription provided more detailed articulatory information, which would have been missed with broad phonetic transcription. Clinically, narrow phonetic transcription should be employed in the assessment of speakers with AOS, otherwise assessment findings could provide a misleading clinical picture in terms of selecting a treatment approach (i.e., sound-specific treatment approach vs non-sound-specific treatment approach).

This was the first study to analyse the group performance of 11 individuals with AOS and aphasia across sampling times. This investigation focused on monosyllabic words with target phonemes in the initial word position that were selected for analysis due to previous research identifying patterns of errors associated with different phonemes (Mauszycki et al., 2007; Shuster & Wambaugh, 2000; Wambaugh et al., 2004). Generalisation of findings from the current study are restricted to the phonemes studied and cannot be generalised to phonemes not studied. However, additional information could be gathered regarding performance for the group as well as individual speakers by analysing all phonemes from each exemplar. Another issue related to generalisation is the nature of the speaking task (i.e., controlled speaking task) employed to elicit stimuli. Certainly, external validity is limited in terms of generalisation to other speaking tasks; however, the methods utilised are similar to tasks that would be used in a clinical setting for evaluation and treatment of speakers with AOS and aphasia.

Despite these limitations, this investigation provided subtle articulatory detail via narrow phonetic transcription that would otherwise have been overlooked. Subsequent research examining additional phonemes (i.e., target phoneme or each phoneme in tokens) in a variety of stimuli (e.g., words with a varying number of syllables) would be useful in gaining a better understanding of nature of AOS with concomitant aphasia. Future research should include examination of both group and individual performance of speakers with AOS by combined methods of analysis (i.e., narrow phonetic transcription combined with acoustic or physiologic methods) to provide additional information regarding motor control during speech tasks.

Manuscript received 23 July 2009
Manuscript accepted 25 October 2009

# REFERENCES

Aichert, I., & Ziegler, W. (2004). Syllable frequency and syllable structure in apraxia of speech. *Brain and Language*, *88*, 148–159.

Ballard, K. J., Grainer, J. P., & Robin, D. A. (2000). Understanding the nature of apraxia of speech: Theory, analysis, and treatment. *Aphasiology*, *14*(10), 969–995.

Croot, K. (2002). Diagnosis of AOS: Definition and criteria. *Seminars in Speech and Language*, *23*(4), 267–279.

Dabul, B. (2000). *Apraxia Battery for Adults-2*. Austin, TX: Pro-Ed.

Deal, J. L., & Darley, F. L. (1972). The influence of linguistic and situation variables on phonemic accuracy in apraxia of speech. *Journal of Speech and Hearing Research*, *15*, 639–653.

Duffy, J. R. (2005). *Motor speech disorders: Substrates, differential diagnosis, and management* (2nd ed.). St. Louis, MO: Elsevier Mosby.

Haley, K., & Gottardy, G. (2007). *Variability considerations for word intelligibility testing in aphasia and apraxia of speech*. Presentation at the annual Clinical Aphasiology Conference, Scottsdale, AZ.

Haley, K. L., Wertz, R. T., & Ohde, R.N. (1998). Single word intelligibility in aphasia and apraxia of speech. *Aphasiology*, *12*(7, 8), 715–730.

Johns, D. F., & Darley, F. L. (1970). Phonemic variability in apraxia of speech. *Journal of Speech and Hearing Research*, *13*, 556–583.

Jones, D. (2003). *Cambridge English pronouncing dictionary* (16th ed., P. Roach, J. Hartman, & J. Setter, Eds.). Cambridge, UK: Cambridge University Press.

Kertesz, A. (1982). *The Western Aphasia Battery*. New York: Grune & Stratton.

Knock, T. R., Ballard, K. J., Robin, D. A., & Schmidt, R. A. (2000). Influence of order of stimulus presentation on speech motor learning: A principled approach to treatment for apraxia of speech. *Aphasiology*, *14*(5, 6), 653–668.

LaPointe, L. L., & Horner, J. (1976). Repeated trials of words by patients with neurogenic phonological selection-sequencing impairment (apraxia of speech). *Clinical Aphasiology*, *6*, 261–277.

LaPointe, L. L., & Johns, D. F. (1975). Some phonemic characteristics of apraxia of speech. *Journal of Communication Disorders*, *8*, 259–269.

Mauszycki, S. C., Dromey, C., & Wambaugh, J. L. (2007). Variability in apraxia of speech: A perceptual, acoustic and kinematic analysis of stop consonants. *Journal of Medical Speech-Language Pathology*, *15*, 223–242.

Mauszycki, S. C., & Wambaugh, J. L. (2006). Perceptual analysis of consonant production in multisyllabic words in apraxia of speech: A comparison across repeated sampling times. *Journal of Medical Speech-Language Pathology*, *14*, 263–267.

McNeil, M. R., Odell, K., Miller, S. B., & Hunter, L. (1995). Consistency, variability, and target approximation for successive speech repetitions among apraxic, conduction aphasic, and ataxic dysarthria speakers. *Clinical Aphasiology*, *23*, 39–55.

McNeil, M. R., Robin, D. A., & Schmidt, R. A. (2008). Apraxia of speech: Definition, differentiation, and treatment. In M. R. McNeil (Ed.), *Clinical management of sensorimotor speech disorders* (2nd ed., pp. 249–268). New York: Thieme.

Mines, M., Hanson, B., & Shoup, J. (1978). Frequency of occurrence of phonemes in conversational English. *Language and Speech*, *21*, 221–241.

Nicholas, L. E., & Brookshire, R. H. (1993). A system for quantifying the informativeness and efficiency of the connected speech of adults with aphasia. *Journal of Speech and Hearing Research*, *36*, 338–350.

Odell, K., McNeil, M. R., Rosenbek, J. C., & Hunter, L. (1990). Perceptual characteristics of consonant production by apraxic speakers. *Journal of Speech and Hearing Disorders*, *55*, 345–359.

Odell, K., McNeil, M. R., Rosenbek, J. C., & Hunter, L. (1991). Perceptual characteristics of vowel and prosody production by apraxic, aphasic and dysarthric speakers. *Journal of Speech and Hearing Research*, *34*, 67–80.

Raven, J., Raven, J. C., & Court, J. H. (1998). *Coloured Progressive Matrices*. Oxford, UK: Oxford Psychologist Press, Ltd.

Schmidt, R. A. (1975). A schema theory of discrete motor learning. *Psychological Review*, *82*, 255–260.

Schmidt, R. A., & Lee, T. D. (1999). *Motor control and learning: A behavioral emphasis* (3rd ed.). Champaign, IL: Human Kinetics.

Shriberg, L., Kwiatkowski, J., & Hoffman, K. (1984). A procedure for phonetic transcription by consensus. *Journal of Speech and Hearing Disorders*, *51*, 309–324.

Shriberg, L. D., & Kent, R. D. (2003). *Clinical phonetics* (3rd ed.). Boston: Allyn & Bacon.

Shuster, L., & Wambaugh, J. L. (2000). Perceptual and acoustic analysis of speech sound errors in apraxia of speech accompanied by aphasia. *Aphasiology*, *14*(5, 6), 635–651.

Shuster, L., & Wambaugh, J. L. (2003). *Consistency of speech sound errors in apraxia of speech accompanied by aphasia*. Presentation at the annual Clinical Aphasiology Conference, Orcas Island, WA.

Skenes, L. L., & Trullinger, R. W. (1988). Error patterns during repetition of consonant-vowel-consonant syllables by apraxic speakers. *Journal of Communication Disorders*, *21*(3), 263–269.

Van der Merwe, A. (2008). A theoretical framework for the characterisation of pathological speech sensorimotor control. In M.R. McNeil (Ed.), *Clinical management of sensorimotor speech disorders* (2nd ed., pp. 3–29). New York: Thieme.

Wambaugh, J. L., Duffy, J. R., McNeil, M. R., Robin, D. A., & Rogers, M. (2006). Treatment guidelines for acquired apraxia of speech: A synthesis and evaluation of the evidence. *Journal of Medical Speech-Language Pathology*, *14*(2), xv–xxxiii.

Wambaugh, J. L., Nessler, C., Bennett, J., & Mauszycki, S. C. (2004). Variability in apraxia of speech: A perceptual and VOT analysis of stop consonants. *Journal of Medical Speech-Language Pathology*, *12*, 221–227.

Wertz, R. T., LaPointe, L. L., & Rosenbek, J. C. (1984). *Apraxia of speech in adults: The disorder and its management*. Orlando, FL: Grune & Stratton.

Yorkston, K. M., & Beukelman, D. R. (1981). *Assessment of intelligibility of dysarthric speech*. Austin: Pro-Ed.

APHASIOLOGY, 2010, 24 (6–8), 856–868

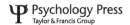

# Automated analysis of the Cinderella story

Brian MacWhinney and Davida Fromm

*Carnegie Mellon University, Pittsburgh, PA, USA*

Audrey Holland

*University of Arizona, Tucson, AZ, USA*

Margaret Forbes

*Carnegie Mellon University, Pittsburgh, PA, USA*

Heather Wright

*Arizona State University, Tempe, AZ, USA*

*Background*: AphasiaBank is a collaborative project whose goal is to develop an archival database of the discourse of individuals with aphasia. Along with databases on first language acquisition, classroom discourse, second language acquisition, and other topics, it forms a component of the general TalkBank database. It uses tools from the wider system that are further adapted to the particular goal of studying language use in aphasia.
*Aims*: The goal of this paper is to illustrate how TalkBank analytic tools can be applied to AphasiaBank data.
*Methods &Procedures*: Both aphasic (*n* = 24) and non-aphasic (*n* = 25) participants completed a 1-hour standardised videotaped data elicitation protocol. These sessions were transcribed and tagged automatically for part of speech. One component of the larger protocol was the telling of the Cinderella story. For these narratives we compared lexical diversity across the groups and computed the top 10 nouns and verbs across both groups. We then examined the profiles for two participants in greater detail.
*Conclusions*: Using these tools we showed that, in a story-retelling task, aphasic speakers had a marked reduction in lexical diversity and a greater use of light verbs. For example, aphasic speakers often substituted "girl" for "stepsister" and "go" for "disappear". These findings illustrate how it is possible to use TalkBank tools to analyse AphasiaBank data.

*Keywords:* Lexicon; Narrative; Computer analysis.

In 2005, a group of 25 aphasiologists met to organise a proposal for a shared database on aphasia. This database was configured to operate within the framework of the larger TalkBank system that provides methods for studying a variety of language types, including child language development (childes.psy.cmu.edu), second language learning (talkbank.org/BilingBank), conversation analysis (talkbank.org/CABank),

Address correspondence to: Brian MacWhinney, Carnegie Mellon University, Department of Psychology, 5000 Forbes Avenue, Pittsburgh, Pennsylvania 15213, USA. E-mail: macw@cmu.edu

This project is funded by NIH_NIDCD grant R01-DC008524 (2007–2012).

http://www.psypress.com/aphasiology     DOI: 10.1080/02687030903452632

phonological development (childes.psy.cmu.edu/PhonBank), legal discourse (talkbank. org/Meeting/SCOTUS), classroom discourse (talkbank.org/ClassBank), and others. The overall goal of TalkBank is to construct a shared database of multimedia data on human communication. Within the larger project, AphasiaBank focuses on the construction of a structured database that will permit the evaluation of individual differences and treatment effects in aphasia. Funding for the development of Aphasia-Bank was provided by NIDCD and work has been progressing on the construction of this database since 2007.

AphasiaBank collects and analyses video and audiotaped samples of the discourse of aphasic and non-aphasic participants across a wide range of tasks. One aim of AphasiaBank is to assist in the improvement of treatment for aphasia. To accomplish this, it is necessary to solidify the empirical database supporting our understanding of communication in aphasia. The eight specific aims of AphasiaBank include: protocol standardisation, database development, analysis customisation, measure development, syndrome classification, qualitative analysis, development of recovery process profiles, and evaluation of treatment effects. To advance these goals, an additional group meeting was held to formalise a shared protocol that is now available at http://talkbank.org/AphasiaBank. This protocol includes two free speech elicitation tasks, four picture description tasks, one story narrative (Cinderella), and one procedural discourse task. In addition there is a repetition test, a verb naming test (Thompson, 2010), and the Boston Naming Test (Kaplan, Goodglass, & Weintraub, 2001). All of these tasks and tests are recorded using high-definition video and transcribed in the CHAT format (MacWhinney, 2000), with specific extensions for aphasic language. The transcripts and videos, which are password protected, can be accessed and downloaded by consortium members. Because each utterance in the transcripts is directly linked to the audio, it is possible to replay transcripts and follow along using continuous playback both over the web and locally. Participant information includes scores on the Western Aphasia Battery (WAB; Kertesz, 2007), clinical reports, and 54 demographic variables.

In this paper we focus on just one segment of this larger protocol: the telling of the Cinderella story. Within this segment we further constrain our focus to the study of patterns of lexical use in these narratives. The purpose of this paper is to provide an illustration of how one can examine substantive issues in aphasiology using this database and the CLAN programs (MacWhinney, 2000) for data analysis.

The Cinderella story has frequently been used in aphasia research (Faroqi-Shah & Thompson, 2007; Rochon, Saffran, Berndt, & Schwartz, 2000; Stark & Viola, 2007; Thompson, Ballard, Tait, Weintraub, & Mesulam, 1997). Both Berndt, Wayland, Rochon, Saffran, and Schwartz (2000) and Thompson et al. (1997) have developed general systems for scoring narrative productions that have been applied to the Cinderella transcripts of individuals with aphasia. The Cinderella story was included in the AphasiaBank protocol primarily because of its demonstrated utility, and because of its general familiarity in Western cultures. However, a surprising oversight in past research has been the lack of a non-aphasic standard for comparison. Without a baseline for how non-aphasic speakers narrate Cinderella, it is difficult to understand how measures of severity relate to normal expectations, and to evaluate the extent to which aphasic speakers can recover function.

The various analyses of production in the Cinderella task have focused primarily on the construction of measures of morphosyntactic control. These measures include a wide diversity of counts of grammatical structures, inflectional processes, and sentence patterns. However, with the exception of a recent analysis by Gordon (2008), there has been relatively little attention to the analysis of the use of specific lexical items that play a role within the story of Cinderella. The study of lexical patterns in narrative has been a core topic in language acquisition studies (Malvern, Richards, Chipere, & Purán, 2004; Snow, Tabors, Nicholson, & Kurland, 1995; Tingley, Berko Gleason, & Hooshyar, 1994). Many of the methods for studying lexical patterns from this research tradition can be applied directly to the study of lexical usage in participants with aphasia. In order to take a closer look at the patterns of lexical usage in this task, we implemented a method that allowed us to contrast the patterns of lexical usage of normal participants with those of aphasic participants.

## METHOD

The elicitation of the Cinderella story used the following procedure. First, participants were asked if they remembered the story of Cinderella. Then they were given a 25-page Cinderella picture book (Grimes, 2005). The text on each page of the book was covered with white duct tape to make it impossible to read. Participants paged through the book at their own pace, looking at each picture. Then the book was removed and participants were asked to tell the story of Cinderella in their own words. There was no time limit placed on their story telling. The investigator refrained from making any comments at all during the story telling. All of the productions were videotaped with audio recording that used a separate sound system.

### Participants

Aphasic participants were recruited from the Adler Aphasia Center in Maywood, New Jersey, and from various venues in Tucson, Arizona, and non-aphasic participants all came from an ongoing study of normal discourse under the direction of one of the authors (HW). The aetiology for aphasia was stroke in all cases but one, which was a gunshot wound. All had been aphasic for a minimum of 6 months and a maximum of 16 years. The non-aphasic participants were screened for memory impairment (Folstein, Folstein, & Fanjiang, 2002), mood disorders, and history of stroke or other neurological conditions. The mean ages of the two groups were not significantly different. All participants had vision and hearing adequate for testing and were native speakers of standard American English. The criteria for inclusion of participants in AphasiaBank are at http://talkbank.org/AphasiaBank/inclusion.doc. Table 1 summarises demographic and other information on participant characteristics. The four participants with residual anomia tested above the cutoff on the WAB, but continued to experience and demonstrate word-finding difficulties.

### Transcription

The Cinderella narratives were transcribed in the CHAT transcription format (MacWhinney, 2000). CHAT is a transcription format that has been developed over the last 30 years for use in a variety of disciplines, including first language acquisition, second language acquisition, classroom discourse, conversation analysis, etc. The CHAT transcription format is designed to operate closely with a set of programs called CLAN, which is also described in MacWhinney (2000). The CLAN programs

TABLE 1
Participant characteristics

|  | Non-aphasic participants (n = 25) | Aphasic participants (n = 24) |
|---|---|---|
| Age range (yrs) | 23–80 (mean = 58) | 30–80 (mean = 64) |
| Gender | 16 females, 9 males | 8 females, 16 males |
| Handedness | right = 23 | right = 21 |
|  | left = 1 | left = 3 |
|  | ambidextrous = 1 |  |
| Education range (yrs) | 12–20 (mean = 15) | 12–25 (mean = 16) |
| WAB aphasia type |  | Anomic = 7 |
|  |  | Residual Anomia = 4 |
|  |  | Conduction = 6 |
|  |  | Broca = 3 |
|  |  | Wernicke = 3 |
|  |  | Transcortical Motor = 1 |

permit the analysis of a wide range of linguistic and discourse structures. Transcription in CHAT is facilitated by a method called Walker Controller, which allows the transcriber to continually replay the original audio record. This method is built into the CLAN program (MacWhinney, 2000) and the editing of transcripts relies on the CLAN editor facility. One direct result of this process is that each utterance is then linked to a specific region of the audio or video record. This linkage can be useful for verification of transcription accuracy and for later phonological, gestural, or conversational analysis. A second highly trained transcriber checked over the accuracy of each transcription and the two transcribers reached complete agreement on all features of the coding and transcription. Table 2 is a sample Cinderella story from participant Adler06a. This sample is a segment of a much larger transcript for the entire 1-hour interview.

The transcript includes various word-level error codes (e.g., [* wu] which indicates that the error is a real word and that the intended word is unknown) and utterance-level codes (e.g., [+ jar] for jargon) developed specifically for typical aphasic

TABLE 2
Cinderella CHAT transcript

@G: Cinderella
*PAR: &uh a little bit I think, yeah.
*PAR: was [//] what was the name ?
*PAR: Secerundid [: Cinderella] [* nk].
*PAR: she was &uh &b angel for legwood@n. [+ jar]
*PAR: she was &uh &f for fendle@n for someone else. [+ jar]
*PAR: the other children [/] &r &d children for her are three children or whatever . [+ es]
*PAR: with her it was very closed [* wu] walking [* wu] in generalis@n . [+ jar]
*PAR: &th &th &p pezzels@n are going for the party.
*PAR: and she was &f fen@n people [* wu] for prezzled@n (.) for the present [* wu]. [+ jar]
*PAR: the present &t (...) was s(up)posed to be &uh thirty [/] &t &uh thirty or something. [+ es]
*PAR: she &ch &er had a ranned@n from home she &ha huddled [* wu]. [+ jar]
*PAR: the &uh (..) people were +//.
*PAR: they found her letter.
*PAR: and <the pezzes@n> [//] &w the other people wed [* wu] they found her.
*PAR: found her for the prezzled@n and the calls this one so. [+ jar]

TABLE 3
Cinderella CHAT transcript with %mor line included

@G: Cinderella
*PAR: &uh a little bit I think, yeah .
%mor: det|a adj|little n|bit pro|I v|think co|yeah .
*PAR: was [//] what was the name ?
%mor: pro:wh|what v:cop|be&PAST&13S det|the n|name ?
*PAR: Secerundid [: Cinderella] [* nk] .
%mor: n:prop|Cinderella .
*PAR: she was &uh &b angel for legwood@n . [+ jar]
%mor: pro|she v:cop|be&PAST&13S n|angel prep|for neo|legwood .
*PAR: she was &uh &f for fendle@n for someone else . [+ jar]
%mor: pro|she v:cop|be&PAST&13S prep|for neo|fendle prep|for pro:indef|someone post|else .
*PAR: the other children [/] &r &d children for her are three children or whatever . [+ es]
%mor: det|the qn|other n|child&PL prep|for pro|her v:cop|be&PRES det:num|three n|child&PL
      conj:coo|or pro:wh|whatever .
*PAR: with her it was very closed [* wu] walking [* wu] in generalis@n . [+ jar]
%mor: prep|with pro|her pro|it v:cop|be&PAST&13S adv:int|very part|close-PERF
      part|walk-PROG prep|in neo|generalis .
*PAR: &th &th &p pezzels@n are going for the party .
%mor: neo|pezzels aux|be&PRES part|go-PROG prep|for det|the n|party .
*PAR: and she was &f fen@n people [* wu] for prezzled@n (.) for the present [* wu] . [+ jar]
%mor: conj:coo|and pro|she v:cop|be&PAST&13S neo|fen n|person&PL prep|for neo|prezzled
      prep|for det|the n|present .
*PAR: the present &t (.).was s(up)posed to be &uh thirty [/] &t &uh thirty or something . [+ es]
%mor: det|the n|present v:cop|be&PAST&13S adj|supposed inf|to v:cop|be det:num|thirty
      conj:coo|or pro:indef|something .
*PAR: she &ch &er had a ranned@n from home she &ha huddled [* wu] . [+ jar]
%mor: pro|she v|have&PAST det|a neo|ranned prep|from n|home pro|she v|huddle-PAST .
*PAR: the &uh (..) people were +//.
%mor: det|the n|person&PL v:cop|be&PAST +//.
*PAR: they found her letter .
%mor: pro|they v|find&PAST pro:poss:det|her n|letter .
*PAR: and <the pezzes@n> [//] &w the other people wed [* wu] they found her .
%mor: conj:coo|and det|the qn|other n|person&PL v|wed pro|they v|find&PAST pro|her .
*PAR: found her for the prezzled@n and the calls this one so . [+ jar]
%mor: v|find&PAST pro|her prep|for det|the neo|prezzled conj:coo|and det|the
      n|call-PL det|this pro:indef|one conj:subor|so .

language characteristics. It also includes conventional markings used by the CHAT
program for repetitions ([/]), revisions ([//]), word fragments and fillers (&), replace-
ments ([: *intended word*]), and pauses (.). The AphasiaBank website has links to a
two-page sheet summarising guidelines for transcription, an error-coding document,
a more detailed transcription training manual, and the complete CHAT and CLAN
manuals.

The sample given in Table 2 is given again in fuller form in Table 3. The difference
between Table 2 and Table 3 is that the latter includes additional material regarding
part of speech tagging on the %mor line. This line gives the part of speech for each
word and then provides a complete lexical analysis of the word into prefixes, stems,
suffixes and clitics. It also marks whether inflectional categories are transparently
analytic (as in English –ing) or fusional (as in many irregular forms), and it analyses
compounds into the parts of speech of their components.

Computation of the %mor line can be done automatically, using the MOR program (Parisse & Le Normand, 2000; Sagae, Davis, Lavie, MacWhinney, & Wintner, 2007) which is included as a part of CLAN. The reader can verify that, in this example passage, all of the tags are accurate, with the exception of the last word of the last sentence that should have been tagged as an adverb. Overall, the accuracy of MOR tagging for AphasiaBank transcripts is above 98%. Although the tagger was trained on material derived from normal adult productions, it performs remarkably well at the task of tagging aphasic language.

## RESULTS

To study the relative frequency of lexical items within the Cinderella story-telling task, we used a series of commands from the CLAN programs. CLAN is a single application that works on both Windows and Mac OS X (it can be downloaded from childes.psy.cmu.edu/clan). The program includes a text editor with various transcription and playback functions. There is also a commands window into which the user can type single-line commands for data analysis. The analyses presented here depend primarily on the use of these commands. In order to pull out the Cinderella story segments from the larger transcripts, we used the CLAN command called GEM. This command relies on the presence of an @G marker of the type that can be seen in the first line of Table 2 and Table 3. The specific form of the GEM command that we used was:

gem +sCinderella +t∗PAR +n +d1 +f ∗.cha

Figure 1 illustrates how this command was typed into the CLAN commands window. The result of the use of this command was a file that contained the material in Table 2. We extracted files of this type for each of our 24 aphasic and 25 non-aphasic transcripts.

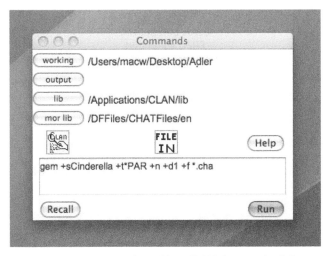

**Figure 1.** GEM command typed into CLAN Commands window.

## LEXICAL FREQUENCY ANALYSIS

To construct a lexical frequency analysis, we used the FREQ command to compute the frequencies of word form occurrences on the %mor line for each of the two folders of transcripts. The command for this was:

freq +t%mor  t* +s@r-*,o-% +u +o +fS *.gem.cex

This command has eight segments. The meanings of each are as follows:

| | |
|---|---|
| freq | this calls up the FREQ command |
| +t%mor | this includes information from the %mor line |
| –t* | this excludes any information on the main line |
| +s@r-*,o-% | find all stems and ignore all other markers |
| +u | merge all specified files together |
| +o | sort output by descending frequency |
| +fS | send output to file |
| *.gem.cex | run the command on all of the files with the .gem.cex extension |

Table 4 shows the first lines of the output with the highest-frequency words in the stories from individuals with aphasia. This analysis is based on tallies of the intended word. Analyses of errors are beyond the scope of the current paper.

A similar analysis was computed for the non-aphasic speakers. Non-aphasic speakers generated 839 different word types and a cumulative total of 13,309 tokens; participants with aphasia generated 526 word types and a cumulative 5330 tokens. Table 5 summarises these findings and provides type token ratios, their ranges and means.

Examination of the word totals showed that, for each group, roughly 1/3 of the words occurred only once, another 1/3 from two to four times, with the remaining 1/3 occurring five times or more. Although this wide range of lexical diversity is of interest in itself, the core ideas of the Cinderella story appear to be captured in the 306 words that occurred at least five times in the non-aphasic sample. These words included

TABLE 4
CLAN output from
FREQ command

489 and
323 the
300 be
170 she
133 to
118 it
116 a
106 they
97 go
93 I
80 Cinderella
80 not
78 do
75 her
69 he

TABLE 5
TTR results

|  | Non-aphasic speakers (n = 25) | Aphasic speakers (n = 24) |
|---|---|---|
| Total # of different word types used | 839 | 526 |
| Total # of tokens | 13302 | 5539 |
| TTR – mean # of types | 165.2 | 77.54 |
| range | 68–329 | 21–155 |
| TTR – mean # of tokens | 532.26 | 222.45 |
| range | 123–1347 | 38–705 |
| TTR – mean | .35 | .41 |
| range | .24–.56 | .17–.72 |

TABLE 6
The 10 most frequent nouns for the two groups

| Non-aphasic speakers (n = 25) | Aphasic speakers (n = 24) |
|---|---|
| Cinderella | Cinderella |
| ball | girl |
| prince | ball |
| slipper | prince |
| mother, stepmother | mother, stepmother |
| dress | home |
| daughter, stepdaughter | man |
| fairy | slipper |
| godmother | shoe |
| sister, stepsister | sister, stepsister |

nouns, verbs, adjectives, and adverbs. For purposes of this paper, we are considering only the nouns and verbs of the non-aphasic sample as constituting a target lexicon for the Cinderella data. This initial lexicon is given in the Appendix. It is the lexicon against which the stories of the participants with aphasia will be compared.

Table 5 has already alerted readers to the comparative paucity of aphasic tokens and types, and the analysis of the aphasic narratives also presents no big surprises. As a group, speakers with aphasia provided only 2/3 as many different word types as did the non-aphasic speakers, with less than half the number of tokens. As can be seen in the Appendix, 80 nouns and 71 verbs were used at least five times by non-aphasic speakers. In comparison, speakers with aphasia used 34 nouns and 36 verbs five times or more, reflecting the far more restrictive lexical diversity imposed by aphasia. Nevertheless, 76% the nouns they did use also appeared in the non-aphasic lexicon.

Tables 6 and 7 present the 10 most frequently occurring nouns and verbs in the non-aphasic lexicon and the aphasic comparison. Interestingly, the most frequently occurring nouns in both the non-aphasic and the aphasic samples have six words in common. The aphasic stories included the words *man, shoe, girl,* and *home,* which are not as tightly and specifically linked to the Cinderella story, as are the words *dress, fairy, stepdaughter,* and *godmother* that appear in the non-aphasic top 10. Nevertheless, read aloud, both noun lists sound almost like an agrammatic synopsis of the Cinderella plot. It is also of interest that none of the most frequent nouns in the non-aphasic transcripts contains even a faintly abstract noun. In fact, the entire non-aphasic lexicon has only a few nouns that could possibly be construed as abstract (*love, life, course*).

TABLE 7
The 10 most frequent verbs for the two groups

| Non-aphasic speakers (n = 25) | Aphasic speakers (n = 24) |
|---|---|
| be | be |
| go | go |
| have | do |
| get | have |
| come | get |
| do | say |
| say | know |
| try | find |
| marry, remarry | work |
| know | come |

Verbs (see Table 7) are equally interesting. There are 7 verbs in common among the "top 10", and all 33 verbs used by speakers with aphasia were found in the non-aphasic lexicon. Gordon (2008) tracked the usage of 11 light verbs (*be, have, come, go, give, take, make, do, get, move*, and *put*). All of these, with the exception of *move* and *get*, occurred in the aphasic sample, whereas only six of them appeared in the non-aphasic lexicon. The fact that the non-aphasic verb lexicon was more than twice as large as the sample provided by speakers with aphasia supports the argument that speakers with aphasia are in general more reliant on light verbs, showing more limited diversity for verbs. It is important to remember that this sample of speakers with aphasia has only a few individuals with Broca aphasia and many more with anomic and conduction aphasia.

## Error analysis

This analysis of the Cinderella lexicon has focused on the semantics of the words in the story. We also used CHAT codes to track neologisms and paraphasias (although the analysis of these error patterns is outside our current scope, a description of AphasiaBank error coding categories can be found at http://talkbank.org/AphasiaBank/errors.doc). However, it may be interesting to consider just a simple example of how these errors can be tracked using CLAN commands. Specifically, the following command was used to trace variant forms of production of the word *Cinderella*:

freq + s"Cinderella" + t* PAR + u*gem.cex

This command tracks both correct uses of *Cinderella* and uses of incorrect forms with the replacement code [: Cinderella] when the intended target was *Cinderella*. The results included paraphasic errors such as: *Cinderenella, Cinderlella, Cilawella, Cilawilla and Cilawillipa* and the example in line 4 of Table 2, *Secerundid*.

## Example applications

What might be the value of lexical analysis for the study of aphasic language? At present, the analysis of discourse is largely descriptive and largely dependent on features of the discourse that are of theoretical interest to the researcher. Carefully constructed lexicons of discourse samples in measures that have general use, such the Cinderella story, would make it possible to assess the severity of an individual's discourse processing deficits in a standardised way. Knowing how much and in what ways an aphasic individual's discourse performance differs from those of non-aphasic speakers on a given task could provide a real-world approach to assessment and provide guidelines and targets for treatment. For example, the simple illustration explicated here might suggest that work on developing more precise expressions for light verbs could be beneficial both in extending a linguistic repertoire, and for moving an individual closer to normal language usage. But, more generally, what would we learn from comparing a discourse sample from a speaker with aphasia to a very well-developed narrative lexicon?

To illustrate the application of these findings, we will take a closer look at the Cinderella lexicons for two speakers with aphasia. Speaker 1 has severe Wernicke's aphasia as a result of his stroke, (WAB AQ = 28.2). He is 4 years post-onset of his aphasia, and has received both individual and group therapy since that time. Speaker 2, although scoring above the WAB cut-off for aphasia, has persistent mild word-finding problems. He also displays many hesitancies and false starts of the type that characterise speakers with anomia. One of the researchers (ALH) has followed this individual since his stroke approximately 10 years ago. Throughout the decade he has received extensive individual and group treatment, and has made significant progress in rehabilitation. These two fluent speakers represent extremes of the aphasia severity scale, and not only should contrast with each other in their Cinderella narratives, but Speaker 2 should also more closely approximate the non-aphasic speech sample than he does the aphasic sample overall. If there is merit in comparing such individuals to non-aphasic speakers, then their similarities and differences from the normal lexicon should become apparent.

Following the same procedures used to gather the group data for the comparisons presented in Table 2 and 3, these speakers' individual lexicons were extracted from the larger sample. Speaker 1's total speech output was 107 words, representing 59 different word types. Accordingly, his TTR (.55) is considerably higher than the aphasic mean TTR. In fact, Speaker 1 used 42 words of his 107-word narration only once. Largely, this reflects his unfocused and neologistic output. (Table 2 includes a coded sample of his speech.) However, the TTR measure fails to correct for sample size. This problem with TTR is corrected by the VOCD command (Malvern et al., 2004). Using the version of VOCD built into CLAN, we found that his lexical diversity score was 45.95. However, seven of his "words" were in fact neologisms for which no clear referent could be identified. Only three nouns (*Cinderella, home, party*) and three verbs (*go, have, think*) appear in the non-aphasic lexicon.

In contrast, Speaker 2's narrative was both longer and much more clearly related to the lexicon of the non-aphasic speakers. It included 96 word types and 263 tokens, with a resultant TTR of .36 and lexical density of 31.11, almost precisely the non-aphasic mean for TTR and lexical density. Even though his narrative was relatively brief, it provided a substantially correct summary of the Cinderella story. (It is interesting to note that it also contained words that were not in the non-aphasic lexicon at all, but were used appropriately. These included *lowly, envious*, and *smitten*.)

## DISCUSSION

The purpose of this paper has been to introduce readers to the value of developing an archival database for aphasic language for both research and teaching purposes. This analysis illustrated the use of a few of the many analytic tools available through AphasiaBank and how they might be applied to the development of a lexicon for a narrative task that has been used frequently in aphasia research.

Eventually, the AphasiaBank database will support a much broader set of research and clinical applications. Narrative tasks of this type can be repeated across months or years to study the course of recovery from aphasia. Or we may consider the value of pre- and post-treatment samples to measure the effects of some specified treatment on lessening the impairment of aphasia. In related work, we have also developed auto-mated methods (Sagae et al., 2007) to analyse and evaluate syntax in aphasia.

These are big questions but there are smaller, but no less interesting, questions that can be asked of the AphasiaBank database. For example, what are the attributes of neologistic errors of speakers with aphasia that permit listeners to grasp its mean-ing? Are they phonologic or contextual? Do they depend on shared knowledge or are they independent of it? It is not the purview of this paper to provide a laundry list of such questions but merely to suggest that the AphasiaBank database can be used to explore many issues such as these.

Manuscript received 21 July 2009
Manuscript accepted 29 October 2009
First published online 20 April 2010

## REFERENCES

Berndt, R., Wayland, S., Rochon, E., Saffran, E., & Schwartz, M. (2000). *Quantitative production analysis: A training manual for the analysis of aphasic sentence production.* Hove, UK: Psychology Press.

Faroqi-Shah, Y., & Thompson, C. K. (2007). Verb inflections in agrammatic aphasia: Encoding of tense features. *Journal of Memory and Language, 56,* 129–151.

Folstein, M., Folstein, S., & Fanjiang, G. (2002). *Mini-mental State Examination.* Lutz, FL: Psychological Assessment Resources, Inc.

Gordon, J. (2008). Measuring the lexical semantics of picture description in aphasia. *Aphasiology, 22,* 839–852.

Grimes, N. (2005). *Walt Disney's Cinderella.* New York: Random House.

Kaplan, E., Goodglass, H., & Weintraub, S. (2001). *Boston Naming Test* (2nd ed.). Austin, TX: Pro-Ed.

Kertesz, A. (2007). *Western Aphasia Battery Revised.* San Antonio, TX: Psychological Corporation.

MacWhinney, B. (2000). *The CHILDES Project: Tools for Analysing Talk* (3rd ed.). Mahwah, NJ: Lawrence Erlbaum Associates Inc.

Malvern, D. D., Richards, B. J., Chipere, N., & Purán, P. (2004). *Lexical diversity and language develop-ment.* New York: Palgrave Macmillan.

Parisse, C., & Le Normand, M. T. (2000). Automatic disambiguation of the morphosyntax in spoken language corpora. *Behavior Research Methods, Instruments, and Computers, 32,* 468–481.

Rochon, E., Saffran, E., Berndt, R., & Schwartz, M. (2000). Quantitative analysis of aphasic sentence production: Further development and new data. *Brain and Language, 72,* 193–218.

Sagae, K., Davis, E., Lavie, E., MacWhinney, B., & Wintner, S. (2007). High-accuracy annotation and parsing of CHILDES transcripts. In *Proceedings of the 45th Meeting of the Association for Computa-tional Linguistics.* Prague: ACL.

Snow, C. E., Tabors, P. O., Nicholson, P., & Kurland, B. (1995). SHELL: Oral language and early literacy skills in kindergarten and first-grade children. *Journal of Research in Childhood Education, 10,* 37–48.

Stark, J. A., & Viola, M. S. (2007). Cinderella, Cinderella! Longitudinal analysis of qualitative and quantitative aspects of seven tellings of Cinderella by a Broca's aphasic. *Brain and Language, 103,* 234–235.

Thompson, C. K. (2010). *Northwestern assessment of verbs and sentences – experimental version.* Evanston, IL: Northwestern University Press. Manuscript in preparation.

Thompson, C. K., Ballard, K. J., Tait, M. E., Weintraub, S., & Mesulam, M. (1997). Patterns of language decline in non-fluent primary progressive aphasia. *Aphasiology*, *11*, 297–321.

Tingley, E., Berko Gleason, J., & Hooshyar, N. (1994). Mothers' lexicon of internal state words in speech to children with Down syndrome and to nonhandicapped children at mealtime. *Journal of Communication Disorders*, *27*, 135–156.

# APPENDIX

## Cinderella lexicon of nouns and verbs for non-aphasic participants (in order of decreasing frequency)

*Nouns (n = 80)*

| | | |
|---|---|---|
| Cinderella | horse | life |
| ball | clock | man |
| prince | kingdom | dance |
| slipper | chore | door |
| mother, stepmother | king | end |
| dress | love | footman |
| daughter, stepdaughter | story | princess |
| fairy | wife | gown |
| godmother | castle | hair |
| sister, stepsister | invitation | maid |
| glass | person | night |
| home | servant | room |
| girl | day | dog |
| time | palace | family |
| house | wand | piece |
| pumpkin | Prince Charming | scene |
| midnight | clothes | son |
| mouse | course | step |
| carriage | cat | stroke |
| foot | land | word |
| father | magic | ballroom |
| shoe | party | child, stepchild |
| coach | stair | meantime |
| lady | thing | messenger |
| animal | friend | o'clock |

*Verbs (n = 71)*

| | | |
|---|---|---|
| be | think | see |
| go | appear, disappear, reappear | bring |
| have | strike | give |
| get | send | start |
| come | tell | must |
| do | wear | decide |
| say | excite | fall |
| try | put | pass |
| marry, remarry | realise | talk |
| know | make | want |
| make | let | ask |
| work | like | belong |
| fit | find | hear |
| find | invite | keep |
| see | become | push |
| take | help | sit |
| dance | meet | tear |
| leave | remember | happen |
| run | clean | end |
| lose | fall | happen |
| live | need | mean |
| look | treat | strike |
| turn | cry | |

APHASIOLOGY, 2010, 24 (6–8), 869–886

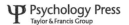

# Implementing and evaluating aphasia therapy targeted at couples' conversations: A single case study

Ray Wilkinson

*University of Manchester, UK*

Karen Bryan

*University of Surrey, Guildford, UK*

Sarah Lock

*Eden Rehabilitation Centre, Cooroy, Queensland, Australia*

Karen Sage

*University of Manchester, UK*

*Background*: In recent years conversation has become an area of interest for aphasia therapy, with several studies using conversation analysis (CA) to target and evaluate therapy. Most of these studies have focused on the main conversation partner of the person with aphasia, and in particular have targeted the partner's pedagogic behaviours in relation to the person with aphasia. Evaluations of therapy have primarily taken the form of qualitative analyses of change in conversational behaviours.
*Aims*: This single-case intervention study aims to advance research into interaction-focused intervention for aphasia in the following ways: by targeting intervention at the person with aphasia and the main conversation partner as a couple; by focusing on conversational behaviours where the person with aphasia can be seen to be restricted by the conversational actions of the conversation partner, in particular by recurrent questioning using closed questions and yes/no interrogatives; and by using a novel combination of qualitative and quantitative approaches to evaluate the intervention.
*Methods & Procedures*: CA was used to target and evaluate interaction-focused intervention for a couple where one partner has aphasia. Evidence for change was evaluated using qualitative and quantitative evidence of change in conversational behaviours; evidence from naïve raters of pre- and post-intervention conversation extracts; and interview/other feedback from the conversation partner.
*Outcomes & Results*: There was evidence that the intervention had changed the couple's conversational behaviours. In particular, the conversational behaviours of the non-aphasic partner were in general less restricting for the person with aphasia in that she was now using fewer questions and more instance of other types of turns, such as paraphrases. Following intervention the person with aphasia had also changed in that he was now producing turns that had more sentences, or attempts at sentences, and which developed the topic of talk across several of his turns.

---

Address correspondence to: Ray Wilkinson, Neuroscience and Aphasia Research Unit (NARU), School of Psychological Sciences, University of Manchester, Zochonis Building, Oxford Road, Manchester M13 9PL, UK. E-mail: ray.wilkinson@manchester.ac.uk

This research was funded by the Tavistock Trust for Aphasia.

http://www.psypress.com/aphasiology                    DOI: 10.1080/02687030903501958

*Conclusions*: The study provides evidence that directly targeting the conversational behaviours of the person with aphasia and/or a main conversational partner can produce positive change, and can achieve this in a way that is ecologically valid. In particular, it highlights the usefulness of targeting conversational behaviours that are proving to be maladaptive for the participants. It provides further evidence that creating change in the non-aphasic partner's conversational behaviour may facilitate change in the person with aphasia's conversational and linguistic performance.

*Keywords:* Aphasia; Therapy; Conversation; Couples.

The ultimate aim of therapy for people with spoken language impairments due to aphasia is to improve their ability to communicate and interact with significant others in daily life. One way in which this issue has begun to be addressed is by focusing aphasia therapy on conversation (Hopper, Holland, & Rewega, 2002; Kagan, Black, Duchan, Simmons-Mackie, & Square, 2001; Simmons-Mackie, Kearns, & Potechin, 2005). There have been a small but growing number of aphasia therapy studies that have drawn on the method and findings of conversation analysis (CA) (Hutchby & Wooffitt, 2008) in order to implement therapy targeted at the everyday conversational behaviours of the person with aphasia and a significant other (usually a spouse) and to evaluate that therapy (see Wilkinson, submitted, for an overview of these interaction-focused intervention studies). In this paper we present the findings of a single-case therapy study that used CA as the basis for targeting and evaluating intervention.

This study adds to the existing literature in a number of ways. First, the person who has been the target for therapy in these interaction-focused therapy studies has typically been the non-aphasic conversation partner (Booth & Perkins, 1999; Lesser & Algar, 1995; Simmons-Mackie et al., 2005; Turner & Whitworth, 2006). In this study therapy was targeted at, and carried out with, the person with aphasia and the wife of the person with aphasia as a couple. While some other conversation-focused therapy studies have targeted both partners as a couple (e.g., Boles, 1997; Cunningham & Ward, 2003), these studies involved differences from the one presented here. The conversations recorded in the Cunningham and Ward (2003) study, for example, were less "naturally occurring" than those used in our study. Topics were suggested to the participants before their conversations and the participants were encouraged to use props such as magazines, catalogues and an atlas that had been left for their use. In the Boles (1997) study the therapy provided for four couples where one partner had aphasia was based primarily on linguistic analyses of word frequency, utterances in T-units, and repair-type behaviours of each participant. The analysis in the study presented here focuses on how the couple collaborate on a turn-by-turn basis to produce interactional sequences of talk together, with a particular focus on question–answer sequences.

Second, a main theme of previous studies has been to work with the non-aphasic partner to cut down or stop using certain pedagogic behaviours in conversation that have led to displays of negative emotions such as upset, frustration, or embarrassment in the couple's conversations (for exceptions, see Lesser & Algar, 1995, and Sorin-Peters, 2004). These pedagogic behaviours have included test questions (i.e., the non-aphasic partner asking questions to which he/she already knows the answer) (Burch, Wilkinson & Lock, 2002), and "correct production sequences" (Lock, Wilkinson, & Bryan, 2001), i.e., stretches of talk where the non-aphasic partner encourages the person with aphasia to produce the correct version of a word, even when it is clear that both partners know what the target is (Booth & Perkins, 1999;

Booth & Swabey, 1999; Lock et al., 2001; Turner & Whitworth, 2006; Wilkinson et al., 1998). In this study we report intervention targeted at a different issue, i.e., where the couple post-onset of aphasia have developed a restricted style of talking that masks the competence of the person with aphasia and does not allow him (or in other circumstances, her) opportunities to make significant use of his remaining linguistic resources.

Third, since CA is primarily a qualitative approach that does not straightforwardly incorporate quantitative analysis (Schegloff, 1993), some therapy studies using CA have used a qualitative approach as the method of evaluating the intervention (Burch et al., 2002; Turner & Whitworth, 2006; Wilkinson et al., 1998). Here we use a novel combination of qualitative and quantitative approaches to evaluate the intervention, which provides more robust evidence of positive change than a qualitative approach alone.

## METHOD

### Participants

The couple who took part in this study will be referred to as "Len" and "Jane". At the time of the study Len was 66 and had had a left cerebro-vascular accident (CVA) 18 months previously. He presented with a Broca-type aphasia and a right hemiplegia, and was able to walk with care and write with his non-preferred (left) hand. Jane, his wife, was 63. Both were retired teachers.

### Conversation data: assessment and intervention

Jane recorded the couple's conversation at home on two separate occasions prior to the intervention (termed here "Conversation 1" and "Conversation 2") and once after it ("Conversation 3"). The length of the two sets of conversation recordings prior to the intervention was 15 minutes 10 seconds and 9 minutes 28 seconds respectively, giving 24 minutes 38 seconds in total. The length of the conversation recorded after the therapy was 37 minutes 36 seconds. In each case the recording was made up of more than one conversation. The conversational data were analysed using CA methods and findings as outlined in Lock et al. (2001) with a particular focus on features of turn taking, turn construction, topic and repair (see Hutchby & Wooffitt, 2008, for a description of these phenomena). Excerpts of around 8–10 minutes were transcribed in order to allow a more detailed analysis of certain sections (for CA transcription symbols see Hutchby & Wooffitt, 2008; in the transcripts presented here, words in round brackets mark where those words are misproduced due to sound production problems and/or are unclear to the transcriber).

There were eight intervention sessions, which took place once a week at the couple's home and lasted between 1 and 2 hours. The intervention focused on changing the conversational behaviours of both Len and Jane and included:

- Jane to use open questions more often; to repeat or paraphrase what Len had just said; and to use minimal turns in the form of continuers (Hutchby & Wooffitt, 2008) such as "mm hm".
- Len to use the possibilities afforded by Jane's changes in conversational behaviour to add something new to the topic and to take an active role in conversation (for example, correcting Jane).

TABLE 1
Raw scores on subtests of the Comprehensive Aphasia Test (CAT)
(Swinburn et al., 2004, pre-publication version)

|  |  | Pre-intervention scores | Post-intervention scores |
|---|---|---|---|
| Cognition | Ravens coloured progressive matrices | 8/12 | 8/12 |
|  | Pyramids and palm trees | 6/10 | 8/10 |
|  | Verbal fluency | 4 | 5 |
|  | Visual recognition | 10/10 | 10/10 |
|  | Ideomotor apraxia | 7/12 | 6/12 |
|  | Picture description | 5/10 | 6/10 |
|  | Arithmetic | 5/6 | 4/6 |
| Language | Auditory comprehension: single words | 24/30 | 22/30 |
|  | Written comprehension: single words | 26/30 | 24/30 |
|  | Auditory comprehension: sentences | 11/16 | 13/16 |
|  | Written comprehension: sentences | 10/16 | 15/16 |
|  | Repetition: single words | 8/32 | 6/32 |
|  | Naming: noun pictures | 9/48 | 10/48 |
|  | Reading: single words | 7/48 | 4/48 |

## Results of other clinical assessments used

Len was assessed on a range of clinical aphasia assessments. The results of the relevant assessments are presented below.

*Comprehensive Aphasia Test (CAT): Cognitive and linguistic sections.* The CAT (Swinburn, Porter, & Howard, 2004: used here in a pre-publication version) was administered twice; at the same time as Conversation 1 (pre-intervention) and at the same time as Conversation 3 (post-intervention). The cognitive and linguistic sections of the CAT showed no change post-intervention. Table 1 shows the pre- and post-intervention scores on the subtests of the CAT split between cognitive and linguistic functions, and clearly reflects a lack of change in these skills.

This is as expected, since at 18 months post-onset most significant spontaneous recovery of language is likely to have taken place and since no aspect of this intervention was targeted at changing Len's linguistic impairments. One finding from the CAT, which was significant for the interaction-focused intervention, was that on the spoken picture description task Len was able to produce sentences or attempt sentence structure. In the pre-intervention administration of the task Len described the picture in this way: "a man asleep and the /rai/ is (*points*) it . . . (ah) cup (*points to book*) /dɪk/ /kɒts/ /frɒt/ (cat) goin in the /blefə/ the gates are falling and recorder it on . . . a plant". Len's output here has far more grammatical structure than is evident in his conversational talk with Jane.

*Conversation Analysis Profile for People with Aphasia (CAPPA).* The CAPPA (Whitworth, Perkins, & Lesser, 1997) interview was carried out with Len and Jane together on the three occasions when conversations were collected from the couple. The CAPPA allows the interview responses to be quantified and compared pre- and post-intervention. Figure 1 shows the comparison of how the couple viewed changes in Len's conversation before and after intervention compared to his pre-morbid conversation. It suggests that, after the intervention, the couple's impressions were

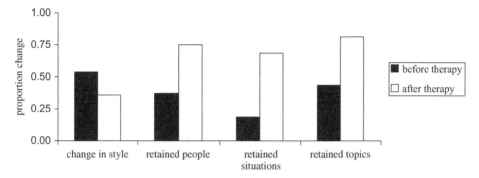

**Figure 1.** Conversation analysis profile for people with aphasia: Changes compared to pre-morbid conversation.

that Len was able to speak with more people in a wider range of places and on a wider range of topics.

## Quantitative comparisons of pre- and post-intervention conversations

Conversation analysis (CA) was used in this study to compare the sequential patterns of talk in the couple's conversations pre- and post- intervention. As well as this qualitative analysis of change we also evaluated change post-intervention by carrying out quantitative comparisons of the pre- and post-intervention conversations.

*Using pre- and post-intervention conversational extracts for quantitative comparison.* Since the pre- and post-intervention conversational data were of different length, for the quantitative analysis we compared two continuous conversational extracts, one from Conversation 2 (pre-intervention data) and one from Conversation 3 (post-intervention data). To select the best extract from the pre-intervention conversation data (Conversations 1 and 2), all of those data (i.e., 24 minutes 38 seconds in total) were divided up into eight segments of roughly equal length (these were roughly equal length because some segments coincided with natural breaks, such as the beginning or end of a conversation). Three speech and language therapists independently rated the eight video-recorded segments in terms of which one showed the best examples of the conversational behaviours that were later to be the targets for therapy. All three independently chose the same segment. In order to compare this segment with a segment from the post-intervention conversation, excerpts of both were transcribed into written extracts of an equal number of turns (35 turns). These pre- and post-intervention extracts are presented below as Extracts 2 and 3 respectively.

One way in which these pre-and post-intervention conversation extracts were used was to carry out a quantitative comparison of the conversational behaviours that had previously been examined qualitatively across the two conversations. Another way in which they were used was that they were presented to 15 outside raters (clinical speech and language therapists) for them to rate. The rationale and method for this part of the study will now be discussed.

*Ratings of the pre- and post-intervention conversation sections by naïve raters.* We were interested in finding out whether the changes that had been identified by the researchers on this project, who were familiar with the participants, the conversational data, and the conversation-analytic investigation of those data, could also be identified by raters who were naïve to all of these phenomena. There were two primary motivators for this part of the study. The first was the possibility that we, as the research team who were so closely aligned to the data, might be unconsciously identifying and arguing for particular changes between the pre- and post-intervention conversation data that were not evident to others outside the research project. This is one possible risk of using qualitative data analysis when arguing for change as a result of the intervention. The second motivator was to examine the following question: If naive raters could see a change in the two conversation extracts at a gross level, would they also be able to identify the presence of specific behaviours that made up that overall appearance of difference between the two extracts?

Specifically, the questions we examined were:

1. Could 15 naive speech and language therapists select, from the two extracts of conversational data, which extract was taken from the pre-intervention conversation and which from the post-intervention conversation?
2. Was there a significant difference between the two extracts in terms of the conversational behaviours identified by the naïve raters?

*Selection of speech and language therapists to carry out the two task analyses.* A total of 15 local speech and language therapists were recruited to take part in the analysis. On average the group had been qualified for 11.20 years (*SD* 9.63), with a range from 1 year to 37 years. The average time spent working with people with aphasia varied from 1 year to 27 years with a mean of 9.63 years (*SD* 9.53).

*Method for two task analyses.* The first task required of the therapists was to watch the two video extracts from which the two 35-turn conversation transcriptions had been made, and to decide which extract was before intervention and which after. Therapists were not told what sort of intervention was provided. Therapists watched both extracts twice and were asked to write down which one they believed was from the pre-intervention conversation and which from the post-intervention conversation. They were also invited to comment on why they had selected their choice if they wished to do so. Their choices were then removed and collected before the second task was carried out.

The therapists were then told what the intervention had consisted of and were given written transcripts of the two extracts on which to mark down, using a number or letter code, their observations of specific conversational behaviours. These were subdivided into three behaviours from Jane (use of open questions; use of repeats or paraphrases of what Len had just said; use of minimal turns such as "mm hm") and two behaviours from Len (adding something new to the topic; taking an active role in conversation in some other way, e.g., by correcting Jane). The therapists again watched each video extract twice, first to note down Jane's behaviours and then on the second viewing to note Len's behaviours.

## Interview and other feedback from Jane

Following the intervention Jane was interviewed about her experiences of taking part in the project. Post-intervention, Jane also spontaneously wrote the research team a letter about Len's progress. Both of these forms of feedback provide insights into

Jane's view of the couple's experience of the intervention programme and will be presented below.

# RESULTS

## Conversation pre-intervention

A strongly recurring pattern throughout the two pre-intervention conversations was question and answer sequences where Jane asked a question, Len produced or attempted to produce an answer, and Jane followed Len's answer with a further question. Extract 1 (from Conversation 1) is an example of the type of talk made up of questioning sequences that recur throughout the two pre-intervention conversations.

Extract 1: Pre-intervention conversation (from Conversation 1).

```
01  Jane:   did you have a good walk?
02  Len:    (4.5) ((Len turns from Jane and looks forward; goes as if to speak then stops))
03  Jane:   did you enjoy your walk?
04  Len:    °yes°
05  Jane:   was it very hot?
06  Len:    yes.
07  Jane:   did you see anybody?
08  Len:    (0.5) uh: no. yeah, (1.9) (man) with a dog.
09  Jane:   you saw the man with the dog uhm (.)°whats his name. not Bill. can't
            remember what his name is°. right. was he going for a walk with the dog?
10  Len:    no
11  Jane:   oh ⌈(right)
12  Len:       ⌊(he's) coming (down).
13  Jane:   he was coming down, ⌈right.
14  Len:                        ⌊yeah
15  Jane:   and uhm you didn't see Glen or Ellen?
16  Len:    (0.2) y:es,
17  Jane:   oh right. who did you see?
18  Len:    (hh) (1.5) ⌈(two) uh
                       ⌊ ((holds up two fingers))
19  Jane:   you saw them both.
20  Len:    yeah
21  Jane:   oh right. and what was- was Ellen going to the shops?
22  Len:    no,
23  Jane:   what was she doing?
```

The fact that so many of Jane's turns are questions can be seen to be constraining for Len in a number of ways. As a first pair part of an adjacency pair (Hutchby & Wooffitt, 2008), questions are constraining in that they place the recipient of the question in the position of being expected to produce a certain type of action in the next turn, i.e., a second pair part in the form of an answer (Schegloff, 2007). If we examine the form of Jane's questions, however, it can be seen that Len is even more constrained. Many of the questions are in the form either of "wh"-type questions which demand a specific piece of information (as in turn 17: "who did you see?") or, in particular, are what Raymond (2003) terms "yes/no interrogatives" (turns 01, 03,

05, 07, 09, 15, 21, 23). These are a type of question that constrains the linguistic form available to the answerer, in that the expected form of an answer would contain a "yes" or "no" (or an equivalent token such as "uh huh" or "nope" etc.) (Raymond, 2003). As such, utterances produced in response to these questions may typically display evidence of what Schegloff (1996) terms "positionally sensitive grammar", i.e., where the grammar of the utterance can be seen to be affected by its sequential position within the conversation, such as here in its role as an answer to a particular type of question.

Answerers can, of course, "escape" from these constraints of action and form to some extent. They may, for example, produce an answer to a yes/no interrogative that does not contain a "yes"- or "no"-type token (Raymond, 2003), or produce another action as well as, or instead of, the answer requested by the question. However, such responses are likely to entail more linguistic work (see Raymond, 2003), and this might be difficult for Len to achieve on a regular basis.

As such, the majority of Len's turns in these conversations are answers to Jane's questions, as is evident in Extract 1. In terms of the linguistic form of Len's utterances in the pre-intervention conversations, it is notable that he uses few sentences or attempted sentences in his talk. This is despite the fact that he is able to produce, or attempt to produce, sentences in other types of speech activity, such as the CAT picture description. In Extract 1, for instance, he produces one sentence ("(he's) coming (down)" in turn 12). Most typically, however, his utterances use a minimal form sufficient to produce an answer. Thus he regularly answers yes/no interrogatives with a "yes" or a "no" alone (turns 4, 6, 16, 20, 22) and "wh"-type questions with the minimal required information (turn 18). Where he does elaborate, it is typically where there is an expectation to do so (see Raymond, 2003), such as when his answer is different from that anticipated by Jane's question (turns 08 and 10/12), although even in this situation his response is often limited to "yes" or "no" (e.g., turn 16).

In response to Len's turns, it is notable that Jane in her next turn regularly produces another question. This may occur either by itself (turns 03, 05, 07, 23) or after some other kind of action earlier in her turn (turn 09, 17, 21). As such, there is a strong sequential pattern in these pre-intervention conversations of question-answer-question or question-answer-response/question, which means that Len is almost constantly in the role of answerer and has very little opportunity to break out of that role in the talk. As a result of this, Len's role in terms of determining the content, direction, and topical development of these two conversations is a minimal one. Rather, his role in these and other aspects of these conversations is passive and responsive, with Jane constantly taking the initiating actions (such as asking questions and initiating and developing the topics of talk).

Extract 2 is the one from the two pre-intervention conversations that was judged by all three raters to be the "best", i.e., it is this section that the raters felt showed an overall better balance in the conversation, with Len producing more sentences and Jane's talk being less restrictive for Len:

Extract 2: Pre-intervention conversation (from Conversation 2).

01 Jane:  so when I went (.) ehm (0.4) to the hospital with Nana this morning (0.8) what did you do

02 Len:  I went eh (0.4) (wa ge gu) walk

03 Jane:  you went for a walk (0.4) ehm (0.4) what time did you get up

04 Len:   (6.0) eh (se woo) (1.3) (wah) (0.6) °t-t-⌈(tu)°
05 Jane:                                      ⌊before eight o'clock?
06 Len:   (0.7) yes ((*nods*))
07 Jane:  got up before eight o'clock (0.8) right and em (0.4) did you do your
          breakfast or did Andrew do it for⌈you
08 Len:                                     ⌊°ooh° I did it
09 Jane:  you did it right did you make yourself a cup of tea=
10 Len:   =ye:s= ((*nods*))
11 Jane:  =good=
12 Len:   =ooh (.) and I made (.) Andrew (.) (cup of) (.) tea
13 Jane:  you m(h)ade Andrew a cup of t(h)ea heh heh (.) did you take it up
14 Len:   no
15 Jane:  heh heh heh ok(h)ay so he came down⌈for his cup of tea
16 Len:                                      ⌊yeah
17 Jane:  (0.5) so (.) what did you do then
18 Len:   (1.4) went out for a walk
19 Jane:  you went out for a walk (0.4) ehm (.) where did you go
20 Len:   ooh (.) I-I (0.8) I: (0.6) went (.) to: (.) the: (0.7) ((*points with finger, tuts
          and looks to Jane*))
21 Jane:  (°right°) did you go up as far as Sou⌈thfield?
22 Len:                                       ⌊°y-ah! °((*points at Jane*)) y-no
23 Jane:  you went to the end of Brig⌈don'sLane?
24 Len:                             ⌊ye:s ((*nods*)) ye:s
25 Jane:  right okay you went to the end of Brigdon's⌈Lane
26 Len:                                             ⌊ yeah (0.4) <(and) I
          came back>
27 Jane:  and you came back
28 Len:   yeah
29 Jane:  right straight back?
30 Len:   ooh I: ((*points forward*)) k- (1.6) I: (.6) (wata) (0.6) ((*unintelligible
          speech*)) ((*points left*)) (chaylim) (0.8) eh (cemetery)
31 Jane:  you walked around the c⌈emetery
32 Len:                         ⌊yes ((*nods*))
33 Jane:  ⌈a long way round?
34 Len   ⌊I- yes
35 Jane:  mm (0.4) did you go to look at grandad's grave?

Examples of Len producing, or attempting to produce, sentences are seen, for instance, in turns 02, 08, 12, 18, 20 (incomplete due to the final location reference missing), 26 and 30 (although partly unintelligible and perhaps missing a verb). In part, this larger number of sentences and attempted sentences may be linked to Jane's production of more "open" (and hence less restrictive) questions in forms such as "what did you do" (turn 01) and "what did you do then" (turn 17). Len can also produce a sentence that is more than, or in addition to, the minimal form necessary at that point in the conversation, for example in his response to Jane's question in turn 30.

Significantly for the form of intervention that was later carried out with Len and Jane, one place where Len produces a sentence was in response to a non-question form by Jane, for example in turn 12 where he produces a sentence following Jane's assessment "good" in turn 11. Thus, on one of the relatively few occasions when Jane did not respond to an answer by Len with another question, Len was able to produce a turn that added to the topic and to what he had just previously said (in turn 10), and to do so in the form of a sentence. On two occasions, Jane also produced a paraphrase of what Len had just said rather than a new question (turns 27 and 31).

While Extract 2 shows some positive features compared to Extract 1, there are also many similarities between the two extracts. For example, Jane is still largely using her turns to produce questions (turns 01, 03, 05, 07, 09, 13, 15, 17, 19, 21, 23, 29, 33, 35). Len is still largely in the role of providing answers to questions. With the limited exceptions noted above, he is also contributing relatively little to the topical development and direction of the conversation.

## Intervention

The intervention had three interlinked aims; two relevant for Jane and one relevant for Len. These aims emerged out of the investigation of the two pre-intervention conversations using CA and through discussion with the couple.

1. Jane would make greater use of forms to initiate sequences other than yes/no interrogatives and "closed" wh-type questions. The purpose of this change in Jane's conversational style was to make it less constricting for Len, and thus to provide him with more choices about the content and form of his turns (e.g., whether they should take the form of a sentence, or even more than one sentence).
2. Jane would respond to some of Len's turns with a repeat or paraphrase of his turn, or with a minimal turn such as "mm hm" (Hutchby & Woofitt, 2008) rather than with another question. The purpose of this change was to provide Len with opportunities to add to his prior turn if he wished, and thus be more active in topic development in the conversation by building up more extended talk on a topic across his turns at talk.
3. Len would attempt to use the extra opportunities for talk that Jane's changes in conversational style would provide in order to contribute more to the conversation where relevant.

The intervention followed the three-stage therapy process described in the *SPPARC* (Lock et al., 2001). This involved:

1. working to raise the couple's/non-aphasic partner's awareness of relevant conversational behaviours in general (by, for example, using handouts, role plays, written exercises or video clips, and transcripts of other couples from the SPPARC);
2. working to raise their awareness of their own relevant patterns of conversational behaviours (by, for example, using video clips and transcripts from the couple's own conversations);
3. discussing and practising various strategies for changing relevant conversational behaviours (by, for example, using role plays in the therapy sessions or asking the non-aphasic partner to try a new behaviour between sessions and keep a written record of its success or otherwise for discussion at the next therapy session).

In the case of question behaviours, for example, Jane was introduced to findings about turns and sequences (such as questions and answers) using handouts adapted from those used in the *SPPARC* (Lock et al., 2001) that focused on different types of questions and the constraining effects on the recipient.

To raise her awareness of her own patterns of questioning, Jane and the speech and language therapist observed selected video clips of Jane's questioning behaviours from the video recordings of the pre-intervention conversations. Handouts were also made for Jane, which included examples of her different types of questions and their effect on Len's responses. In discussion with the couple, Jane said that she felt her pattern of asking questions was helping Len to talk. She felt that she had "always been a bit of a teacher" and that this was behind some of her conversational behaviours observed on the video. In response the therapist suggested that, while Jane's style of asking many questions was indeed giving Len a space in the conversation to say something, he might be able to say more if he was given other types of opportunity to do so at certain points within conversation. The therapist discussed with Jane that she might want to take on less of a "teacher" role in conversation with Len. As a couple, they discussed an option whereby Jane would change her current style of talking to provide Len with opportunities to produce longer turns. It was stressed that if Len wanted to say more at these points in the conversation he then could do, but if he did not, Jane should not pressure him to speak. Len agreed with these points.

Strategies for change included paper and pen exercises where Jane had to analyse written versions of a range of questions she used in the pre-intervention conversations and decide which type of question each was (i.e., whether yes/no interrogative or another type of question). Jane was also encouraged to try different types of turns at home to initiate sequences (i.e., different types of questions, and statement forms instead of question forms) and also different types of turns in response to Len's turns (i.e., minimal turns or paraphrases of what Len had said rather than a further question). She was also encouraged to keep notes about what the effect of these different types of turn appeared to be on Len's talk. Jane and the therapist also engaged in role-plays together where the therapist took the part of Len, and Jane tried out different types of sequence-initiating and responsive turns in real time with the therapist. The therapist also videoed a role play between Jane and Len trying out their target conversational behaviours, and fed back to them about this. Each of these activities to facilitate change was preceded and followed by discussions between the therapist and the couple, in particular Jane, about the phenomenon being practised and how the participants felt about it.

Other parts of the intervention for the couple, which are not discussed here, included working to reduce the use of test questions by Jane and attempts to facilitate Len's writing skills within conversation.

## Conversation post-intervention

In the post-intervention conversation there was evidence that the couple had changed their conversational behaviours in line with the aims of the intervention. Here we will provide four forms of evidence for these changes. These are: (1) qualitative changes in the sequential patterns in the pre- and post-intervention conversations; (2) quantitative comparisons of samples from the pre- and post-intervention conversations; (3) ratings by naïve speech and language therapists comparing samples from the pre- and post-intervention conversations; and (4) interview and other feedback from Jane on the couple's conversations post-intervention. These will now be presented in turn.

*Qualitative changes in the sequential patterns in the pre- and post-intervention conversations.* There was evidence in the post-intervention conversation that the couple were now producing sequences of talk that differed from those seen anywhere in the pre-intervention conversations, and which were in line with the conversational behaviours discussed with the couple and practised by them during the intervention. An example of this can be seen in Extract 3:

Extract 3: Post-intervention conversation (from Conversation 3).

```
01  Jane:   tell me about your walk.
02  Len:    (2.0) I eh (1.9) I've eh (4.7) I (0.7) eh (walked)⌈(past the) (0.5) (cemetery)
                                                             ⌊((points outside))
                (1.1) I (saw Glen)
03  Jane:   (1.1) you walked (.) past the cemetery (.) you s⌈aw Glen
04  Len:                                                    ⌊(saw Glen)
                (0.5) and he⌈(was) (0.7) (coming down)
                            ⌊((gestures towards himself))
05  Jane:   Glen was coming down.=
06  Len:    =yeah. (0.5) and he⌈have (bwocks) with him
                               ⌊((gestures carrying something))
                (0.9) a (with) eh- (0.4) °(him)° (1.0)⌈°eh°
07  Jane:                                             ⌊he had a box⌈with him
08  Len:                                                           ⌊NO::: a bag.
09  Jane:   he had a⌈bag with him right?,
10  Len:            ⌊°ye:s° (1.2) ((gestures carrying something)) and he was (2.1)
                (going out) (0.5) t-to, (2.2) to eh, (2.6) ) oh (anyone oski) the (0.3) eh
                (0.5) (kowers but eh lays), ((laughs)) and k-heh heh and ((laughing))
                (0.5) he was (0.7) eh s: saying (0.6) eh (par) (0.5) eh (.7) ooh ((waves hand))
                (0.9) (at) ((laughs)) eh (1.1) ooh ((makes gesture on lap-tray))
11  Jane:   (1.5) eh he had a bag with him was he going shopping?
12  Len:    no⌈((pointing))
13  Jane:     ⌊coming home from the⌈shops.
14  Len:                           ⌊no he was (0.9) he (wa) (ts)
                (0.9) and he (wat) (.) talked to me about the (wales)?
15  Jane:   he talked to⌈you- he talked to you about Wales (.) right?
16  Len:                ⌊yeah
                (0.3) and he (said), (0.7) but that wa- wasn't (3.1) (ay) eh (1.6)
17  Jane:   and he said that,
18  Len:    ah ah: ((growls and does dismissive gesture)) and he said
                eh (.) I (want aint a par) (0.8)⌈ca:r.
19  Jane:                                       ⌊car. (0.4) right
20  Len:    and he ((gestures pointing)) got (0.2) in the (.) (opposish).
21  Jane:   he went in the car⌈(.) and he parked it opposite.
22  Len:                      ⌊no:
23  Jane:   (0.7) no (0.4) did⌈you say opposite (0.5) heh⌈heh
24  Len:                      ⌊((growls))                ⌊(ay)
                (0.8) ((moves hand left and right)) the (1.0) (cartin) (0.3) (poshtit)
25  Jane:   (1.0) say that bit again=
26  Len:    =(e) (0.3) (wo) (.) (ps tk) ah (0.9) (2 syllables) (1.2) I (wo) (2 syllables)
                (1.9) they (.) pa:k (.) it opposite.
```

27  Jane:   (0.6) o-ppo-⌈site.
28  Len:                    ⌊ yeah ((*nods*))
29  Jane:   they parked the car oppo⌈site?
30  Len:                              ⌊ (enh) (.) yeah ((*nods*))
31  Jane:   right (.) somebody was in his space, was he annoyed?
          (0.5)⌈ heh heh (.) heh
32  Len:          ⌊((*gestures 'don't know'*)) °no no°
33  Jane:   no but he parked the car opposite.=
34  Len:    =°yeah°=
35  Jane:   =right (0.9) ehm had he been out in the car today then.

In turn 01 Jane starts the sequence not with a question but with a topic elicitor in the form of a statement ("tell me about your walk"). This is a non-restrictive form, which allows Len a range of choices about the content of his turn and what form it might take. It is also notable that following Len's turns Jane regularly responds with non-question forms, e.g., with a paraphrase or partial repeat of what she understands Len to have just said (turns 03, 05, 07, 21, 27), or with a repeat/paraphrase and a tag such as "right" (either with or without rising intonation) (turns 09, 15, 19). These turns by Jane are "other-oriented" (i.e., oriented to Len) in that they do not forward the conversation by Jane choosing to add some new topical content to the conversation (e.g., through a new question). Rather, these turns repeat or paraphrase something Len has just said and leave it to him to add something new to what he has previously said, and thus to direct the topical content of the conversation. Even though they are not paraphrases of what Len has just said, a similar phenomenon of other-orientation is seen in a number of Jane's other turns (i.e., the partial paraphrase/prompt in turn 17; the request for a repeat in turn 25; the re-statement of an already agreed element of the telling in turn 33).

The result of Jane's conversational behaviours is that Len has far greater opportunities to choose the content and form of his turns and to make use of the lexical and grammatical resources that he has available and which were evident, for example, in the CAT picture description. Len regularly takes these opportunities. For example, many of his turns contain sentences or attempts at sentences (turns 02, 04, 06, 10, 14, 16, 18, 20, 24, 26). In two cases his turns contain two or more sentences or attempts at sentences (turns 02 and 10), a phenomenon that never occurred in the two pre-intervention conversations. One way to consider this change in Len's grammatical production is in terms of Schegloff's (1996) notion of positionally sensitive grammar: while Jane's style of turn design in the pre-intervention conversations was restricting Len's ability to use the linguistic resources that he had available to him, the style she was now adopting post-intervention was less restrictive and allowed Len more opportunities to use these resources. These changes highlight the importance of considering language production, not simply in terms of an individual speaker, but rather in terms of that speaker within the context of other participants and *their* contributions to the conversation. It may be particularly important to analyse what type of utterance(s) occurred immediately prior to the speaker with aphasia's talk and to consider how the linguistic forms and social action evident in that talk might have been affected by the prior utterance(s).

Most notably, Len is now taking an active role in the conversation in ways that were not evident in the two pre-intervention conversations. First, he regularly actively develops the topic of the conversation in general and of his prior turn(s) in particular. This topical development carried out by Len can be seen across the following turns: Len informing Jane about where he walked and about meeting Glen (turn 02); that Glen was coming down and had a box with him (turns 04 and 06); other facts about Glen including what he said to Len (turns 10); this included talking about the Welsh rugby match (turn 14); something about his (Glen's) car (turn 18); and something about Glen parking his car opposite (turns 20, 24, and 26). This type of topical development by Len is quite unlike anything seen in his talk in the pre-intervention conversations and is directly linked to the changes in Jane's conversational behaviours. Len is also active in that he twice initiates a correction of Jane's understandings of what he has said (turns 08 and 22).

*Quantitative comparisons of extracts from the pre- and post-intervention conversations.* Based on the qualitative analyses provided above, Table 2 provides an overview of quantitative comparisons of the key conversational behaviours from the pre- and post-intervention extracts (i.e., Extracts 2 and 3). The comparison is made first in terms of how many of each speaker's turns contain an example of a key conversational behaviour. In both the pre- and post-intervention conversation samples Jane has 18 turns and Len has 17 turns.

Table 2 shows how the number of turns by Jane that contain questions to Len decreases from 78% to 22%. Correspondingly, the number of her turns that do not contain questions to Len rises from 22% to 78%. The differences in Len's sentence production, or attempted sentence production, are as follows. The number of his turns that contain at least one sentence, or attempted sentence, rises from 41% to 59%, while the number of these turns that contain two or more sentences and/or attempted sentences rises from 0% to 17%. (It is notable that it is not only this pre-intervention excerpt that contains no example of this phenomenon; rather, there are no turns by Len in the whole 24 minutes 38 seconds of the pre-intervention conversational data that contain two or more sentences or attempts at sentences). What this quantitative analysis does not capture, however, is the way in which Len's more grammatically complex utterances are now used post-intervention to develop the topic of talk in a manner that is quite different from anything observed in the pre-intervention data.

*Ratings by naïve speech and language therapists comparing sections from the pre- and post-intervention conversations*
*Activity 1: Which section is pre- and which post-intervention?* Of the 15 therapists, 14 correctly identified which section was from the pre-intervention conversation and which from the post-intervention conversation.

TABLE 2
Quantitative comparisons of extracts from the pre- and post-intervention conversations

| Key conversational behaviour in extract of conversation | Number pre-intervention | Number post-intervention | Percentage pre-intervention | Percentage Post intervention |
|---|---|---|---|---|
| Jane: turns that contain questions to Len | 14/18 | 4/18 | 78% | 22% |
| Jane: turns that do not contain questions to Len | 4/18 | 14/18 | 22% | 78% |
| Len: turns containing at least one sentence or attempted sentence | 7/17 | 10/17 | 41% | 59% |
| Len: turns that contain two or more sentences and/or attempted sentences | 0/17 | 2/17 | 0% | 12% |

TABLE 3
Mean (*SD*) for all selected conversation behaviours
pre- and post-intervention

|  | Before therapy | After therapy |
|---|---|---|
|  | *Mean (SD)* | *Mean (SD)* |
| Total | 11.07 (4.10) | 23.84 (4.49) |
| Jane | 6.93 (2.60) | 13.53 (2.03) |
| Len | 4.13 (2.85) | 10.33 (3.33) |

Total across the 35 turns and subtotals for Jane and Len.

*Activity 2: Was there a significant difference between the two sections in terms of the conversational behaviours identified by the naïve raters?* Table 3 shows the mean values and standard deviations for the number of times the therapists identified the five conversational behaviours in the pre- and post-intervention extracts (i.e., Jane using open questions, using repeats or paraphrases of what Len had just said, and using minimal turns such as "mm hm"; Len adding something new to the topic, and taking an active role in conversation in some other way, e.g., by correcting Jane). There was a significant change in the mean for all the behaviours (Wilcoxon matched pairs test: W = 60, two-tailed $p$ = .0007) suggesting that the targeted therapy behaviours were observed in the conversation more in the post-intervention section than the pre-intervention section. The second part of the table indicates that this change was driven by both Jane's and Len's change in conversational behaviours as both showed significant differences in their pre- and post-intervention means (Jane: Wilcoxon matched pairs test: W = 60, two-tailed $p$ = .0007; Len: Wilcoxon matched pairs test: W = 52.50, two-tailed $p$ = .0011).

*Post-intervention programme interview and other feedback from Jane on the couple's conversation post-intervention.* In the post-intervention programme interview with Jane she commented on the changes she and Len had made in conversation due to the intervention they had received.

> [On changes in her style of talking with Len] In my way of thinking about how do I talk to Len, I've changed in that way. As I've said, with the questions, with the statements, and he then had to think of something to say because, I wasn't going to go on and spoon feed him all the way along the line, which I think I did . . . And I think that's why when you said to me, "right, hang back a bit, let him do this", that he improved because of this. I mean he would start to talk and I would immediately jump in, and say so and so and so and so, you know, instead of letting him continue, slowly, in his own way.
>
> [On changes in Len's language/conversation] He only spoke in word answers, I should say he had used sentences on about five occasions only in all that time that he'd had the stroke. But now he was beginning to use complete sentences.

A few months after the completion of the intervention programme, Jane also wrote an unsolicited letter to the research team to update them on Len's progress. Relevant sections are included below:

> The main difference in Len's conversation since last June is that he now uses sentences daily instead of one word requests or answers. Len speaks to our son and my mother and his weekly telephone call to his brother is much less of a chore for Len. He attempts

more conversation with friends. When Sarah first set up the recorder and stated that she wanted us to record our conversation my heart dropped. We <u>had</u> no conversation as I understood it. I would talk to Len constantly and apart from making sure that he understood me, I was content to leave it at that. When Len needed to tell me something we played "twenty questions" until I understood his needs. When we studied the tape we were both very surprised to see that Len was able to answer some questions. He gained in confidence through this experience and has gone from strength to strength. The initial sounds are sometimes wrong but Len is forming complete sentences, in his head, and attempts to talk in complete sentences. Len finds it easier to initiate a conversation relating to his needs . . .

## CONCLUSION

The focus of a significant number of previous research studies of interaction-focused intervention has been on changing pedagogic behaviours adopted by the conversation partner, such as test questions or correct production sequences (Booth & Perkins, 1999; Booth & Swabey, 1999; Burch et al., 2002; Lock et al., 2001; Turner & Whitworth, 2006; Wilkinson et al., 1998). In this study we have discussed how an intervention programme was implemented and evaluated for a couple where the conversation partner had adopted a strongly recurrent pattern in conversation of using questions (in particular yes/no and closed questions) as a means of interacting with her husband with aphasia. This style of interaction was restrictive for the couple since, for example, it placed the person with aphasia in the position of recurrently providing answers, in particular short and linguistically limited answers such as "yes", "no" or a single word, and resulted in him adding little to the topical development of the talk. The fact that these conversational contributions by the person with aphasia recurrently displayed so few sentence structures or attempts at sentence production was notable since he was able to produce these in a picture description task.

The study provided evidence that interaction-focused intervention, which targeted particular conversational behaviours, particularly of the non-aphasic partner, was able to effect change in the conversational behaviours of both speakers. This included a larger production of sentences and attempted sentences by the person with aphasia. A result of this intervention was to allow the person with aphasia to use remaining linguistic resources in conversation, in particular grammatical resources, which had previously been suppressed by the conversational style adopted by the non-aphasic conversation partner (see also Simmons-Mackie et al., 2005).

The study used a novel combination of qualitative and quantitative approaches in order to evaluate the intervention. We suggest that this combination provides more robust evidence of positive change than would be provided by qualitative evidence of conversational change alone. There were four forms of evidence: both qualitative and quantitative evidence of change in the conversational behaviours produced by both the speaker with aphasia and the conversation partner; evidence from ratings by naïve speech and language therapists comparing sections from the pre- and post-intervention conversations; and evidence from the main conversation partner provided by an interview and an unsolicited letter.

The study highlights the importance for clinicians and aphasiologists of collecting everyday conversational data from the person with aphasia and a main conversation partner as part of an intervention programme. Without this form of data it is not possible to know which types of conversational behaviours one or both speakers may have adopted in everyday life in their attempts to adapt to conversations in the light of the person with aphasia's linguistic limitations. In some cases, one or more of the participants may adopt behaviours that appear to be maladaptive in that they, for example, highlight the person with aphasia's linguistic incompetence and lead to displays of negative emotion such as upset (Lock et al., 2001), or, as here, significantly restrict the person with aphasia's ability to use their remaining linguistic resources. This study suggests that when couples present with these maladaptive behaviours in conversation, these might be considered a priority for a therapy programme. One reason for this is that it may be easier and quicker to create noticeable change in participants' linguistic behaviour (including the person with aphasia's linguistic behaviour) by changing these maladaptive behaviours than by attempting to teach new linguistic or communicative behaviours. Since these maladaptive behaviours can often lead to negative emotions for participants, such as frustration or upset, dealing with these psychosocial issues first may also provide a more solid basis for the subsequent teaching and learning of new linguistic and/or communicative skills.

Finally, this study adds to a growing body of evidence showing that directly targeting the conversational behaviours of the person with aphasia and/or a main conversational partner can provide evidence of positive change. Notably, this change is ecologically valid in that it is evident not only within clinical testing or in interaction with a clinician or other professional, but rather can be seen in the participants' spontaneous conversational behaviour within their everyday lives.

Manuscript received 24 July 2009
Manuscript accepted 16 November 2009
First published online 17 May 2010

## REFERENCES

Boles, L. (1997). Conversation analysis as a dependent measure in communication therapy with four individuals with aphasia. *Asia Pacific Journal of Speech, Language and Hearing, 2*, 43–61.

Booth, S., & Perkins, L. (1999). The use of conversation analysis to guide individualised advice to carers and evaluate change in aphasia: A case study. *Aphasiology, 13*(4–5), 283–304.

Booth, S., & Swabey, D. (1999) Group training in communication skills for carers of adults with aphasia. *International Journal of Language and Communication Disorders, 34*(3), 291–310.

Burch, K., Wilkinson, R., & Lock, S. (2002). A single case study of conversation-focused therapy for a couple where one partner has aphasia. *British Aphasiology Society Therapy Symposium Proceedings 2002* (pp. 1–12). London: British Aphasiology Society.

Cunningham, R., & Ward, C. (2003). Evaluation of a training programme to facilitate conversation between people with aphasia and their partners. *Aphasiology, 17*(8), 687–707.

Hopper, T., Holland, A., & Rewega, M. (2002). Conversational coaching: Treatment outcomes and future directions. *Aphasiology, 16*(7), 745–761.

Hutchby, I., & Wooffitt, R. (2008). *Conversation analysis: Principles, practices and applications* (2nd ed.). Cambridge, UK: Polity Press.

Kagan, A., Black, S. E., Duchan, J. F., Simmons-Mackie, N. N., & Square, P. (2001). Training volunteers as conversation partners using 'Supported Conversation for Adults with Aphasia' (SCA): A controlled trial. *Journal of Speech, Language and Hearing Research, 44*, 624–638.

Lesser, R., & Algar, L. (1995) Towards combining the cognitive neuropsychological and the pragmatic in aphasia therapy. *Neuropsychological Rehabilitation, 5*, 67–96.

Lock, S., Wilkinson, R., & Bryan, K. (2001). *SPPARC (Supporting Partners of People with Aphasia in Relationships and Conversation): A resource pack*. Bicester, UK: Speechmark Press.

Raymond, G. (2003). Grammar and social organization: Yes/no interrogatives and the structure of responding. *American Sociological Review, 68*, 939–967.

Schegloff, E.A. (1993). Reflections on quantification in the study of conversation. *Research on Language and Social Interaction, 26*(1), 99–128.

Schegloff, E. A. (1996). Turn organization: One intersection of grammar and interaction. In E. Ochs, E.A. Schegloff, & S. A. Thompson (Eds.), *Interaction and grammar*. Cambridge, UK: Cambridge University Press.

Schegloff, E. A. (2007) *Sequence organization in interaction*. Cambridge, UK: Cambridge University Press.

Simmons-Mackie, N. N., Kearns, K. P., & Potechin, G. (2005). Intervention of aphasia through family member training. *Aphasiology, 19,* 583–593.

Sorin-Peters, R. (2004). The evaluation of a learner centred training programme for spouses of adults with chronic aphasia using qualitative case study methodology. *Aphasiology, 18*(10), 951–975.

Swinburn, K., Porter, G., & Howard, D. (2004). *Comprehensive Aphasia Test* (CAT). Hove, UK: Psychology Press.

Turner, S., & Whitworth, A. (2006). Conversational partner training programmes in aphasia: A review of key themes and participants' roles. *Aphasiology, 20,* 483–510.

Whitworth, A., Perkins, L., & Lesser, R. (1997). *Conversation Analysis Profile for People with Aphasia*. London: Whurr.

Wilkinson, R. (2009). Conversation analysis and aphasia therapy. *International Journal of Language and Communication Disorders*. Manuscript submitted for publication.

Wilkinson, R., Bryan, K., Lock, S., Bayley, K., Maxim, J., Bruce, C., et al. (1998). Therapy using conversation analysis: Helping couples adapt to aphasia in conversation. *International Journal of Language and Communication Disorders, 33,* 144–149.

APHASIOLOGY, 2010, 24 (6–8), 887–901

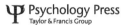

# Rethinking repetition in therapy: Repeated engagement as the social ground of learning

Julie A. Hengst

*University of Illinois at Urbana-Champaign, IL, USA*

Melissa C. Duff

*University of Iowa, Iowa City, IA, USA*

Alexis Dettmer

*University of Illinois at Urbana-Champaign, IL, USA*

*Background*: Clinical aphasiologists have long attended to *repetition* in aphasia classification and used it in treatment. Within traditional approaches, repetition has been conceptualised narrowly as the ability to produce relatively immediate, verbatim reproductions of target behaviours; treatment protocols have relied heavily on drill, eliciting client repetition of targets. In sharp contrast, sociocultural theories conceptualise repetition as a fundamental, pervasive feature operating at every level of language use. Repetition thus includes partial and paraphrased as well as verbatim repetitions, across time as well as immediate. These theories also stress the communicative functions of repetition. With respect to learning, sociocultural theories emphasise the way such loosely structured, diverse patterns of repetition emerge in, and are prompted by, *repeated engagement* in meaningful activities.

*Aims*: This study (1) presents a sociocultural approach to repetition in conversation; (2) illustrates that approach through analysis of a clinician–client pair's repeated productions of labels for 30 target cards during a 10-session pilot treatment; and (3) offers detailed examples of how the pair's repeated engagement with target cards across sessions might support learning.

*Methods & Procedures*: This study utilises situated discourse analysis of a pilot barrier task treatment (10 sessions) in which the clinician and client (a 67-year-old man, with mild anomia and severe amnesia) worked together as partners to identify and place target cards. At the end of each session researchers interviewed the clinician–client pair to identify their agreed-upon target labels (ATL) for the cards. Analysis of card label repetition included: (1) identification of all verbal labels used for target cards during game play; and (2) coding labels as matching or not matching the ATL, and as either a first or repeated use of that label during that sequence.

*Outcomes & Results*: Analysis confirmed that repetition was pervasive. The client–clinician pair routinely repeated their own or each other's referencing expressions during the

Address correspondence to: Julie A. Hengst, Department of Speech and Hearing Science, University of Illinois, 901 S. Sixth Street, Champaign, IL, 61821., USA. E-mail: hengst@illinois.edu

This research would not have been possible without the support and work of many people. Our thanks go first to the client, "Dave", and his family, and to Melissa Bostwick, CCC-SLP, for her assistance in coordinating the study. In addition we appreciate the careful work and many hours spent collecting, transcribing, and coding the data by student lab assistants: Stephanie Bay, Mary Bremer, Keri Buma, Lisa Cardella, Michelle Dailey, Kristen Hammons, Laura Savicki, and Laura Schmidke.

http://www.psypress.com/aphasiology                    DOI: 10.1080/02687030903478330

task, collaboratively developing specific, meaningful, and increasingly succinct labels from chains of conversational repetition (within, between, and across trials). Critically, this repetition occurred without clinician-directed repetition of isolated treatment targets. *Conclusions*: This examination of repetition suggests that marshalling *conversational repetition* through *repeated engagement* offers a theoretically and empirically grounded framework for reconceptualising language intervention. Furthermore, memory research offers useful guidance in understanding the role of repetition across multiple types of learning, which we propose can guide SLPs in when to deploy drill-based and/or conversational repetition to best achieve specific treatment goals.

*Keywords:* Conversational repetition; Repeated engagement; Memory and learning; Language therapy; Aphasia; Amnesia.

Clinical aphasiologists have long attended to *repetition*, both as a diagnostic sign in aphasia classification and as a key strategy in treatment. Grounded primarily in a speech chain model of communication (Denes & Pinson, 1993), these conceptualisations of repetition have focused narrowly on relatively immediate and verbatim reproductions of specified verbal or motor targets—e.g., *a listener correctly perceiving the target, deconstructing its motoric elements and accurately reproducing the original target*. Diagnostically, the disruption of neurological pathways supporting the ability to repeat motor targets can lead to patterns of language production that are over-repetitive (e.g., palilalia, echolalia) or under-repetitive (e.g., conduction aphasia). Clinically, repetition has long been considered integral to effective therapy programmes, and providing patients with repeated stimuli and/or with guided repetition (drill) is widely understood to support learning by reinforcing behaviours and/or strengthening neuro-pathways that underlie target skills. Recent attention has focused on the importance of repetition in motor skill acquisition and treatment of motor speech disorders (e.g., Maas et al., 2008), and some researchers have begun to apply motor learning principles to language rehabilitation (e.g., Maher et al., 2006; Pulvermüller et al., 2001). However, a potential pitfall of modelling language therapy on motor learning principles is the intrinsic tie of motor learning to non-declarative memory systems. Whereas successful language use requires the *flexible*, creative construction of *new utterances* with new partners in new contexts, non-declarative memory systems support representations that are *inflexible* and *routinised* (not novel).

To address the limits of traditional approaches to repetition, we have turned to sociocultural theories of communication that conceptualise *repetition* as a fundamental and flexible aspect of everyday language use. Grounded in the basic premise that language use is *dialogic*—i.e., that people produce and understand discourse through chains of situated experience with words, phrases, and actions (Wertsch, 1991)—sociocultural perspectives focus on the diverse and creative uses of repetition typical of everyday talk as speakers routinely draw on and *repurpose* words, actions, and practices from other times and places (see Hengst, Duff, & Prior, 2008; Prior, Hengst, Roozen, & Shipka, 2006; Tannen, 1989). Sociocultural theories also posit a central role for repetition in learning, emphasising the way loosely structured and diverse patterns of repetition emerge in, and are prompted by, individuals' *repeated engagement* in meaningful, goal-directed activities. The concept of *repeated engagement* points to the contextual framing of repetition (not just target behaviours), the varied ways in which repetition may support communicative success (not just accurate productions), and the multimodal character of repetition (with repeated elements including speech acts, conversational routines, and complex semiotic configurations not just isolated language forms). Whereas traditional clinical approaches to learning make verbatim repetition the focal goal of treatment, a sociocultural approach begins with structuring meaningful, goal-directed activity (the repeated engagement) in which repetition will emerge and be marshalled around the demands of the task and the participants' motivated uptakes of the task.

In order to illustrate the application of sociocultural theories to the identification and use of repetition in clinical settings, this article introduces this theoretical framework and offers a situated discourse analysis of a client and clinician's use of repetition during a pilot treatment study. The background section briefly reviews research on conversational repetition and barrier task protocols, including the pilot treatment study that serves as the data set for this current analysis of repetition. The method section outlines the specific procedures employed in this analysis of the client–clinician pair's use of conversational repetition and repeated engagement with target card labels, and the results section presents both a quantitative summary of the pair's use of repetition in this task, and detailed accounts across all 10 sessions of the pair's repeated engagement with two specific cards. Finally, we discuss the clinical implications we see emerging from sociocultural theories of repetition and repeated engagement.

## BACKGROUND

### Patterns of repetition in conversation

Tannen (1989) describes repetition as a fundamental building block of everyday conversation. Theoretically, she notes the centrality of repetition to classical rhetoric and poetics (e.g., the many linguistic tropes that feature forms of repetition or patterned transformations of an original) as well as to current sociocultural accounts of language. Descriptively, she notes the variability of conversational repetition in form and function. To capture the diversity of forms, Tannen identifies three broad dimensions that characterise variations in the relationships between an original utterance and its repetition. The first dimension addresses the *temporal relationship* with the original—i.e., whether the repetition is *immediate*, occurring shortly after the original; *delayed* by minutes, hours, or days; or *unspecified* (e.g., a proverb). The second focuses on the *source*, or who is being repeated—i.e., whether *self, other* (and if *other*, whether a *specific* or *generalized* other), or a *mixed* pattern, such as choral production. The third attends to *what* is being repeated (e.g., sounds, words, phrases, prosody, meaning) and the *exactness* of repetition (e.g., from identical and complete to partial, paraphrased or transformed repetitions of the original). Tannen also argues that repetition is deployed locally to meet conversational functions (e.g., emphasising points, confirming understandings), and more broadly to signal ongoing involvement among conversational partners. Thus, the value placed on any dimension (e.g., accuracy of what is being repeated) or instance of repetition is based on the communicative work of the participants in deploying that repetition. Finally, research points to the pervasiveness of conversational repetition. Indeed, our preliminary study of conversational repetition and amnesia (Erickson, Hengst, & Duff, 2008) documented frequent conversational repetition (2.48 to 2.92 repetitions per spoken turn) and, surprisingly, found no differences in the frequency or pattern of conversational repetition deployed by participants with and without amnesia.

In stark contrast to the complexities of conversational repetition, repetition elicited during clinician-directed drill is designed to be limited both in form and function. Using Tannen's dimensions, repetition typical of drills usually takes the form of *immediate, verbatim,* and *other* repetitions such as when clients are given model targets to reproduce. In addition, such targets are intentionally stripped of communicative functions, and the frequency of repetition is limited to clinical activities in which accuracy of repetition can be clinically supported.

## Repeated engagement and barrier task protocols

The barrier protocol has a long history as a learning task designed to provide participants with repeated opportunities to engage with target material. Typically, barrier tasks involve two people sitting across from one another, with their view of each other completely obscured. Each person is assigned a role (director or matcher), with the director providing verbal clues to the matcher on how to, for example, match a set of pictures to specific locations on a board. Research has documented change over repeated trials in the way speakers adjust their utterances in response to the listeners' knowledge and social roles and in how speakers and listeners collaborate on the development and use of specific references (see Clark, 1992; Yule, 1997). Studies have consistently found that referencing expressions simplify and shorten across trials.

We redesigned Clark's (1992) barrier task protocol to align it with sociocultural theories and to investigate collaborative referencing between pairs in which one individual had an acquired cognitive-communication disorder (amnesia, aphasia). This redesign included a partial barrier to allow nonverbal as well as verbal communication, a greater number of referencing opportunities, and use of familiar partners (e.g., a family member). Our research has found that participants display creative language use and robust learning—evidenced across trials by pairs' completion of the task, decreased overt collaboration around identification of cards, and development of more concise labels (Duff, Hengst, Tranel, & Cohen, 2006, 2008, 2009; Hengst, 2003, 2006).

That our barrier task protocol was effective in promoting rapid and robust learning, even in patients with severe declarative memory impairments, suggests that these collaborative sessions constitute a powerful learning environment. Although memory research has shown that drill-based repetition can promote semantic learning even in individuals with amnesia, the amount learned is much less than healthy participants (e.g., O'Kane, Kensinger, & Corkin, 2004), and the effort it takes is much greater (e.g., requiring as many as 10 times more learning trials than non-memory impaired participants; Bayley & Squire, 2002). In contrast, the amnesia participants in our barrier task protocol displayed an entirely normal rate of acquisition (Duff et al., 2006), suggesting that simple repetition of card labels cannot account for this striking success.

So what does account for the pairs' successful learning? Although the barrier task was not designed to elicit repeated behaviours from participants, it was designed to support participants' repeated engagement in managing the target cards as they completed the activity (i.e., identifying and placing target cards). Successful collaborative referencing was rewarded (e.g., correctly placing cards) regardless of how the pairs referenced the cards, and the researchers made no attempt to direct the participants to use any specific words or phrases. Within this protocol, conversational repetition was common, both during task trials (as pairs negotiated card labels and confirmed card selections) and between trials (as some pairs told stories or teased one another about card labels). From a sociocultural perspective, it is this meaningful, goal-directed, and collaborative repetition of labels that accounts for the robust learning seen within this protocol.

As an initial step towards translating the successful learning found in the research protocol into a clinical intervention, we undertook a pilot treatment study using our collaborative barrier task (Hengst, Duff, Buma, & Bay, 2006; Hengst et al., 2008). A critical goal was to determine if a clinician could assume the collaborative partner role that was filled in the research design by the clients' routine communication partners. Designed for a patient with amnesia and mild aphasia, the pilot also expanded the number of referencing targets from 12 to 30 and extended the protocol from 4 to 10 sessions. On all measures the pilot was a success—the client–clinician pair completed all trials, accurately placed cards (98.9% accuracy overall), and developed specific labels for all 30 targets. A fidelity analysis documented that the clinician successfully adopted a collaborative partner role during the trials (for details see Bay, 2007; Bay, Hengst, & Duff, 2008). The current analysis follows up the findings of the pilot study by examining the client–clinician pair's use of conversational repetition of card labels during these treatment sessions.

## METHOD

This study presents a situated discourse analysis of conversational repetition of card labels during the 10-session pilot treatment study discussed above. Here we describe the dataset and then detail the procedures developed to identify and code repetition across sessions.

### Participants and dataset analysed

Four people participated in the pilot study: Melissa, the second author, was the clinician-partner for Dave, the client-participant; Lori, a graduate student, was the clinician-moderator who managed the sessions (providing instructions, setting up the director's board, scoring accuracy of card placements); and Julie, the first author, took the lead in managing the research. At the time of the study, Dave (a 67-year-old administrator with a doctoral degree) was medically stable and 8 months post a series of left hemisphere strokes. MRI revealed lesions in left temporal, parietal and occipital lobes, left pons, and genu of left internal capsule. Neuropsychological testing (at 5 months post-onset) revealed a mild anomic aphasia (Boston Naming Test 53/60), moderate-severe deficits in executive functioning (Wisconsin Card Sorting Task = 1 Category; 41 perseverative errors) and average intellectual functioning (Wechsler Adult Intelligence Scale-III Full Scale IQ = 107). Dave had a severe memory impairment (Wechsler Memory Scale-III General Memory Index = 69) and displayed incomplete retrograde amnesia spanning 4 years, impaired prospective memory, and difficulty carrying on conversations about current events.

In each of the 10 treatment sessions, which averaged 45 minutes (range 33–55), six barrier task trials were completed. Sessions began by reviewing the purpose of the study and the pair's success during the previous session, and discussing any memory/ word finding problems Dave reported during the past week. Dave and Melissa then completed the barrier task trials, with Lori (clinician moderator) giving instructions and arranging the director's board before, and checking accuracy of the matcher's board after each trial. Dave and Melissa alternated director/matcher roles each trial and were instructed to work together to arrange the matcher's cards in the same order as the director's board, to have fun and communicate freely, but to not look over the barrier at each other's boards. Cards included 30 referencing targets (10 each of familiar people, local street intersections, and area buildings), with two colour photographs used for each target; each target was used in four sessions. At the end of each session, Dave and Melissa were asked to report the most specific and useful label for each card, which was recorded as their agreed-upon target label (ATL) for the session.

Throughout the pilot we explained that the goal of the study was to investigate the therapeutic value of conversational repetition of referential labels through repeated engagement in a meaningful task. We developed a point system, with 1 point awarded for each card correctly placed on the matcher's board (12 possible points per trial) and a second for each time the pair referenced the card using their ATL (12 possible points per trial). To support Dave's goal of improving his word finding, we encouraged him to work with Melissa to develop and use specific or proper names for the cards, and to see the game as an opportunity to practise these labels by repeating them often. We anticipated that the matcher would use repetition to confirm labels (e.g., Barack Obama; Okay, Barack Obama). However, Dave and Melissa did not consistently use repetition this way. So, during the fourth session, we added a point for the matcher's repetition of the director's label, increasing the total possible points to 36 per trial. Although Lori provided summary feedback on their use of conversational repetition, she was not in the room during game trials. Thus, any prompting to repeat labels during trials came directly from the pair (e.g., *You have to say it for us to get full points*).

## Analysing conversational repetition of referencing expressions

All 10 sessions were videotaped and transcribed. Each barrier task trial consisted of 12 relatively discrete *card placement sequences* (CPSs), for which we could confidently relate *referencing expressions* to specific cards. Thus for coding we only identified expressions used to reference cards during CPSs (i.e., not those that occurred between trials or during interviews). Across 10 sessions this yielded a total of 2022 referencing expressions for further analysis.

## Coding conversational repetition of card labels during barrier task trials

Two coding teams, using consensus procedures (at least three passes through the data and resolution of all disagreements), coded all labels in one of four categories: *agreed-upon target label* (ATL), *non-agreed-upon target label* (NATL), *repetition of agreed-upon target label* (R-ATL), and *repetition of non-agreed-upon target label* (R-NATL). Broadly, the first two codes (ATL, NATL) compared referencing expressions to the ATL for the card in that session; the second two codes (R-ATL, R-NATL) compared referencing expressions to others within the same CPS. Thus the first use of an ATL by either Dave or Melissa within a CPS was coded ATL, with any subsequent uses within that CPS coded R-ATL. The first use of any other referencing expression for the target card within a CPS was coded as NATL and any subsequent uses coded R-NATL.

Reflecting the diversity of conversational repetition (e.g., from identical and complete to transformed or partial repetitions), our coding included exact matches (e.g., *Oliver Sacks*; *Oliver Sacks*) and close approximations that involved changes in word order (e.g., *Missy and Julie*; *Julie and Missy*), inclusion/deletion of adjectives (e.g., *restaurant with green benches*; *restaurant with two benches*), partial productions (e.g., *Hessel Boulevard*; *Hessel and Elm*), and expansions (e.g., *a man with a beard*; *a man with glasses and a beard*). In order for expressions to be coded as an ATL or repetition, it needed to include key elements and/or at least half of the original expression. If coders did not agree on a match, the referencing expression was coded NATL.

## Analysing repetition outside barrier task trials

To examine chains of repetition across trials and sessions, two other analyses were completed. First the four ATLs identified during the interviews for each of the 30 targets were compared, and the consistency of ATL expressions used across sessions is reported in the results. Second, the transcript segments that occurred before, after, and between barrier task trials were reviewed for instances of referencing expressions (ATLs and NATLs) identified during CPS. This analysis supported the interpretive accounts for two specific cards presented in the results.

# RESULTS

The barrier task design supported conversational repetition of the emerging labels with little direction from the clinician-moderator. In this section we summarise the results of the repetition coding, which documents the amount of immediate conversational repetition of referencing expressions used during the 60 barrier task trials. Using situated discourse analysis we trace patterns of conversational repetition for two referencing targets. We also briefly document the patterns of more distant, or delayed conversational repetition that extended well beyond the immediate interactions around identifying and placing target cards within each trial.

## Conversational repetition of referencing expressions

Coding results (see Table 1) revealed three general findings. First, while completing the trials Dave and Melissa verbally referenced the cards more often than would be predicted by the treatment protocol alone. Minimally, in a streamlined CPS the director provides an initial reference for each card and the matcher repeats it to confirm the target card (i.e., 12 initial references and 12 repetitions per trial, or 144 references per session). However, Dave and Melissa averaged 202.2 (range of 196 to 222) referencing expressions per session, or 40% more than this minimal amount of referencing supported by the design alone. The second finding was that Dave and Melissa routinely repeated their own, or each other's, referencing expressions more than the anticipated 72 times. Overall, just under half (88.3, or 44%) of the referencing expressions Dave and Melissa used per session were coded as repetitions (R-ATL or R-NATL), with the remainder (113.9, or 56%) coded as first sayings (ATL or NATL). Third, by comparing referencing expressions to the ATL, analysis indicated that Dave and Melissa were not simply using any reference, but

TABLE 1
Referencing expressions for target cards

| Session (card sets) | ATL | NATL | R-ATL | R-NATL | TOTAL |
|---|---|---|---|---|---|
| 1 (A1, A2) | 71 | 70 | 26 | 36 | 203 |
| 2 (A3, A4) | 82 | 46 | 41 | 12 | 181 |
| 3 (A5, A1) | 75 | 58 | 45 | 30 | 208 |
| 4 (A2, A3) | 75 | 20 | 102 | 2 | 199 |
| 5 (A 4, A5) | 75 | 30 | 83 | 14 | 202 |
| 6 (B1, B2) | 81 | 14 | 98 | 3 | 196 |
| 7 (B3, B4) | 79 | 45 | 88 | 10 | 222 |
| 8 (B5, B1) | 77 | 36 | 90 | 6 | 209 |
| 9 (B2, B3) | 81 | 14 | 98 | 3 | 196 |
| 10 (B4, B5) | 79 | 31 | 86 | 10 | 206 |
| TOTAL | 775 | 364 | 757 | 126 | 2022 |

Number of referencing expressions for target cards within card placement sequences which were coded as the agreed-upon target label (ATL), a non-agreed-upon label (NATL), as an immediate repetition (R-) of the ATL or NATL. Totals presented for each of the ten treatment sessions (with 72 card placements per session). (Note: Target cards were organised into sets, with six referencing targets in each of five numbered sets, and the perspectives for each photograph identified by letters. Thus, sets A1 and B1 contained different photographs of the same six targets. Cards sets were alternated each session.)

were collaborating to focus on consistent, specific, and meaningful labels. On average, the majority (153.2, or 76%) of referencing expressions per sessions were coded as first or repeated productions of the ATL (77.5 ATL, 75.7 R-ATL), whereas only 49 (24%) were coded as NATL (36.4 NALT, 12.6 R-NALT). Across sessions referencing expressions coded as (R-)NATL declined while references coded as (R-)ATL increased.

### Referencing target cards: Two examples

*Oliver Sacks.* The first example, which documents referencing of the *Oliver Sacks* cards, is striking because the referencing expressions were very stable and repetitions were mostly verbatim repetitions of the ATL. Although Dave and Melissa both knew of Oliver Sacks and later reported having read several of his books, for the first three trials they had not yet identified one card as a photo of him (see Appendix for a list of referencing expressions used across the first six trials). Thus they used referencing expressions that described the photo (e.g., D: *A picture of someone . . .*) and described the man pictured (e.g., M: *Fellow has a beard*; D: *Man with glasses and beard*; M: *Guy with beard . . . looking pensive*). After the third trial Dave asked Lori (clinician-moderator) about the card, and Lori told them it was a photo of Oliver Sacks, to which Dave responded: *Oh I should have recognised him.* For the remaining three trials of that session Dave and Melissa used *Oliver Sacks* as the only referencing expression for this card. Indeed, *Oliver Sacks* was a remarkably stable label for this target. In all four post-session interviews Dave and Melissa quickly agreed that *Oliver Sacks* was their label, and with only two exceptions, it was the only referencing label used initially by directors and repeated by matchers during the remaining 18 trials. The two exceptions were during the first trials for the second and fourth session using the card. Dave was directing and could not recall the name, a fact that he folded into the NATL (D: *Forgot the guy's name, uh with a beard*; D: *Guy whose name I've forgotten*). In both cases, Melissa had no trouble identifying the target card and offering their ATL (M: *Oliver Sacks?*), which Dave without prompting confirmed by repeating exactly (D: *Oliver Sacks*). Overall, across the 24 CPS with this target, Dave and Melissa produced 53 referencing expressions, 21 were coded as ATL, 21 as R-ATL, 6 as NATL, and 5 as R-NATL.

*University and Walnut.* In contrast, this second example illustrates variability in referencing expressions and the transformative character of conversational repetition. The target reference here is a downtown intersection of two main streets, *Walnut Street* and *University Avenue*. Dave and Melissa found the intersection targets the most difficult to identify (e.g., confusing one intersection for another) and the most difficult to label succinctly (e.g., unsure of street names). This particular target was no exception (see Appendix for a list of referencing expressions used in first 12 trials for this target). Dave and Melissa knew both of these streets by name and were quite familiar with the downtown area shown in the photographs. However, in the foreground of the photographs was a third street, a small street (Chester Street) that many area residents would have difficulty naming, and in the distance was the point where Walnut Street splits from Neil Street (with each forming one-way streets in opposite directions through downtown). Across the four sessions Dave and Melissa quickly identified and accurately placed the target card; however, while doing so they used many different referencing expressions detailing what was pictured including street names (e.g., University, Neil, Walnut), buildings (e.g., Inman Hotel, Esquire), and other descriptions (e.g., three-way intersection; yellow car). In total Dave and Melissa produced 90 referencing expressions for this target during these 24 trials (almost twice as many as the 48 that would be predicted by the task itself or the 53 used for the *Oliver Sacks* cards). Of these, 24 were coded as ATL, 25 as R-ATL, 28 as NATL, and 13 as R-NATL. In the first trial Dave initiated referencing with a NATL that he immediately repeated and expanded (D: *An intersection. An intersection with a yellow car.*). Melissa also offered several NATL that she or Dave repeated, and one ATL (M: *University and Neil?*) which she partially repeated twice and fully repeated once (*University. I think it's Neil. University and Neil.*). This pattern of Dave and Melissa producing multiple different referencing expressions and repeating them partially or with qualifications was common across trials with this card. The difficulty they had settling on a specific and accurate label for this target was also evident in post-session interviews—across the four sessions they identified three different ATL (i.e., *University and Neil...two cars*; *Corner with the Inman Hotel*; *Neil and Walnut;*) two of which were inaccurate since *Neil Street* was not part of this intersection. Interestingly, during the interview at the end of the second session Dave, Melissa, Lori, and Julie discussed this card, beginning with Dave reporting *I called it the Inman Hotel*, and Melissa adding *But we talked about the intersection being Neil and University . . . we usually said both*. Lori, while checking her master list, offered the correct street names *Actually, Dr Hengst has Neil and Walnut ...I mean–excuse me University and Walnut*. Melissa and Lori discussed which streets are actually in the photo, and Lori assures Melissa that *Walnut is actually the main one . . . I actually took that this morning*. Dave questioned if this label choice was okay *You don't like Inman Hotel*, and Julie responded *that would be a fine label*. The discussion then shifted to stories about downtown bars and coffee shops, before moving to the next card.

## Patterns of repetition of referencing expressions across trials and sessions

The discourse analysis of referencing specific cards presented above not only illustrates the way that the pair used immediate repetition of referencing labels of their own and each other's references during the card placement sequences, but also highlighted the way that conversational repetition extended well beyond the immediate interactions of the card placement sequences. Indeed, conversational repetitions coded here were anchored in chains of interactions Dave and Melissa had with each other and the researchers across trials and sessions as they discussed specific cards— pointing out what was confusing about naming them, celebrating their success in placing them, and telling stories related to the people or places pictured. The post-session interviews were designed to encourage such repeated conversational engagement with the targets (see *University and Walnut* example above). In addition, our analysis of the transcripts documented that Dave and Melissa discussed specific cards at the beginning of two sessions before trials even began, and after 24/60 trials (see *Oliver Sacks* example above). Through documentation of chains of interactions, we begin to see how during the barrier task trials Dave and Melissa productively leveraged or transformed conversational repetitions of referencing expressions from earlier interactions to meet the goals of the barrier task.

Once Dave and Melissa settled on specific and meaningful labels for the targets, they consistently reused them in later trials and sessions. This was apparent not only in the higher percentage of referencing expressions coded as (R-)ATL across trials and sessions (see Table 1), but also in the stability of referencing expressions identified as ATL across sessions. For 29/30 referencing targets, Dave and Melissa reported the same ATL in all four interviews: for 16 targets the wording was exact (e.g., *Oliver Sacks*) or only altered word order (e.g., *Missy and Julie*; *Julie and Missy*), and for 13 there was a stable key element (e.g., *Campbell Hall*; *Lobby of Campbell Hall*). The ATL changed across interviews for only one target (see *University and Walnut* above). In addition, analysis documented that Dave and Melissa often repeated some or all of a specific NATL in later trials, such as with *Oliver Sacks* (see Appendix) when they repeated the same descriptive reference (e.g., *Fellow has a beard*; *Man with glasses and the beard with hand on his chin*; *Guy with a beard*). Similarly, for the *University and Walnut* target they repeatedly referred to the large building in the photograph (e.g., *A big five story building on the left*; *With the big building on the left*), which in the second session was transformed into the ATL (*Corner with the Inman Hotel*). This last example points to more distant dialogic histories that routinely shape, or provide resources for, referencing. The Inman Hotel, built in downtown Champaign in 1915, is an historic landmark that has been part of the public discourse for years; well known to area residents, it is listed on the National Registry of Historic Places, and its original name has been partially retained—The Inman Plaza—by the current owners.

## DISCUSSION

The barrier task provided repeated opportunities within a treatment protocol for Dave to engage meaningfully and successfully with these 30 treatment targets. Analysis documents that Dave and Melissa routinely repeated their own and each other's referencing expressions throughout the protocol, and that they leveraged chains of conversational repetition (within, between, and across trials) into succinct labels. Moreover, this repetition was achieved without any sustained clinician-directed or guided repetition of isolated treatment targets. Thus, this examination of repetition leads us to the conclusion that marshalling *conversational repetition* through *repeated engagement* in everyday tasks offers a theoretically and empirically grounded framework for reconceptualising language intervention.

## Repeated engagement is not equal to repeated behaviours

The first key to reconceptualising language intervention from this sociocultural approach is a recognition that repeated engagement is not the same as repeated behaviours. To take an analogy, a clinical focus on repeated behaviours is much like practising scales on a piano, whereas repeated engagement involves something more like playing music on the piano or, for that matter, engaging in musical performances with various audiences and in different forums. Drill divorces repetition from histories of use and is functionally simple; the function of repetition in drill is simply to repeat, to perform the drill successfully. In contrast, repeated engagement works to build histories of use (like playing music and performing) and is marked by functional complexity. The analysis presented here shows conversational repetition supporting multiple functions, such as confirming cards within task, recalling earlier card placement sequences to locate a reference, complying with the rule to repeat, talking about each other's labelling of cards, sharing experiences about the people, locations, and intersections depicted, and engaging in humour, verbal play, or ironic critique. What looked most like repeated behaviours was the Oliver Sacks example (see Appendix), where Dave and Melissa produced sequences like *Oliver Sacks, Oliver Sacks, Oliver Sacks.* What is critical to recognise, however, is that this series of immediate, verbatim repetitions was the *motivated end point* of a chain of repeated engagements, not the given starting point that it would be in drill. The power of repeated engagement is that it is flexible in form and heterogeneous in function whereas repeating behaviours involves fixed forms oriented to a narrow clinical function (much like practising scales). Although certain types of automaticity and motor routines can be effectively supported by drill, this perspective argues that mastery of language-in-use and communication depends on repeated engagement in complex activities, where forms are flexibly and creatively deployed across time and functions are multiple and emergent.

## Repeated engagement as the ground of social learning

A second key in reconceptualising the place of repetition in clinical practice is to relate the role of repetition in learning to a broader conceptualisation of memory. Memory research demonstrates that repetition promotes learning (Verfaellie, Rajaram, Fossum, & Williams, 2008). But, just as the functionally and anatomically distinct memory systems in the brain uniquely support acquisition and use of different types of knowledge (e.g., non-declarative memory supporting skill acquisition; declarative memory supporting vocabulary, facts, autobiographical events), these memory systems also differ in their support of different types of repetition. Guided repetition (or drill) of isolated behaviours disproportionately engages the non-declarative memory system. This system supports representations of experience that are *individual (non-relational)* and such memories are isolated as they are encoded only with processors engaged during learning; consequently, these representations are *inflexible* and can only be retrieved within the restrictive range of stimuli and situations of the original learning (Eichenbaum & Cohen, 2001). While drill-based repetition of individual behaviours is effective in mastering those isolated skills, for the reasons outlined above, generalisation tends to be poor. Attention to the nature and limitations of non-declarative memory suggests it is not a candidate system for supporting complex, flexible, communication.

Repeated engagement within meaningful activities and with repeated discursive resources (e.g., words, conversational routines, goal-oriented collaborations) places significant demands on declarative memory. Two hallmark features of declarative memory provide the capability to manage the functional complexity necessary for successful communication and social learning. First, declarative memory supports the *flexible expression* of memory, permitting knowledge to be accessible across processing systems (as when a rich, multi-sensory autobiographical memory is evoked by the sight of a familiar face or the sound of a familiar song) and to be used in novel situations (Eichenbaum & Cohen, 2001). Second, declarative memory supports *relational (non-individual) representations* permitting encoding and retrieval of historical chains of situated experience (that is, the co-occurrences of people, places, words, phrases, actions, and so on) constituting the larger record of one's experience (Eichenbaum & Cohen, 2001).

Our collaborative barrier task protocol builds in flexibility, optimising opportunities for repeated engagement within a goal-directed communicative activity. These sessions are in stark contrast to traditional experimental studies and the gold standards in neuropsychological assessment of memory—consider the use of guided repetition in word list learning tasks or errorless learning protocols, which call for rote learning and later verbatim reproduction. That we have shown here and in our experimental work that repeated engagement confers benefits in memory and learning, even in patients with declarative memory impairments, suggests that repeated engagement is critical in social learning and in intervention.

## Designing clinical activities to support conversational repetition and repeated engagement

Critical to rethinking repetition is a theoretical understanding of how to harness this theory and marshal the robust power of everyday learning and communicative practices. We are not, for example, arguing that the barrier task alone, uniquely, or in any configuration represents a realisation of this theory, so what is critical? We discussed earlier how we redesigned the barrier task research protocol to align it with sociocultural theories and then further adapted that redesigned protocol for the specific clinical intervention with Dave. The first step then is design. Clinicians would need to design activities that draw on the repeated engagement of everyday learning; that is, (a) that allow for complex, functional communication; and (b) that involve mutual and emergent structuring of interaction as opposed to clinician-directed drill. The second step is shifting the role of clinician to seriously take up the role of a communicative partner—a skilled partner and one with multiple goals, including clinical targets, but a partner rather than a drill leader and assessor (Hengst & Duff, 2007; Hengst et al., 2008). The third step involves a shift in attitudes and trusting the process to work. We need to trust that we can get repetition, including immediate verbatim repetition, without directed drill. People will repeat conversationally, even engage in verbatim repetition, through repeated engagement in everyday activities, and they will do much more as well. The flip side of this argument is that the use of guided repetition that works on isolated forms should be used sparingly and refined for specific goals. We believe that current memory research can offer useful guidance in understanding the place of both types learning so that we can strategically and skilfully work with our clients to optimise the reorganisation of their communicative practices and systems after brain damage.

Manuscript received 24 July 2009
Manuscript accepted 9 November 2009
First published online 19 April 2010

## REFERENCES

Bay, S. (2007). *A fidelity analysis of an in-frame treatment approach using a barrier task protocol: A case study of a patient with aphasia and amnesia*. University of Illinois, Urbana-Champaign.

Bay, S., Hengst, J.A., & Duff, M.C. (2008). *A fidelity analysis of in-frame therapy*. Paper presented at the American Speech Language Hearing Association Convention.

Bayley, P., & Squire, L. (2002). Medial temporal lobe amnesia: Gradual acquisition of factual information by nondeclarative memory. *Journal of Neuroscience*, *22*(13), 5741–5748.

Clark, H.H. (1992). *Arenas of language use*. Chicago: University of Chicago Press.

Denes, P., & Pinson, E. (1993). *The speech chain: The physics and biology of spoken language*. New York: W. H. Freeman & Company.

Duff, M.C., Hengst, J.A., Tranel, D., & Cohen, N.J. (2006). Development of shared information in communication despite hippocampal amnesia. *Nature Neuroscience*, *9*, 140–146.

Duff, M.C., Hengst, J.A., Tranel, D., & Cohen, N.J. (2008). Collaborative discourse facilitates efficient communication and new semantic learning in amnesia. *Brain and Language*, *106*(1), 41–54.

Duff, M.C., Hengst, J.A., Tranel, D., & Cohen, N.J. (2009). Hippocampal amnesia disrupts verbal play and the creative use of language in social interaction. *Aphasiology*, *23*(7), 926–939.

Eichenbaum, H., & Cohen, N.J. (2001). *From conditioning to conscious recollection: Memory systems of the brain*. New York: Oxford University Press.

Erickson, C., Hengst, J.A., & Duff, M.C. (2008). *Conversational repetition and amnesia*. . Paper presented at the American Speech-Language-Hearing Association (ASHA).

Hengst, J.A. (2003). Collaborative referencing between individuals with aphasia and routine communication partners. *Journal of Speech, Language, and Hearing Research*, *46*, 831–848.

Hengst, J.A. (2006). "That mea::n dog": Linguistic mischief and verbal play as a communicative resource in aphasia. *Aphasiology*, *20*(2/3/4), 312–326.

Hengst, J.A., & Duff, M.C. (2007). Clinicians as communication partners: Developing a mediated discourse elicitation protocol. *Topics in Language Disorders*, *27*(1), 37–49.

Hengst, J.A., Duff, M.C., Buma, K.F., & Bay, S. (2006). *Targeting collaborative referencing: Translating research into clinical practice*. Paper presented at the American Speech-Language-Hearing Association Annual Convention.

Hengst, J.A., Duff, M.C., & Prior, P.A. (2008). Multiple voices in clinical discourse and as clinical intervention. *International Journal of Language and Communication Disorders*, *43*(S1), 58–68.

Maas, E., Robin, D., Hula, S., Feedman, S., Wulf, G., Ballard, K., et al. (2008). Principles of motor learning in treatment of motor speech disorders. *American Journal of Speech-Language Pathology*, *17*, 277–298.

Maher, L., Kendall, D., Swearengin, J., Rodriguez, A., Leon, S., Pingel, K., et al. (2006). A pilot study of use-dependent learning in the context of constraint induced language therapy. *Journal of International Neuropsychological Society*, *12*(6), 843–852.

O'Kane, G., Kensinger, E., & Corkin, S. (2004). Evidence for semantic learning in profound amnesia: An investigation with patient H.M. *Hippocampus*, *14*, 417–525.

Prior, P.A., Hengst, J.A., Roozen, K., & Shipka, J. (2006). 'I'll be the sun': From reported speech to semiotic remediation practices. *Text & Talk*, *26*(6), 733–766.

Pulvermüller, F., Neininger, B., Elbert, T., Mohr, B., Rockstroh, B., Koebbel, P., et al. (2001). Constraint-induced therapy of chronic aphasia after stroke. *Stroke*, *32*, 1621–1626.

Tannen, D. (1989). *Talking voices*. Cambridge, UK: Cambridge University Press.

Verfaellie, M., Rajaram, S., Fossum, K., & Williams, L. (2008). Not all repetition is alike: Different benefits of repetition in amnesia and normal memory. *Journal of International Neuropsychological Society*, *14*(3), 365–372.

Wertsch, J.V. (1991). *Voices of the mind*. Cambridge, MA: Harvard University Press.

Yule, G. (1997). *Referential communication tasks*. Mahwah, NJ: Lawrence Erlbaum Associates Inc.

# APPENDIX

The two tables below list the referencing expressions for two different treatment targets used by Dave (D) and Melissa (M) during portions of the treatment protocol. The first table lists referencing expressions for the first six trials with the person target *Oliver Sacks* (photo card cards #17/18), and the second table lists referencing expressions for the first 12 trials of the intersection target University and Walnut (cards #11/12). The ATL for the session is in the top row, and codes (ATL, NATL, R-ATL, and R-NATL) for each expression are in the last column.

| Session 1 | ATL (Card #17) Oliver Sacks | Code |
|---|---|---|
| Trial 1 | D: A picture of someone and you know he looks remarkably familiar. | NATL |
|  | D: Fellow has a beard. | NATL |
|  | M: Fellow with the beard. | R-NATL |
|  | M: He's got a beard and glasses. | R-NATL |
|  | M: Man with glasses. | R-NATL |
| Trial 2 | M: Man with glasses and the beard with hand on his chin. | NATL |
|  | D: Man with glasses and beard. | R-NATL |
| Trial 3 | D: Guy with a beard. | NATL |
|  | M: Guy with a beard ..looking pensive. | R-NATL |
| Trial 4 | M: Oliver Sacks. | ATL |
| Trial 5 | D: Oliver Sacks. | ATL |
|  | M: Oliver Sacks. | R-ATL |
| Trial 6 | M: Oliver Sacks. | ATL |

| Session 1 | ATL (Card #11) University and Neil ..two cars | Code |
|---|---|---|
| Trial 1 | D: An intersection. | NATL |
|  | D: An intersection with a yellow car. | R-NATL |
|  | M: City? | NATL |
|  | D: City | R-NATL |
|  | M: It doesn't look like a parking lot. | NATL |
|  | D: No, no parking lot. | R-NATL |
|  | M: A big five story building on the left. | NATL |
|  | M: University and Neil? | ATL |
|  | M: It looks like downtown. | NATL |
|  | M: Esquire? | NATL |
|  | M: Esquire. | R-NATL |
|  | M: University. | R-ATL |
|  | M: I think it's Neil. | R-ATL |
|  | M: University and Neil | R-ATL |
| Trial 2 | M: Picture of the intersection. | NATL |
|  | M: University and I think it's Neil Street. | ATL |
|  | M: With the big building on the left. | NATL |
|  | D: Two cars in the picture? | ATL |
| Trial 3 | D: A street scene probably Urbana:: ..Two cars visible. | ATL |
|  | M: University and Neil . . . Down by Esquire. | ATL |
| Trial 4 | M: Intersection of University and Neil. | ATL |
|  | D: Two cars in the road? | ATL |

(*Continued*)

## APPENDIX
*(Continued)*

| | | |
|---|---|---|
| Trial 5 | D: Street scene in Champaign . . . with two cars visible. | ATL |
| | M: University and Neil. | ATL |
| Trial 6 | M: University and Neil . . . with the big building on the left. | ATL |
| Session 3 | ATL (Card #11) Corner with the Inman Hotel | Code |
| Trial 1 | D: University and First street. | NATL |
| | D: Large building:: yellow car. | NATL |
| | M: University and I think that's Neil. | R-NATL |
| | D: University. | R-NATL |
| | M: The Esquire::: and all those bars on the left side. | NATL |
| Trial 2 | M: University and Neil. | NATL |
| | M: Neil, you pass the Esquire: and Radio Maria .1. the flower shop. | R-NATL |
| | M: University and Neil. | R-NATL |
| | M: I think it's Neil. | R-NATL |
| | M: I know it's University. | R-NATL |
| Trial 3 | D: Ancient Inman Hotel building. | ATL |
| | M: University and Neil. | NATL |
| Trial 4 | M: University and Neil. | NATL |
| | M: Old Inman Hotel. | ATL |
| Trial 5 | D: The former Inman Hotel. | ATL |
| | M: The former Inman Hotel. | R-ATL |
| | M: Intersection of University and Neil. | NATL |
| Trial 6 | M: University and Neil | NATL |
| | D: University and Neil | R-NATL |
| | M: University and Neil. | R-NATL |
| | M: Inman Hotel. | ATL |

APHASIOLOGY, 2010, 24 (6–8), 902–913

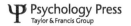

# Social networks after the onset of aphasia: The impact of aphasia group attendance

Candace P. Vickers

*Chapman University, Communication Sciences and Disorders, College of Educational Studies, Orange, CA, USA*

*Background*: Social networks are the context for communication and life participation and are associated with adults' health, well-being, and longevity. Compared to other populations, persons with aphasia have not been included in social network research in the US.
*Aims*: The study aimed to measure and compare 40 participants' social networks and frequency of contact within networks before and after aphasia. It also examined self-ratings of communication/social participation as well as perceived social isolation versus perceived social support. A further aim was to explore the impact of weekly aphasia group attendance on all variables by comparing two groups within the sample: 28 persons attending a weekly aphasia group, and 12 persons not attending an aphasia group.
*Methods & Procedures:* Social network interviews for social network analysis and questionnaire surveys measured the perceptions and experiences of a non-random sample of 40 persons with aphasia in the US. Measures included *Social Networks Inventory* (Blackstone & Hunt-Berg, 2003), *The Friendship Scale* (Hawthorne, 2006), and a pilot tool, *The Survey of Communication and Social Participation* (Vickers & Threats, 2007). Both descriptive and inferential statistics were used to explore the data and compare the aphasia group attendees ($N = 28$) with non-attendees ($N = 12$).
*Outcomes & Results*: Results indicated shrinkage of social networks and reduced frequency of contact with partners after onset of aphasia for the entire group. Independent samples *t* tests revealed significantly higher levels of social participation, and significantly less perceived social isolation and greater social connection for the 28 individuals attending a weekly aphasia group.
*Conclusions*: A major contribution of this study is its direct inclusion of 40 individuals with aphasia in a project in the US that provided quantitative data about social networks before and after aphasia. Results confirm that clinicians should be concerned about potential reduction of social networks and social isolation after aphasia. Data also support the notion of significantly increased social participation and sense of social connectedness for those who attend aphasia groups. The findings point to the need to directly assess aphasic individuals' social networks as the context for life participation through social network analysis. It also suggests that intervention efforts in aphasia therapy would be enhanced by assessing how persons with aphasia perceive their level of social connection as well as their participation in the social environment.

*Keywords:* Social networks; Aphasia; Social participation.

Address correspondence to: Candace P. Vickers, Clinical Faculty in Neurological Disorders, Chapman University, Communication Sciences and Disorders, College of Educational Studies, One University Drive, Orange, CA 92866, USA. E-mail: Candace.Vickers@gmail.com

Thanks are due to the 40 participants with aphasia and their families, as well as to Larry Boles, Jon Lyon, and Travis Threats for helpful comments on the manuscript. The assistance of Darla Hagge at St. Jude Medical Center and Michelle Soo Hoo, honours student at California State University, Fullerton, in collection of data was invaluable.

http://www.psypress.com/aphasiology                    DOI: 10.1080/02687030903438532

According to Gottlieb (1981), the term "social network" denotes the structure of an individual's social contacts. While social networks may constitute the arena for life participation for most people, there are troubling indications that those with aphasia frequently experience social isolation and social exclusion due to attitudinal and environmental barriers (Howe, Worrall & Hickson, 2008; Parr, 2007). Unfortunately, persons with aphasia (PWA) are usually not included in large quantitative social network studies due to their difficulties in communicating (Hilari & Northcott, 2006; Jang, Mortimer, Haley & Graves, 2004). Results of qualitative research indicate reduced social networks after aphasia (Davidson, Worrall & Hickson, 2003; Le Dorze & Brassard, 1995). Quantitative analysis regarding the numbers of partners, frequency of contact, and amount of activity in social networks of persons with chronic aphasia has been reported in Australia (Cruice, Worrall, & Hickson, 2006; Cruice, Worrall, Hickson, & Murison, 2003; Davidson, Howe, Worrall, Hickson, & Togher, 2008), and the United Kingdom (Code, 2003; Hilari & Northcott, 2006). Only three case studies report on the social networks of PWA in the United States (Donham & Lasker, 2007; Simmons-Mackie & Damico, 2001; Trautman Pearson, 2004).

The World Health Organisation's revised classification system, *The International Classification of Functioning, Disability and Health* (ICF) (WHO, 2001), contains two core components that pertain to social network research in aphasia. The first, Functioning and Disability, includes Body Functions and Structures, with a separate category for Activities and Participation. The second, Contextual Factors, includes the environment and personal factors as components that affect individuals' functioning. The ICF asserts that, depending on their presence or absence, environmental factors found in the physical, social, and attitudinal world can serve as barriers or facilitators. For example, an individual with aphasia may attend a social activity yet experience social isolation as an environmental barrier due to the inability or unwillingness of others to appropriately include him or her in interactions (Threats, 2007). Participation is defined as involvement in life situations, which the ICF suggests is a legitimate area of study, research, and assessment as well as intervention. Interpersonal relationships and interactions are domains related to social networks within the activities/participation component of the ICF (WHO, 2001). Clinicians serving PWA can encourage development of social networks in the context of aphasia groups, which are associated with both improved communicative functioning (Elman & Bernstein-Ellis, 1999) and social participation in conversation when trained partners are available (Kagan, Black, Duchan, Simmons-Mackie, & Square, 2001). Aphasia group participation may act as a facilitator by offering PWA chances to experience satisfying interactions in an entirely new social network. Therefore one aim of this study was to determine whether those attending an aphasia group would display enhanced social networks and/or different levels of communication/social participation and social connectedness than those not attending an aphasia group.

This study reports findings with 40 adults with chronic aphasia who were interviewed directly to measure size/functioning of their social networks, communication/social participation and perceived social isolation/social support (Vickers, 2008, 2009). Areas of investigation included: (1) social network size/frequency of contact before and after onset of aphasia; (2) self-ratings of participants for perceived social isolation versus perceived social support; (3) self-ratings of communication and social participation; (4) any significant differences in terms of social networks, perceived social isolation versus perceived social support, and communicative/social participation when comparing two groups within the sample: participants regularly attending an aphasia group and those not attending a group.

## METHOD

### Research design

A total of 40 persons with aphasia responded to social network interviews based on *The Social Networks Communication Inventory* (Blackstone & Hunt-Berg, 2003), as well as two questionnaire surveys: *The Survey of Communication and Social Participation* (Vickers & Threats, 2007) and *The Friendship Scale* (Hawthorne, 2006). Both descriptive and two-tailed inferential statistics were used to explore the data using the computer software package SPSS 14.0 (SPSS, 2005).

### Sampling method

A non-random convenience sample of two groups of participants ($N = 40$) was included. Participants in the first group ($N = 28$), who attended the bi-weekly aphasia group programme created by the author, *Communication Recovery Group* (CRG) (Vickers, 1998, 2004), were invited to participate. CRG served as the site for the experimental group since it offers up to 3 hours of aphasia groups weekly. Groups led by trained student volunteers and interns emphasise use of natural conversation through multi-modality communication (e.g., talking, writing, gesturing, and drawing), and the development of new social networks within the group is a priority (Vickers & Hagge, 2005). Participants for the comparison group ($N = 12$) (non-attendees of CRG) were recruited through referral from colleagues, or recruitment flyers sent to both medical and university training settings, or hand-delivered to community centres serving stroke survivors. Individuals who had not attended *CRG* or any other aphasia group program for at least 10 years were also invited to participate.

### Participants

The study included 21 male and 19 female community-dwelling participants already discharged from outpatient speech language therapy: $N = 40$; mean age = 66.15 ($SD = 12.25$). Inclusion criteria were: chronic/stable aphasia of at least 6 months, judged by SLP as having adequate hearing, vision, and language skills to participate, and no history of psychiatric disorders, rapidly progressing dementia or other degenerative neurological condition. Most participants were married or partnered (78%) and 65% were White/Anglo, with at least five other ethnicities represented in the remainder of the group. All had completed high school and 78% had completed at least 2 years of college. Occupational history indicated that 85% were "white-collar" workers prior to onset of aphasia. Participants had received a mean of 7.47 months ($SD = 10.89$) outpatient speech/language therapy prior to the study and 14 had attended speech language therapy in the university training setting after discharge for an average of 17.66 months ($SD = 25.14$). Aphasia group participants within the sample ($N = 28$) had attended a mean of 111.20 ($SD = 111.48$) hours of group treatment. Of 40 participants, 11 of the 28 aphasia group attendees, and 1 of the 12 non-attendees were also attending individual speech language therapy in university training settings at the time of the study.

## Aphasia severity rating

A clinician with 30 years experience rated participants' aphasia with the Aphasia Severity Rating Scale from the *Boston Diagnostic Aphasia Examination* (BDAE) (Goodglass & Kaplan, 1983) using a semi-standardised interview (Visch-Brink et al., 2005). Individuals were engaged in informal conversation about their week or week-end, and asked to describe the BDAE "Cookie Theft" picture. Table 1 summarises demographic, physical, and functional status variables for each group. Participants self-reported their conditions with support from families as needed. Aetiologies in the CRG group included 24 individuals with left CVA, 3 with CVA due to aneurysm, and 1 with a rare vascular condition causing repeated haemorrhages. The comparison group included 9 individuals with left CVA, 2 with CVA due to aneurysm, and 1 with craniotomy for left hemisphere brain tumour.

## Consent process

Three Institution Review Boards in California approved the study: California State University, Fullerton, Claremont Graduate University, and St. Jude Medical Center, and informed consent was obtained directly from 39 of the 40 participants with aphasia. Procedures incorporated Kagan and Kimelman's (1995) suggestions for increasing access for PWA during the consent process. At the request of participants,

TABLE 1
Summary of participant characteristics: CRG and comparison groups

| Variable | CRG (N = 28) | | Comparison group (N = 12) | |
| --- | --- | --- | --- | --- |
| | Total N | % of N | Total N | % of N |
| *Gender* | | | | |
| Female | 12 | 43 | 7 | 58 |
| Male | 16 | 57 | 5 | 42 |
| *Marital status* | | | | |
| Unmarried | 6 | 21 | 4 | 33 |
| Married or partnered | 22 | 78 | 8 | 67 |
| *Age* | | | | |
| Mean (*SD*) | 64.43 (11.71) | | 70.2 (13.04) | |
| *Number of left hemisphere strokes/brain injuries* | | | | |
| Mean (*SD*) | 1.75 (.967) | | 1.17 (.389) | |
| *Number of months post onset aphasia* | | | | |
| Mean (*SD*) | 81.39 (45.83) | | 70 (54.30) | |
| *Hearing problem* | | | | |
| | 9 | 32 | 3 | 25 |
| *Visual problem related to stroke/brain injury* | | | | |
| | 8 | 28 | 4 | 33 |
| *Mobility problem related to stroke/brain injury* | | | | |
| | 21 | 75 | 9 | 75 |
| *Conditions related to stroke/brain injury (e.g., heart conditions, seizures)* | | | | |
| | 15 | 54 | 7 | 58.3 |
| *Total related conditions* | | | | |
| Mean (*SD*) | .893 (.994) | | 1.0 (1.35) | |
| *Aphasia Severity Rating (from BDAE) * (Ratings reverse coded)* | | | | |
| Mean (*SD*) | 3.96 (1.23) | | 4.25 (.754) | |

a total of 26 individuals considered as significant others signed informed consent forms designed for them so that they could assist as needed during social network interviews.

## Procedure

Social network interviews held in homes or before/after group therapy sessions lasted from 2 to 3 hours total over two sessions to minimise fatigue and ensure that the "before aphasia" and "after aphasia" social networks would be discussed about a week apart. Communication support strategies (Garrett & Beukelman, 1992; Kagan et al., 2001) to enhance language comprehension and expression were utilised as needed throughout the consent process and all assessments.

*Survey of Communication and Social Participation* (Vickers, 2008; Vickers & Threats, 2007): A newly developed 47-item questionnaire tracked demographic, physical, and rehabilitation variables as well as communication and social participation. Codes from the activities/participation section of the ICF were used to develop a simple research tool that explored participants' self-ratings of ability to communicate in daily situations, as well as the frequency of social participation in the community for activities such as eating in restaurants with friends and family. Other questions inquired about whether participants had made new social contacts in the post-aphasia state, and how often they socialised with various categories of partners. Survey questionnaire items were read to participants at a relaxed rate as they followed visually and the examiner pointed to choices for responding. The questionnaire has not yet been standardised and is currently undergoing modifications in line with strategies recommended by Dalemans, Wade, van den Heuvel, and de Witte (2009).

*Social network measurement*: The *Social Networks Communication Inventory* (Blackstone & Hunt-Berg, 2003) documented the social network both before and after aphasia. Participants provided information about their networks using the "Circle of Communication Partners" diagram as follows: Circle 1 = life partners living with the individual; Circle 2 = Good friends and other close family not living with the individual; Circle 3 = Neighbours and acquaintances; Circle 4 = Paid workers; Circle 5 = Universe of unfamiliar partners (Blackstone & Berg, 2003, p. 30). Circle 5 categories included: shopping, restaurants, businesses, religious services, social groups, public speaking, travel, entertainment, and other, and a numerical count of the number of places/opportunities to communicate was taken. The first author of the test confirmed this procedure (S. Blackstone, personal communication, 14 April 2008).

PWA used both speech and writing and collaborated with their families during interviews to provide and confirm social network data. In cases of severe aphasia individuals used yes/no responses and/or pointing to confirm information provided by family members for accuracy. Where family members or caregivers assisted, all information was confirmed with PWA for accuracy through both verbal and multi-modality communication. Many PWA also used address books or other physical reminders to recall names of communication partners. Those who were able to speak fluently enough to generate names of individuals in their networks independently described persons they knew and socialised with before/after the onset of aphasia. When participants could not recall specific names of people for a given section, they were asked to estimate the number of people (e.g., for naming previous co-workers: "Two co-workers") or to describe partners without actually naming them (e.g. for naming a previously known neighbour: "The lady on the corner"). Many partici- pants wrote names of individuals in their networks when they could not say them out loud, or searched through lists of social contacts stored in their calendars, address books, or mobile phones. Others provided information by using pictures from scrap- books or pictures posted on places like refrigerators and throughout the home. The *Social Networks* measurement yielded the total number of partners for each of the five partner sections on the diagram. At each interview, participants also rated fre- quency of contact as follows: 4 = contact two or more times per week; 3 = contact once a week; 2 = occasional contact (monthly or semi monthly); 1 = hardly ever (annually at most). Participants with aphasia with great difficulty speaking pointed at a number rating scale as needed.

The *Friendship Scale* (FS) (Hawthorne, 2006) measured participants' perceived social support versus social isolation. Hawthorne defines perceived social isolation in terms of the subjective sense of living without supports and social contacts. He suggests that *The Friendship Scale* may be useful in health-related quality of life eval- uation studies that need a brief measure of perceived social support or social isola- tion. The FS is a brief six-item questionnaire with reportedly strong internal structures and a Cronbach alpha of 0.83 that was validated with 829 Australian adults, including those with acquired disabilities, over age 60. Examination of FS items suggested the scale might be suitable for use with PWA. Reasons included the following: (1) the FS contains just six items, all worded in present tense about the individual's life over the prior 4 weeks; (2) items are brief, averaging 8.3 words per statement; (3) three items pertain directly to the individual's perspective on commu- nication with others while the other three allow disclosure of emotion about amount and type of interactions; (4) data facilitating interpretation of the FS with PWA are available (Hawthorne, 2008). For ease of reading by people with aphasia, all FS items and their response categories were typed in 20-point bold font using double spacing. Items such as "I had someone to share my feelings with" (Hawthorne, 2006, p. 541) were read aloud to most participants as they followed visually. Response options for each of the questions are: Almost always; Most of the time; About half the time; Occasionally; and Not at all. Each question uses a 5-point Likert scale (Range = 0–4), with scoring advice for certain items to be reverse coded.

## RESULTS

### Demographic, physical, and rehabilitation variables

Independent samples $t$ tests found no significant differences between the aphasia group attendees (CRG) and non-attendees (Comparison Group) for demographic variables such as age, gender, driving status, marital status, employment status, edu- cation level, and income level. Additional tests found no significant differences for average months post stroke onset or brain injury, hearing status, vision status, mobility problem status, presence of other physical problems, total number of other physical problems, and aphasia severity. There was a significant difference between groups for mean number of strokes and/or brain injuries $t(38) = -2.719, p < .010$). Cross tabs comparison confirmed that the highest mean for strokes or brain injuries occurred among the aphasia group attendees. No significant differences between groups were found for rehabilitation variables such as amount of outpatient speech- language therapy received in a medical setting, but differences were found for number of months of college-based speech-language therapy, $t(38) = -2.847, p <$ .007. The CRG group contained 12 individuals currently attending therapy at a college or university setting compared to 2 people who did so in the comparison group.

## Social network size results

Calculations yielded social network size differences for the before and after aphasia conditions for the entire group of 40 participants. Social network size was calculated for life partners, good friends/close relatives, and acquaintances, yielding a mean size of 75.35 ($SD = 87.90$) prior to aphasia and 39.50 ($SD = 19.90$) after aphasia. A second tally combined life partners, good friends/close relatives, and unfamiliar partners for a mean network size of 45.05 ($SD = 24.25$) prior to aphasia and 36.78 ($SD = 21.23$) after aphasia. There were no significant differences for network size in terms of gender for either tally. Two-tailed paired samples $t$ tests indicated significantly fewer social network contacts after aphasia for the first network tally: life partners/good friends/close relatives, and acquaintances ($M = 35.85, SE = 13.86$) $t(39) = 2.586, p <$ .014; as well as the second network tally: life partners, good friends/close relatives and unfamiliar partners ($M = 8.28, SE = 3.18$) $t(39) = 2.689, p < .010$. Independent samples $t$ tests yielded no significant differences between the two groups for network sizes on either network tally in either the "before" or "after" aphasia conditions.

## Social network "frequency of contact" results

Independent samples $t$ tests (two-tailed) indicated no significant differences between the two groups for frequency of contact with close relatives and good friends, acquaintances and paid workers "before aphasia". CRG participants reported significantly more social contact with life partners in the "before aphasia" condition, $t(38) = -2.32, p < .03$. Paired samples $t$ tests found differences for frequency of contact with partners for the "after aphasia" condition for all 40 participants. Results of two-tailed tests indicated significantly reduced frequency of contact after aphasia with close relatives and friends ($M = 0.266, SE = 0.078$) $t(39) = 3.40, p < .002$, and acquaintances ($M = 0.347, SE = 0.120; t(39) = 2.89; p < .006$). There was also a significant increase in frequency of contact with paid partners after aphasia ($M = -0.372, SE = 0.104$) $t(39) = -3.49, p < .001$. In betweengroups comparisons for frequency of contact within social networks in the "after aphasia" condition, CRG participants ($N = 28$) reported spending significantly more time after aphasia with friends, $t(38) = -2.180, p < .04$, with acquaintances, $t(38) = -3.86, p < .001$, and with paid workers, $t(38) = -2.23, p < .032$. The latter finding may be due to the higher mean number of total strokes and brain injuries found among the CRG participants ($p < .052$).

## Survey of communication and social participation

There were no significant differences for mean scores for any of the communication-related variables between the two groups. A frequency distribution for all 40 participants indicated that 19 (47.5%) reported not making new friends in the community after aphasia, while 20 (50%) did report making new friends. Independent samples $t$ tests also searched for significant differences in self-ratings of social participation between the aphasia group attendees and non-attendees and found significant differences

TABLE 2
Social participation variables after aphasia

| Variable | Mean (SD) | Independent samples t test |
|---|---|---|
| 1. Attend movies, plays or concerts with friends/family | | |
| CRG (N = 28) | 3.46 (1.20) | $M = 3.46, SE = .227$; |
| | | $t(38) = -3.81, p < .001, r = .53$ |
| Comparison Gp (N = 12) | 1.83 (1.34) | $M = 1.83, SE = .386$ |
| 2. Attend religious services with friends/family | | |
| CRG (N = 28) | 3.07 (1.72) | $M = 3.07, SE = .325$; |
| | | $t(38) = -3.38, p < .012, r = .48$ |
| Comparison Gp (N = 12) | 1.75 (1.29) | $M = 1.75, SE = .372$ |
| 3. Made new friends | | |
| CRG (N = 28) | 1.71 (.658) | $M = 1.71, SE = .124$; |
| | | $t(38) = -2.20, p < .032, r = .34$ |
| Comparison Gp (N = 12) | 1.25 (.452) | $M = 1.25, SE = .131$ |
| 4. Socialise with friends | | |
| CRG (N = 28) | 2.68 (1.81) | $M = 2.68, SE = .341$; |
| | | $t(38) = -1.947, p < .059, r = .30$ |
| Comparison Gp (N = 12) | 1.58 (1.08) | $M = 1.58, SE = .313$ |

between the 28 aphasia group attendees and 12 non attendees for all four social participation variables listed in Table 2.

## Results of The Friendship Scale

Of the 28 aphasia group attendees, 88% responded directly to items on the FS, while 83% of the 12 non-attendees gave responses directly. Five family members provided responses to the *The Friendship Scale* (FS) on behalf of their partners with aphasia. Data gathered directly only from participants is reported first ($N = 35$). The total score on FS yielded insight into participants' perceptions about their interaction within social networks. Possible scores range from 0 to 24 with scores of 15 and below indicating social isolation and higher scores indicating social connection. The mean FS score for the 35 self-reporting participants was 15.06 ($SD = 5.87$). An independent samples $t$ test revealed a significant difference between total scores obtained by the 25 self-reporting aphasia group attendees ($M = 16.44, SD = 5.46$) and the 10 self-reporting non-attendees ($M = 11.60, SD = 1.78$). Levels of perceived isolation were significantly greater in the non-attendees as opposed to aphasia group attendees, $t(33) = -2.35, p < .03$, with an effect size of $r = .38$. Mean score for the aphasia group attendees was consistent with that obtained by 30 individuals with disability and illness in Hawthorne's 2006 study ($M = 16.38$). Individuals not attending an aphasia group obtained a score of 11.60. This score is below that obtained by depressed individuals (14.13) and just below that reported by nursing home residents (12.22) in Hawthorne's 2006 study. An independent samples $t$ test including responses from the five family member proxy respondents also showed significant differences between the groups. Scores for non-attendees indicated more perceived social isolation ($M = 12.25, SE = 1.73$), while CRG participants reported less social isolation ($M = 16.12, SE = 1.01$). The difference was significant, $t(38) = -2.02, p < .050, r = .31$. Due to the fact that 12 of the aphasia group attendees and 2 of the non-attendees were attending college-based speech language therapy at the time of the study, an analysis of covariance was also conducted. Attendance at college-based therapy was not significantly correlated with the FS total score (−.314, $p < .07$), but when held constant in ANCOVA it produced a significant effect ($p < .012$) suggesting an associated benefit for improving social support among the sample. There was also a main effect for CRG attendance with this covariate, which was slightly more significant ($p < .009$), suggesting that group attendance might confer a separate benefit to attendees in terms of decreasing social isolation and improving sense of social support.

## SUMMARY AND CONCLUSION

Results of this study were consistent with previous studies indicating that SLPs should be concerned about possible social isolation and reduced social networks for their clients with aphasia (Code, 2003; Cruice et al., 2003, 2006; Davidson et al., 2003, 2008; Hilari & Northcott, 2006). The data confirmed significant shrinkage of the social network across both friend and acquaintance categories after aphasia. With chronic aphasia there was also loss of communication opportunities due to reduction of unfamiliar partners/settings for interaction and communication. Further, significantly greater perceived social isolation accompanied reduction in social networks in the comparison group as measured by *The Friendship Scale* (Hawthorne, 2006). Results of independent samples *t* tests both with and without family member proxy responses also suggest benefits of attending aphasia groups, with significantly higher levels of social participation, less perceived social isolation, and greater perceived social support for CRG attendees than that reported by non-attendees in the comparison group. While statistical tests revealed no significant differences between aphasia group attendees and non-attendees on most demographic, physical, rehabilitation, and social network variables that could account for the results, individuals choosing to attend aphasia groups may possess unique characteristics that distinguish them from those who do not seek out the group experience. Limitations of the study include use of a non-standardised pilot measurement tool to measure communication and social participation.

Evaluation of the social network addresses the importance of environmental factors by noting numbers and types of relationships for interaction. It also considers the role of personal factors such as current life experiences as part of functional health (WHO, 2001). Such assessment is consistent with outcomes measurements that go beyond measurement of impairments, such as that proposed by the Living with Aphasia: Framework for Outcome Measurement model (A-FROM) (Kagan et al., 2008). For example, while tests such as the *Western Aphasia Battery* track recovery through improved language task performance (Kertesz, 1979), changes such as increased communication and social participation are not routinely measured or reported. Assessment considering participation might view measurement of existing social networks as just as important as assessing for anomia, comprehension problems, or apraxia of speech. In terms of therapy, priority would be given to helping PWA maintain their current social networks as well as to create and sustain new ones (Simmons-Mackie & Damico, 2001). Aphasia groups provide an authentic context for social network development through both forging new relationships within the group in genuine conversational encounters and encouraging transfer of communication skills to settings outside the group (Pound, Parr, Lindsay, & Woolf, 2000). In addition to measures of improved language functioning, outcome of therapy could be assessed through improved scores on measures that highlight increased levels of social and communication participation with a variety of partners in real environments.

If cardiovascular disease continues unabated, many more lives will be affected by aphasia. To promote increased understanding about life with aphasia and encourage support for community-based programmes that enhance social and community integration, more quantitative data regarding the social networks of PWA are needed. Internationally, researchers and policymakers concerned about social isolation of vulnerable older adults are calling for more data and interventions that will address enrichment of social networks in order to promote health and well being (Grundy, 2006; Litwin & Shiovitz-Ezra, 2006; Netuveli, Wiggins, Hildon, Montgomery, & Blane, 2006; Office of Aging, Orange County, California, 2009). Use of measurements based on aspects of the conceptual framework of the ICF can help generate data that may lead to the kind of "evidence-based advocacy" that leads to positive social change for persons with disabilities (WHO, 2001, p. 243). Social network data regarding adults with aphasia are an example of such measurement, and could serve to highlight the issue that some adults with chronic aphasia are at risk for social isolation. Such data could also inform policymakers that the social integration needs of adults with aphasia should be considered along with those of other vulnerable adults in the wider society.

Manuscript received 25 July 2009
Manuscript accepted 26 October 2009
First published online 7 June 2010

## REFERENCES

Blackstone, S., & Hunt-Berg, M. (2003). *Social Networks: A communication inventory for individuals with complex communication needs and their communication partners.* Monterey, CA: Augmentative Communication, Inc.

Code, C. (2003). The quantity of life for people with chronic aphasia. *Neuropsychological Rehabilitation, 13*(3), 379–390.

Cruice, M., Worrall, L., & Hickson, L. (2006). Quantifying aphasic people's social lives in the context of non-aphasic peers. *Aphasiology, 20*(12), 1210–1225.

Cruice, M., Worrall, L., Hickson, L., & Murison, R. (2003). Finding a focus for quality of life with aphasia: Social and emotional health, and psychological well-being. *Aphasiology, 17*(4), 333–353.

Dalemans, R., Wade, D., van den Heuvel, W., & de Witte, L. (2009). Facilitating the participation of people with aphasia in research: A description of strategies. *Clinical Rehabilitation OnlineFirst.* Accessed 7/1/09 at: http://cre.sagepub.com/

Davidson, B., Howe, T., Worrall, L., Hickson, L., & Togher, L. (2008). Social participation for older people with aphasia: The impact of communication disability on Friendships. *Topics in Stroke Rehabilitation, 15*(4), 325–340.

Davidson, B., Worrall, L., & Hickson, L. (2003). Identifying the communication activities of older people with aphasia: Evidence from naturalistic observation. *Aphasiology, 17*(3), 243–264.

Donham, A., & Lasker, J. P. (2007, September). *Partner-dependent techniques for using the Social Networks Inventory: An example of severe aphasia.* Paper presented at Clinical AAC Research Conference, Lexington, KY.

Elman, R., & Bernstein-Ellis, E. (1999). The efficacy of group communication treatment in adults with chronic aphasia. *Journal of Speech, Language and Hearing Research, 42*(2), 411–419.

Garrett, K., & Beukelman, D. (1992). Augmentative approaches to treatment of severe aphasia. In K. Yorkston (Ed.), *Augmentative communication in the medical setting.* Tucson, AZ: Communication Skill Builders.

Goodglass, H., & Kaplan, E. (1983). *The assessment of aphasia and related disorders* (2nd ed.) Philadelphia: Lea & Febiger.

Gottlieb, B. (1981). Social networks and social support in community mental health. In B. Gottlieb (Ed.), *Social networks and social support.* London: Sage Publications.

Grundy, E. (2006). Ageing and vulnerable elderly people: European perspectives. *Ageing and Society, 26*(1), 105–134.

Hawthorne, G. (2006). Measuring social isolation in older adults: Development and initial social validation of the Friendship Scale. *Social Indicators Research, 77,* 521–548.

Hawthorne, G. (2008). *The Friendship Scale and aphasia.* Unpublished raw data.

Hilari, K., & Northcott, S. (2006). Social support in people with chronic aphasia. *Aphasiology, 20*(1), 17–36.

Howe, T., Worrall, L., & Hickson, L. (2008). Observing people with aphasia: Environmental factors that influence their community participation. *Aphasiology, 22*(6), 618–643.

Jang, Y., Mortimer, J., Haley, W., & Graves, A. (2004). The role of social engagement in life satisfaction: Its significance among older individuals with disease and disability. *The Journal of Applied Gerontology, 23*(3), 266–278.

Kagan, A., Black, S., Duchan, J., Simmons-Mackie, N., & Square, P. (2001). Training volunteers as conversation partners using "Supported conversation for adults with aphasia" (SCA): A controlled trial. *Journal of Speech, Language and Hearing Research, 44,* 624–638.

Kagan, A., & Kimelman, M. (1995). Informed consent in aphasia research: Myth or reality? *Clinical Aphasiology, 23,* 65–75.

Kagan, A., Simmons-Mackie, N., Rowland, A., Huijbregts, M., Shumway, E., McEwen, S., et al. (2008). Counting what counts: A framework for capturing real-life outcomes of aphasia intervention. *Aphasiology, 22*(3), 253–280.

Kertesz, A. (1979). *Aphasia and associated disorders: Taxonomy, localization and recovery.* New York: Grune & Stratton.

Le Dorze, G., & Brassard, C. (1995). A description of the consequences of aphasia on aphasic persons and their relatives and friends, based on the WHO model of chronic diseases. *Aphasiology, 9*(3), 239–255.

Litwin, H., & Shiovitz-Ezra, S. (2006). Network type and mortality risk in later life. *The Gerontologist, 46*(6), 735–743.

Netuveli, G., Wiggins, R., Hildon, Z., Montgomery, S., & Blane, D. (2006). Quality of life at older ages: Evidence from the English longitudinal study of aging (wave 1). *Journal of Epidemiology and Community Health, 60,* 357–363.

Office of Aging, County of Orange, California. (2002). *Report on the condition of older adults.* Accessed on 7/12/2009 at http://www.oc.ca.gov/aging/Condition_of_older_adults_report.pdf.

Parr, S. (2007). Living with severe aphasia: Tracking social exclusion. *Aphasiology, 21*(1), 98–123.

Pound, C., Parr, S., Lindsay, J., & Woolf, C. (2000). *Beyond aphasia: Therapies for living with communication disability.* Bicester, UK: Winslow.

Simmons-Mackie, N., & Damico, J. (2001). Intervention outcomes: A clinical application of qualitative methods. *Topics in Language Disorders, 21*(4), 21–36.

SPSS. (2005). *SPSS 14.0 for Windows, graduate student version.* Chicago, IL: SPSS, Inc.

Threats, T. (2007). Access for persons with neurogenic communication disorders: Influences of personal and environmental factors of the ICF. *Aphasiology, 21*(1), 67–80.

Trautman Pearson, J. (2004). Mr R: Communicating with aphasia. *Augmentative Communication News, 16*(1). Retrieved on 6/5/2008 from http://www.augcominc./pdf/Mr_R.pdf

Vickers, C. (1998). *Communication recovery: Group conversation activities for adults.* San Antonio, TX: Communication Skill Builders.

Vickers, C. (2004). Communicating in groups: One stop on the road to improved participation in life for people with aphasia. *Perspectives on Neurophysiology and Neurogenic Speech and Language Disorders, 14*(1), 16–20.

Vickers, C. (2008). *Social networks after the onset of aphasia: The impact of Communication Recovery groups.* Unpublished doctoral dissertation, Claremont Graduate University, Claremont, California.

Vickers, C. (2009, May). *Social networks after the onset of aphasia: The impact of aphasia group attendance.* Poster presented at the annual meeting of the Clinical Aphasiology Conference, Keystone, Colorado.

Vickers, C., & Hagge, D. (2005). Social networks approach for persons with aphasia. *Perspectives on Communication Disorders and Sciences in Culturally and Linguistically Diverse Populations, 12*(3), 6–14.

Vickers, C., & Threats, T. (2007, November). *Measuring increased life participation associated with attending an aphasia group*. Poster session presented at the annual convention of the American Speech Language Hearing Association, Boston, MA.

Visch-Brink, E., El Hachioui, H., Doesborgh, S., Dippel, D., Koudstaal, P., et al. (2005, May). *Recovery of linguistic deficits in stroke patients: A three year follow up study*. Paper presented to Clinical Aphasiology Conference, Sanibel Island, Florida.

World Health Organization (WHO). (2001). *International classification of functioning, disability and health*. Geneva, Switzerland: World Health Organization.

APHASIOLOGY, 2010, 24 (6–8), 914–927

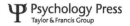

# Measuring the social interactions of people with traumatic brain injury and their communication partners: The adapted Kagan scales

Leanne Togher and Emma Power

*The University of Sydney, NSW, Australia*

Robyn Tate

*The University of Sydney, and Royal Rehabilitation Centre Sydney, NSW, Australia*

Skye McDonald

*The University of New South Wales, Sydney, NSW, Australia*

Rachel Rietdijk

*The University of Sydney, Sydney, NSW, Australia*

*Background*: Considerable attention has been given to the nature of communication impairments of individuals with TBI (Coelho, 2007; Ylvisaker, Turkstra, & Coelho, 2005). However, there have been few data focusing on the way communication partners deal with the often distressing sequelae of TBI.

*Aims*: This study reports inter- and intra-rater reliability of the Adapted Measure of Support in Conversation (MSC) and Measure of Participation in Conversation (MPC) for TBI interactions.

*Method & Procedures*: The MSC and MPC were adapted to reflect theoretical models of cognitive-communication support for people with TBI. A total of 10 casual and 10 purposeful TBI interactions were independently rated by two raters to establish inter-rater reliability and by one rater on two separate occasions to determine intra-rater reliability.

*Outcomes & Results*: Excellent inter-rater agreement was established on the MSC (ICC = 0.85–0.97) and the MPC (ICC = 0.84–0.89). Intra-rater agreement was also strong (MSC: ICC = 0.80–0.90; MPC: ICC = 0.81–0.92). Over 90% of all ratings scored within 0.5 on a 9-point scale.

*Conclusions*: This is the first scale to measure the communication partner during TBI interactions. It shows promise in evaluating communication partner training programmes.

*Keywords:* Traumatic brain injury; Rating scales; Conversation; Assessment; Cognitive-communication.

According to the World Health Organisation, traumatic brain injury (TBI) will surpass many diseases as the major cause of death and disability by the year 2020 (Hyder,

Address correspondence to: Associate Professor Leanne Togher, National Health and Medical Research Council Senior Research Fellow, Speech Pathology, Faculty of Health Sciences, University of Sydney, PO Box 170, Lidcombe, NSW 1825, Australia. E-mail: leanne.togher@usyd.edu.au

This study was supported by a National Health and Medical Research Council (NH&MRC) project grant.

DOI: 10.1080/02687030903422478

Wunderlich, Puvanachandra, Gururaj, & Kobusingye, 2007). It is estimated that 10 million people are affected worldwide annually, leading to a significant pressure on health and medical resources. TBI most often affects young adults who suffer devastating life-long disabilities; however, there is also a higher incidence in early childhood and the elderly (Bruns & Hauser, 2003). Traumatic brain injury (TBI) can result in cognitive communication impairments, which may significantly affect interpersonal relationships (Struchen et al., 2008). Considerable attention has been given to the nature of communication impairments of individuals with TBI (Coelho, 2007; Ylvisaker, Turkstra, & Coelho, 2005); however, there have been few data focusing on the way communication partners deal with the often distressing sequelae of TBI.

In any conversation the person with communication difficulties represents only one side of the interaction. The behaviour of their conversational partner is important, facilitating, or diminishing opportunities for the individual with brain injury to continue the conversation in a successful manner. Indeed, it has been found that TBI individuals are often disadvantaged in interactions because of the way their communication partners interact with them. For example, in a study of telephone conversations where TBI participants requested information from a range of communication partners, they were asked for and were given less information than matched control participants (Togher, Hand, & Code, 1996, 1997a, 1997b). Therapists and mothers never asked people with TBI questions to which they did not already know the answer. Additionally, TBI participants were more frequently questioned regarding the accuracy of their contributions and contributions were followed up less often than matched control participants. Communication partners used patronising comments, flat voice tone, and slowed speech production when talking to people with TBI. This was in contrast to the control interactions, where participants were asked for unknown information, encouraged to elaborate, did not have their contributions checked frequently, and had their contributions followed up. It is therefore important to consider the contributions of the communication partner, as they can be a barrier or facilitator to effective interactions for people with TBI. Examining interactions with everyday communication partners is also consistent with the WHO ICF (WHO, 2001) call to consider environmental and other factors during assessment. As a consequence of increased understanding of the impact of partners on communication, partner training aimed at improving communication support has arisen as an approach to intervention. The difficulty is that few assessment tools have been designed to examine the contributions of communication partners in interactions of people with acquired brain injury.

One exception, developed for use with volunteers in conversations with people with aphasia (PWA) (Kagan, Black, Duchan, Simmons-Mackie, & Square, 2001; Kagan et al., 2004), is the Measure of skill in Supported Conversation (MSC). The MSC rates the uninjured communication partner's ability to (i) acknowledge and (ii) reveal communication competence of the PWA. The Measure of Participation in Conversation (MPC) examines the PWA's ability to participate in the interactional and transactional elements of conversation (Kagan et al., 2004). Kagan et al. (2004, p. 75) states, "The set of measures was deliberately designed to assess aspects of communication on a macro or global level." The motivation behind the measures was to reduce the focus of ratings solely on the person with aphasia and represent the person in the context of another, along with the degree of support their communicative partner provides.

Administration of the MSC and MPC involves the rater scoring a 10-minute videotape of a social interaction between the person with aphasia and their communication partner on a 9-point Likert scale. Psychometric data have been reported (Kagan et al., 2004) attesting to the robust nature of this measure when evaluating the interactions of PWA and volunteer conversational partners. Inter-rater reliability was estimated using intraclass correlations. Intraclass correlations provide a refined estimation of rater reliability, taking into account whether agreement is between the same or different raters (Shrout & Fleiss, 1979). Using this approach, inter-rater reliability on the Patient Participation (MPC) and Partner Support (MSC) Measures ranged between .91 and .96 ($p < .001$). Construct validity was measured by correlating informal clinical judgements by speech pathologists of communicative proficiency with MPC and MSC ratings on 10 individuals with aphasia. There was a significant positive correlation between informal clinical judgement and scores on all categories of the measures for both raters (rater 1: rho ranged from .87 to .95, $p < .01–.001$; rater 2: rho ranged from .83 to .88, $p < .001–.003$).

The structure and main elements of the Kagan scales provide a solid basis for use in examining the interactions of people with TBI. However, the nature of support required in TBI interactions is different. Skills theorised to be important for supporting people with TBI have been developed by Ylvisaker and colleagues including scaffolding, cognitive supports, collaboration, and elaboration techniques (Ylvisaker, Feeney, & Urbanczyk, 1993; Ylvisaker, Sellars, & Edelman, 1998). For example, in teaching collaborative techniques, the following information is given to the communication partner:

*We are doing this together, as a cooperative project.*

*When in conversation, this means that we intend to convey this message to the other person. That is, we take turns, each having a go and helping the other person.*

*Conversation is more about shared meaning than whether content is right or wrong alone.*

*Collaboration is a way of "sharing the floor" in a conversation, making sure that each person contributes as much as they can in the situation, supporting the person with brain injury to participate as much as possible.*

Ylvisaker and colleagues have given specific guidelines regarding how to make a conversation collaborative. These include using collaborative intent, cognitive support, emotional support, positive questioning style, and collaborative turn taking. For example, collaborative intent includes sharing information, using collaborative talk, "Let's think about this", showing an understanding of what was said, inviting the partner to evaluate their contribution, confirming the partner's contribution, showing enthusiasm for contributions, and establishing equal leadership roles. Similarly, Ylvisaker recommends that facilitating elaboration is an effective way to promote the person with TBI's ability to engage in interactions. There are two key ways to do this including, first, elaboration of topics (e.g., introduce and initiate topics of interest which can go further, maintain the topic for many turns, partner contributes many pieces of information to the topic and partner invites elaboration with open-ended questions), and second, elaborative organisation which involves the communication partner providing scaffolding to enable to the person with TBI to organise their ideas in conversation, to make connections when topics change, to make connections among day to day conversational themes, and review organisation of information.

These techniques are currently being evaluating in a multi-centre clinical trial examining communication partner training in improving communication skills for people with severe TBI (Togher, McDonald, Tate, Power, & Rietdijk, 2009). With a paucity of measures to evaluate the contributions of communication partners in addition to those of the person with TBI, we sought to adapt the MSC and MPC to capture the specific conversational supports that were relevant to TBI interactions.

## AIMS OF THE STUDY

This study has the following aims:

1. To describe the modification of the Measure of Support in Conversation (MSC) and Measure of Participation in Conversation (MPC) (Kagan et al., 2004) for people with TBI and their communication partners based on current theoretical perspectives (Ylvisaker et al., 1993).

2. To report on the inter- and intra-rater reliability of these adapted measures using the same conversation text types as will be employed in the clinical trial.

## METHOD

The original MPC and MSC scales are 9-point Likert scales, presented as a range of 0–4 with 0.5 levels for ease of scoring. The scale ranges from 0 (no participation) through 2 (adequate participation) to 4 (full participation in conversation). Within the MPC, there are two subscales encompassing Interaction and Transaction, while the MSC has two subscales including Acknowledging Competence and Revealing Competence. The Revealing Competence subscale is, in turn, composed of three elements that are scored separately and averaged to give the score for this subscale. The elements are: (a) Ensuring the adult understands, (b) Ensuring the adult has a means of responding, and (c) Verification.

Development of the Adapted MPC and MSC scales occurred over approximately a 1-year period in four stages. In stage 1, behavioural descriptors from Ylvisaker et al.'s collaborative/elaborative approach were mapped onto the themes and categories of the original MPC/MSC scales. In stage 2, we undertook a process of deletion of overlapping and irrelevant information to TBI. Next (stage 3), piloting was conducted on scale descriptors and anchors. Both the descriptors and anchors were then modified as the original anchors of the scale ("very poor, adequate, and outstanding") produced binomial results because raters had difficulty differentiating "adequate" and "outstanding". Anchors were therefore changed to: MPC: "No participation / Some participation / Full participation". MSC: "Not supportive / Basic skill in support / Highly skilled support".

In the fourth stage of development the final adapted versions (Appendix 1) were developed after group discussion between the authors and pilot testing on 40 conversational samples of people with TBI from previous studies. Inter- and intra-rater reliability was then examined on 10 casual conversations, and 10 purposeful conversations to cover conversation text types used in the clinical trial.

### Participants

A total of 10 participants and their communication were included in this study. They were part of a larger study of discourse and communication outcomes in individuals with TBI. Table 1 presents demographic and injury-related variables for participants with TBI. Table 2 presents demographic information for the everyday communication partners (ECP) of TBI participants as well as information on the type of relationship between the ECP and person with TBI. All participants with TBI were at least 12 months post onset, and had a severe brain injury as indicated by the duration of their post traumatic amnesia (PTA) (> 24 hours), a social communication disorder on the Pragmatic Protocol (Prutting & Kirchner, 1987), and a cognitive communication disorder based on a severity score below 17 obtained in the Scales of Cognitive Abilities for Traumatic Brain

TABLE 1
Demographics of participants with TBI (P)

| Participant | Sex | Age (years) | Type TBI | Duration of PTA (weeks) | Time Post TBI (years) | Frontal injury on CT scan (Yes/ No) | SCATBI Severity score | Education |
|---|---|---|---|---|---|---|---|---|
| P1 | M | 38 | MVA | 24 | 16.00 | Yes | 9 | High School, TAFE |
| P2 | M | 19 | MVA | 9 | 3.00 | Yes | 8 | High School |
| P3 | M | 24 | Assault | 13 | 4.10 | Yes | 11 | High School |
| P4 | M | 38 | MVA | 40 | 22.00 | Yes | 8 | High School |
| P5 | F | 24 | Pedestrian | 13 | 15.00 | No | 8 | Junior School |
| P6 | M | 30 | MVA | 20 | 10.00 | No | 10 | High School |
| P7 | M | 32 | Fall | >24 | 6.00 | Yes | 10 | High School |
| P8 | M | 35 | MVA | 1.5 days | 5.50 | No | 12 | High School, TAFE |
| P9 | M | 31 | Pedestrian | >20 | 7.10 | No | 9 | High School, TAFE |
| P10 | M | 62 | Assault | 15 | 1.5 | Yes | 7 | High School |

PTA = Post traumatic amnesia.
SCATBI (Adamovich & Henderson, 1992) severity score ranges: 3–6 = Severe, 7–9 = Moderate, 10–13 = Mild, 14–16 = Borderline, ≥ 17 = Average normal.
TAFE = Technical and further education.

TABLE 2
Demographics of everyday communication partners (ECP) of participants with TBI

| Participant | Sex | Age | Education | Time known TBI participant (years) | Type of Friendship | Knew prior to TBI (Yes/ No) |
|---|---|---|---|---|---|---|
| ECP1 | F | 34 | High School, TAFE | 0.50 | Girlfriend | No |
| ECP2 | F | 47 | High School | 19.00 | Mother | Yes |
| ECP3 | M | 42 | High School | 4.50 | Friends | Yes |
| ECP4 | M | 46 | University | 5.00 | Professional carer | No |
| ECP5 | F | 58 | High School | 24.00 | Mother | Yes |
| ECP6 | M | 45 | High School | 6.00 | Carer | No |
| ECP7 | M | 33 | High School | 25.00 | Friends | Yes |
| ECP8 | F | 35 | High School, TAFE | 0.04 | Girlfriend | No |
| ECP9 | M | 34 | High School, TAFE | 20.00 | Friends | Yes |
| ECP10 | F | 60 | High School | 40.00 | Wife | Yes |

Injury (SCATBI) (Adamovich & Henderson, 1992). All participants gave informed written consent to take part in the study.

## Conversational samples

An unstructured 5-minute casual conversational sample and a 5-minute purposeful conversational sample were obtained from each of the 10 participants. The conversations occurred in a quiet room and were videotaped. In the purposeful sample, participants with TBI and their ECP engaged in one of three jointly constructed discourse tasks after instructions from the research clinician. For example:

1. *Together, we want you to come up with a list of situations you are expecting to face over the next four weeks or so where communication is important to you both. It*

*might be something routine like a family dinner or social event. In the next 5 minutes, come up with a list of these situations together and WHY they are important. We have given you a pen and paper and a reminder of the instructions to help.*

2. *We are collecting information about TBI for people with TBI and their families, friends and carers. We would like you to generate five ideas regarding what you have found useful during your recovery. This may be information about: therapy, ways of dealing with stress, depression, practical ideas, how to deal with your family, how to deal with the medical system, financial or legal matters or anything that you wish you had known after your head injury.*

3. *I have a friend who never seems to have a good holiday. Last holiday she went to the Gold Coast and it rained, and there were blue ringed octopuses so she couldn't go in the water. To top it all off she was bitten by sandflies and swelled up like a balloon. Has anything like that happened to you? We'd like you to generate five ideas regarding what you'd recommend to other people going on a holiday. So, simple practical advice about how to choose your holiday as well as advice about dealing with all elements of a holiday.*

## Raters

Two certified practising speech pathologists (EP and RR) were trained in rating the adapted Kagan scales. One rater had over 13 years' clinical experience working with neurogenic communication disorders including TBI. The second rater had 2 years clinical experience working with people with TBI in a specialised community rehabilitation team. Training involved raters familiarising themselves with the scale descriptors and anchor videos. The raters then rated practice videos and discussed any discrepancies before commencing the rating trial.

## Procedure for rating

A total of 10 unstructured casual conversational samples between a person with TBI and their everyday communication partner (ECP) were randomised and rated on the Adapted MSC and MPC scales independently by the two trained raters. Then 10 purposeful conversational samples between a person with TBI and their ECP were randomised and rated by both raters. For intra-rater reliability, Rater 1 (EP) rated the 20 samples 4 months later with re-orientation and training to the scales. The calculations of Walter, Eliasziw, and Donner (1998) indicated 20 samples were required to provide sufficient power to detect fair (ICC $\geq$ 0.4) to excellent (ICC $\geq$ 0.75) levels of reliability (as defined by Cicchetti, 1994). Data were entered in SPSS and reliability analysis was conducted using Intraclass correlation coefficients (Inter-rater reliability: ICC 2, 1, absolute agreement, single measures; Intra-rater reliability: ICC 3, 1, absolute agreement, single measures).

## RESULTS

Results of the inter-rater reliability ratings are presented in Table 3 and intra-rater ratings are presented in Table 4. Inter-rater reliability for both the Adapted MPC and the MSC scales was excellent, with ICCs ranging from .84 to .97. The ICC ratings were comparable with those reported by Kagan et al. (2001, 2004). Intra-rater agreement

TABLE 3

Inter-rater reliability results for Adapted MSC and MPC scales. Intra class correlations (ICC) and confidence interval data for two raters

| | Adapted MPC | | Adapted MSC | |
| --- | --- | --- | --- | --- |
| | *Interaction* | *Transaction* | *Acknowledge competence* | *Reveal competence (average of 3 subscales)* |
| Casual Conversation ($n$ = 10 samples) | ICC = 0.84, $p$ < .01<br>95% CI = 0.47–0.96 | ICC = 0.84, $p$ < .01<br>95% CI = 0.47–0.96 | ICC = 0.97, $p$ < .001<br>95% CI = 0.87–0.99 | ICC = 0.85, $p$ < .001<br>95% CI = 0.53–0.96 |
| Purposeful Conversation ($n$ = 10 samples) | ICC = 0.88, $p$ < .01<br>95% CI = 0.59–0.97 | ICC = 0.89, $p$ < .001<br>95% CI = 0.62–0.97 | ICC = 0.89, $p$ < .001<br>95% CI = 0.63–0.97 | ICC = 0.88, $p$ < .001<br>95% CI = 0.59–0.97 |
| Kagan et al. (2001) / Kagan et al., (2004) (Original scales) | ICC = 0.85 / 0.93 | ICC = 0.73 / 0.94 | ICC = 0.83 / 0.91 | ICC = 0.89 / 0.96 |

TABLE 4

Intra-rater reliability results for Adapted MSC and MPC scales. Intra-class correlations (ICC) and confidence interval data for Rater 1 on two occasions

| | Adapted MPC | | Adapted MSC | |
| --- | --- | --- | --- | --- |
| | *Interaction* | *Transaction* | *Acknowledge competence* | *Reveal competence (average of 3 subscales)* |
| Casual Conversation (*n* = 10 samples) | ICC = 0.92, $p$ < .001<br>95% CI = 0.747–0.98 | ICC = 0.91, $p$ < .001<br>95% CI = 0.57–0.98 | ICC = 0.89, $p$ < .001<br>95% CI = 0.63–0.97 | ICC = 0.80, $p$ < .01<br>95% CI = 0.40–0.95 |
| Purposeful Conversation (*n* = 10 samples) | ICC = 0.81, $p$ < .01<br>95% CI = 0.44–0.95 | ICC = 0.84, $p$ < .01<br>95% CI = 0.49–0.96 | ICC = 0.84, $p$ < .001<br>95% CI = 0.64–0.97 | ICC = 0.90, $p$ < .001<br>95% CI = 0.51–0.98 |

was also strong with ICCs ranging from .80 to .90. Over 90% of all ratings scored within 0.5 on a 9-point scale.

## DISCUSSION

With recent acknowledgement of the need to assess communication performance in real-life contexts (Coelho, Ylvisaker, & Turkstra, 2005) there has been renewed focus on the development of socially valid tools. Two broad approaches have been taken including: (1) report from the person with TBI or a close-other; or (2) direct observation of the communication skills of the person with TBI in real situations. These approaches have resulted in questionnaire tools, such as the La Trobe Communication Questionnaire (Douglas, O'Flaherty, & Snow, 2000) to gain information on perceptions of communicative ability from everyday communication partners, and direct observation of conversations using fine-grained discourse analysis techniques (Turkstra, Brehm, & Montgomery, 2006). Observational assessments range from frequency counts of the occurrences of inappropriate conversational behaviours (Coelho, 2007), and ratings of frequencies of behaviours based on a 4-point scale (Linscott, Knight, & Godfrey, 1996), to an overall rating of language content and communication efficiency (Bellon & Rees, 2006).

Most global conversational proficiency ratings of people with TBI focus either on the person with TBI or on the interaction as a whole (Bond & Godfrey, 1997; Shelton & Shryock, 2007). They do not provide insight into the specific role of the communication partner, and may not be sensitive to the effects of communication partner training. The Adapted MPC and MSC scales provide a tool that specifically focuses on the skills of communication partners in providing conversational support to the person with TBI, and may therefore be sensitive to detecting change following communication partner training. The results of this study lend preliminary support to the psychometric robustness of this scale.

The ICCs in the current study are strong and consistent with those found by Kagan et al. (2004). It should be noted, however, that the high ICCs may have been possible due to the controlled contexts of the conversational samples studied. In Kagan's initial work all conversational partners were volunteers who engaged in semi-structured interactions, whereas in the current study the communication partners represented a variety of relationships types (e.g., carer, mother, friend, girlfriend, wife) but engaged in controlled and potentially predictable discourse. Future research is required to determine the reliability of the Kagan scales with larger sample sizes, other types of communication partners (e.g., unfamiliar conversation partners, volunteers), different discourse types (e.g., service encounters), and other raters (e.g., community clinicians). Our plan is to use the Adapted Kagan scales as a primary outcome measure in a current multi-centre clinical trial to determine whether training communication partners can change acknowledging and revealing competence behaviours and subsequently improve the communicative participation of the person with TBI. While it is recognised that further work is needed to continue to evaluate this scale, the Adapted MPC and MSC scales offers a new way of examining communication partner contributions to TBI interactions.

Manuscript received 16 July 2009
Manuscript accepted 19 October 2009
First published online 3 February 2010

# REFERENCES

Adamovich, B., & Henderson, J. (1992). *Scales of Cognitive Ability for Traumatic Brain Injury (SCATBI)*. Austin, TX: Pro-Ed.

Bellon, M. L., & Rees, R. J. (2006). The effect of context on communication: A study of the language and communication skills of adults with acquired brain injury. *Brain Injury, 20*(10), 1069–1078.

Bond, F., & Godfrey, H. P. D. (1997). Conversation with traumatically brain-injured individuals: A controlled study of behavioural changes and their impact. *Brain Injury, 11*(5), 319–329.

Bruns, J. J., & Hauser, W. (2003). The epidemiology of traumatic brain injury: A review. *Epilepsia, 44*(Supplement 10), 2–10.

Cicchetti, D. V. (1994). Guidelines, criteria, and rules of thumb for evaluating normed and standardized assessment instruments in psychology. *Psychological Assessment, 6*, 284–290.

Coelho, C., Ylvisaker, M., & Turkstra, L. S. (2005). Nonstandardized assessment approaches for individuals with traumatic brain injuries. *Seminars in Speech & Language, 26*(4), 223–241.

Coelho, C. A. (2007). Management of discourse deficits following traumatic brain injury: Progress, caveats, and needs. *Seminars in Speech & Language, 28*(2), 122–135.

Douglas, J. M., O'Flaherty, C. A., & Snow, P. C. (2000). Measuring perception of communicative ability: The development and evaluation of the La Trobe communication questionnaire. *Aphasiology, 14*(3), 251–268.

Hyder, A. A., Wunderlich, C. A., Puvanachandra, P., Gururaj, G., & Kobusingye, O. C. (2007). The impact of traumatic brain injuries: A global perspective. *NeuroRehabilitation, 22*(5), 341–353.

Kagan, A., Black, S. E., Duchan, J. F., Simmons-Mackie, N., & Square, P. (2001). Training volunteers as conversational partners using "Supported Conversation with Adults with Aphasia" (SCA): A controlled trial. *Journal of Speech, Language and Hearing Research, 44*, 624–638.

Kagan, A., Winckel, J., Black, S., Duchan, J. F., Simmons-Mackie, N., & Square, P. (2004). A set of observational measures for rating support and participation in conversation between adults with aphasia and their conversation partners. *Topics in Stroke Rehabilitation, 11*(1), 67–83.

Linscott, R. J., Knight, R. G., & Godfrey, H. P. D. (1996). The Profile of Functional Impairment of Communication (PFIC): A measure of communication impairment for clinical use. *Brain Injury, 10*(6), 397–412.

Prutting, C. A., & Kirchner, D. M. (1987). A clinical appraisal of the pragmatic aspects of language. *Journal of Speech and Hearing Disorders, 52*, 105–119.

Shelton, C., & Shryock, M. (2007). Effectiveness of communication/interaction strategies with patients who have neurological injuries in a rehabilitation setting. *Brain Injury, 21*(12), 1259–1266.

Shrout, P. E., & Fleiss, J. L. (1979). Intraclass correlations: Uses in assessing rater reliability. *Psychological Bulletin, 86*, 420–428.

Struchen, M. A., Clark, A. N., Sander, A. M., Mills, M. R., Evans, G., & Kurtz, D. (2008). Relation of executive functioning and social communication measures to functional outcomes following traumatic brain injury. *NeuroRehabilitation, 23*(2), 185–198.

Togher, L., Hand, L., & Code, C. (1996). A new perspective in the relationship between communication impairment and disempowerment following head injury in information exchanges. *Disability and Rehabilitation, 18*(11), 559–566.

Togher, L., Hand, L., & Code, C. (1997a). Analysing discourse in the traumatic brain injury population:telephone interactions with different communication partners. *Brain Injury, 11*(3), 169–189.

Togher, L., Hand, L., & Code, C. (1997b). Measuring service encounters in the traumatic brain injury population. *Aphasiology, 11*(4/5), 491–504.

Togher, L., McDonald, S., Tate, R., Power, E., & Rietdijk, R. (2009). Training communication partners of people with TBI: Reporting the protocol for a clinical trial. *Brain Impairment, 10*(2), 188–204.

Turkstra, L. S., Brehm, S. E., & Montgomery, E. B. (2006). Analysing conversational discourse after traumatic brain injury: Isn't it about time? *Brain Impairment, 7*(3), 234–245.

Walter, S. D., Eliasziw, M., & Donner, A. (1998). Sample size and optimal designs for reliability studies. *Statistics in Medicine, 17*(1), 101–110.

WHO. (2001). *The International Classification of Functioning, Disability and Health – ICF*. Geneva, Switzerland: WHO.

Ylvisaker, M., Feeney, T. J., & Urbanczyk, B. (1993). Developing a positive communication culture for rehabilitation: Communication training for staff and family members. In C. J. Durgin, N. D. Schmidt, & L. J. Fryer (Eds.), *Staff development and clinical intervention in brain injury rehabilitation* (pp. 57–81). Gaithersburg, MD: Aspen.

Ylvisaker, M., Sellars, C., & Edelman, L. (1998). Rehabilitation after traumatic brain injury in preschoolers. In M. Ylvisaker (Ed.), *Traumatic brain injury rehabilitation. Children and adolescents* (pp. 303–329). Newton, MA: Butterworth-Heinemann.

Ylvisaker, M., Turkstra, L. S., & Coelho, C. (2005). Behavioral and social interventions for individuals with traumatic brain injury: A summary of the research with clinical implications. *Seminars in Speech & Language, 26*, 256–267.

## APPENDIX: ADAPTED MPC AND MSC SCALES

| A. Acknowledging Competence | |
|---|---|
| Natural adult talk appropriate to context | • Feel and flow of natural adult conversation appropriate to context,<br><br>    ○ e.g., social chat vs. interview; respectful approach to verification (verifying that the conversation partner has understood rather than verifying that adult with brain injury knows what they want to say; not over-verifying)<br><br>• Not patronizing (loudness, tone of voice, rate, enunciation)<br><br>• Appropriate emotional tone / use of humour<br><br>• Uses collaborative talk (rather than teaching / testing)<br><br>• Establishes equal leadership roles in the conversation<br><br>• Uses true questions rather than testing questions |
| Sensitivity to partner | • Incorrect / unclear responses handled respectfully by giving correct information in a non-punitive manner<br><br>• Sensitive to TBI's attempts to engage in conversation, Confirms partner's contribution.<br><br>• Encourage when appropriate, Shows enthusiasm for partner's contribution.<br><br>• Acknowledge competence when adult with brain injury is frustrated e.g., "I know you know what you want to say.", Acknowledges difficulties.<br><br>• "Listening attitude", Demonstrates active listening (e.g. acknowledging, back-channelling)<br><br>• Takes on communicative burden as appropriate / making adult with brain injury feel comfortable<br><br>• Communicates respect for other person's concerns, perspectives and abilities<br><br>• Questions in a non-demanding, supportive manner<br><br>• Takes appropriate conversational turns |
| Score MSC Acknow *Comp:* | 0   0.5   1   1.5   2   2.5   3   3.5   4<br><br>Not supportive    Basic skill in support    Highly skilled support |

| A. Acknowledging Competence Anchors | | |
|---|---|---|
| NONE | 0 | Competence of person with TBI **not acknowledged**. Patronising. |
| | 1 | **Minimally acknowledges** competence of person with TBI. |
| BASIC | 2 | Basic level of skill. **Some acknowledgement** of the competence of person with TBI. |
| | 3 | **Mostly acknowledges** the competence of person with TBI. |
| HIGHLY | 4 | Interactionally outstanding. **Full acknowledgement** of the competence of the person with TBI. |

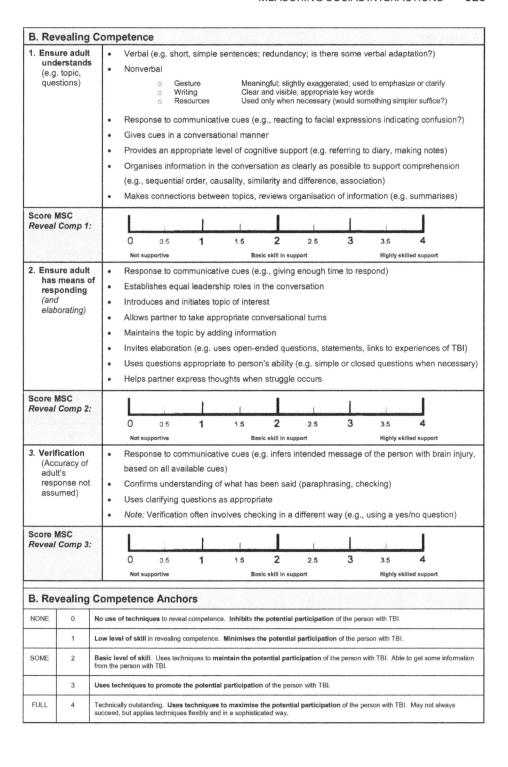

## B. Revealing Competence

| 1. Ensure adult understands (e.g. topic, questions) | • Verbal (e.g. short, simple sentences; redundancy; is there some verbal adaptation?) |
|---|---|

1. **Ensure adult understands** (e.g. topic, questions)

- Verbal (e.g. short, simple sentences; redundancy; is there some verbal adaptation?)
- Nonverbal

  o  Gesture        Meaningful; slightly exaggerated; used to emphasize or clarify
  o  Writing        Clear and visible; appropriate key words
  o  Resources      Used only when necessary (would something simpler suffice?)

- Response to communicative cues (e.g., reacting to facial expressions indicating confusion?)
- Gives cues in a conversational manner
- Provides an appropriate level of cognitive support (e.g. referring to diary, making notes)
- Organises information in the conversation as clearly as possible to support comprehension (e.g., sequential order, causality, similarity and difference, association)
- Makes connections between topics, reviews organisation of information (e.g. summarises)

**Score MSC Reveal Comp 1:**

0    0.5    1    1.5    2    2.5    3    3.5    4
Not supportive          Basic skill in support          Highly skilled support

2. **Ensure adult has means of responding** *(and elaborating)*

- Response to communicative cues (e.g., giving enough time to respond)
- Establishes equal leadership roles in the conversation
- Introduces and initiates topic of interest
- Allows partner to take appropriate conversational turns
- Maintains the topic by adding information
- Invites elaboration (e.g. uses open-ended questions, statements, links to experiences of TBI)
- Uses questions appropriate to person's ability (e.g. simple or closed questions when necessary)
- Helps partner express thoughts when struggle occurs

**Score MSC Reveal Comp 2:**

0    0.5    1    1.5    2    2.5    3    3.5    4
Not supportive          Basic skill in support          Highly skilled support

3. **Verification** (Accuracy of adult's response not assumed)

- Response to communicative cues (e.g. infers intended message of the person with brain injury, based on all available cues)
- Confirms understanding of what has been said (paraphrasing, checking)
- Uses clarifying questions as appropriate
- *Note:* Verification often involves checking in a different way (e.g., using a yes/no question)

**Score MSC Reveal Comp 3:**

0    0.5    1    1.5    2    2.5    3    3.5    4
Not supportive          Basic skill in support          Highly skilled support

## B. Revealing Competence Anchors

| NONE | 0 | No use of techniques to reveal competence. **Inhibits the potential participation** of the person with TBI. |
|---|---|---|
| | 1 | Low level of skill in revealing competence. **Minimises the potential participation** of the person with TBI. |
| SOME | 2 | Basic level of skill. Uses techniques to **maintain the potential participation** of the person with TBI. Able to get some information from the person with TBI. |
| | 3 | Uses techniques to **promote the potential participation** of the person with TBI. |
| FULL | 4 | Technically outstanding. **Uses techniques to maximise the potential participation** of the person with TBI. May not always succeed, but applies techniques flexibly and in a sophisticated way. |

## A. Interaction

| Verbal / vocal | • Does TBI share responsibility for maintaining feel/flow of conversation (incl: appropriate affect)? |
| --- | --- |
| | • Does TBI add information to maintain the topic? |
| | • Does TBI ask questions of ECP which follow-up on the topic? |
| | • Does TBI use appropriate turn-taking (taking their turn, passing turn to ECP appropriately)? |
| | • Does TBI demonstrate active listening (e.g. acknowledging, backchannelling)? |
| | • Does TBI choose appropriate topics and questions for the context? |
| | • Does TBI show communicative intent even if content is poor? |
| Nonverbal | • Does TBI initiate / maintain interaction with CP or make use of supports offered by CP to initiate / maintain interaction? |
| | • Is TBI pragmatically appropriate? |
| | • Does TBI ever acknowledge the frustration of the CP or acknowledge their competence/skill? |
| | • Behaviours might include: <br>    o Appropriate eye contact, use of gesture, body posture and facial expression, use of writing or drawing in any form, use of resource material |

**Score MPC Interaction:**

| 0 | 0.5 | 1 | 1.5 | 2 | 2.5 | 3 | 3.5 | 4 |
| --- | --- | --- | --- | --- | --- | --- | --- | --- |
| No participation at all | | | | Some participation | | | | Full participation |

## A. Interaction Anchors

| NONE | 0 | **No participation at all**. No attempt to engage with communication partner or respond to their interactional attempts. |
| --- | --- | --- |
| | 1 | Person with TBI beginning to take **occasional responsibility for sharing the conversational interaction**, in order to achieve the purpose of the task. |
| SOME | 2 | Person with TBI making **clear attempts to share the conversational interaction some of the time**, in order to achieve the purpose of the task. |
| | 3 | Person with TBI **taking increased responsibility most of the time** for sharing the conversational interaction, in order to achieve the purpose of the task. |
| FULL | 4 | Person with TBI has **full and appropriate participation**. Takes responsibility for sharing the conversational interaction, in order to achieve the purpose of the task. |

## B. Transaction

| Verbal / vocal and Nonverbal | • Does TBI maintain exchange of information, opinions and feelings with CP, by sharing details or by inviting CP to share details? (i.e. is there good content and more than intent alone)? |
|---|---|
| | • Does TBI present information in an organised way? |
| | • Does TBI provide an appropriate amount of information? |
| | • Does TBI ask clarifying questions when necessary? |
| | • Does TBI ever initiate transaction?<br>    • Introducing or referring back to a previous topic<br>    • Spontaneously using a compensatory technique |
| | • Does content of transaction appear to be accurate? (depending on context and purpose of rating, rater would have more/less access to means of verification of information) |
| | • Does TBI use support offered by CP for purpose of transaction? Eg., Referring to a list/diary, using the organization of the conversation provided by CP (e.g. responding to closed choice questions) |

| Score MPC Transaction: | |
|---|---|
| | 0    0.5    **1**    1.5    **2**    2.5    **3**    3.5    **4**<br>No participation at all    Some participation    Full participation |

## B. Transaction Anchors

| NONE | 0 | **No evidence** of person with TBI **conveying content,** in order to achieve the purpose of the task. |
|---|---|---|
| | 1 | Person with TBI occasionally **conveying content**, in order to achieve the purpose of the task. |
| SOME | 2 | Person with TBI is **conveying some content,** in order to achieve the purpose of the task. |
| | 3 | Person with TBI is **conveying content most of the time,** in order to achieve the purpose of the task. |
| FULL | 4 | Person with TBI **consistently conveys content** in order to achieve the purpose of the task. |

APHASIOLOGY, 2010, 24 (6–8), 928–939

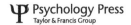

# Distinguishing clinical depression from early Alzheimer's disease in elderly people: Can narrative analysis help?

Laura L. Murray

*Indiana University, Bloomington, IN, USA*

*Background*: Differentiating the reversible cognitive symptoms associated with depression (DEP) from the irreversible dementia associated with early or mild Alzheimer's disease (AD) has proven to be challenging, particularly in elderly individuals. Most previous studies have focused on contrasting the cognitive profiles associated with these disorders, often yielding unreliable clinical differences. Although a limited set of studies have identified significant differences between DEP and early AD groups on both basic and high-level language production and comprehension tasks, none has included spoken discourse measures, and several limitations within these language studies indicate that further research is warranted.

*Aims*: This study examined whether depression is associated with a distinct pattern of discourse changes, and thus whether discourse analyses may help discriminate elderly individuals with DEP from those in the early stages of AD.

*Methods & Procedures*: Groups of elderly participants with DEP, mild AD, or no psychiatric or neurological diagnosis, who were matched for age and education level, completed a spoken narrative task and general cognition and high-level language tests. Quantitative, syntactic, and informativeness aspects of the discourse samples were analysed.

*Outcomes & Results*: Significant group differences were observed on the informativeness discourse measures, with AD participants producing less-informative samples than DEP and control participants. DEP and control groups did not significantly differ on any discourse variable.

*Conclusions*: Including discourse sampling and analyses, with a focus on informativeness, into comprehensive assessment protocols may lead to more accurate discrimination of DEP and early AD in the elderly.

*Keywords:* Dementia; Depression; Discourse analysis; Language.

Despite advances in biomedical assessment procedures, significant overlap in the behavioural and cognitive profiles associated with depression (DEP) and early or mild Alzheimer's disease (AD) in elderly people makes clinical discrimination of these disorders difficult (Caltagirone, Perri, Carlesimo, & Fadda, 2001; Dobie, 2002; Maynard, 2003; Saez-Fonseca, Lee, & Walker, 2007). For instance, both clinical populations demonstrate cognitive decrements in the domains of memory, attention, visuospatial ability, processing speed, and executive functioning as well as behavioural issues such as social withdrawal, anxiety, and apathy (Dobie, 2002; Lantz &

Address correspondence to: Laura Murray PhD, Department of Speech and Hearing Sciences, Indiana University, 200 S. Jordan, Bloomington, IN 47405, USA. E-mail: lmurray@indiana.edu

http://www.psypress.com/aphasiology                    DOI: 10.1080/02687030903422460

Buchalter, 2001; Strang, Donnelly, Grohman, & Kleiner, 2002; Wright & Persad, 2007). Distinguishing these disorders is critical because the cognitive changes associated with DEP are reversible (i.e., they remit with antidepressants), in contrast to the irreversible cognitive consequences of AD.

Unfortunately, because of similar symptoms and because AD can only be definitely confirmed via histopathology findings, misdiagnosis may occur, leading to one or more of the following: (a) prescription of suboptimal or harmful drug and behavioural treatments; (b) provision of inaccurate prognostic information; (c) invalid legal competency rulings; or (d) failure to prevent co-morbidity effects, which in those with untreated depression can include an increased risk of suicide and in those with untreated AD, more rapid disease progression (Alexopoulos, 2003; Caltagirone et al., 2001; Conwell et al., 2000; Dobie, 2002; Lantz & Buchalter, 2001). Diagnostic errors are also problematic given the prevalence of these two disorders (Dobie, 2002). DEP associated with cognitive symptoms, also sometimes referred to as pseudodementia, was found to represent 18% of referrals to a memory clinic, with the diagnosis missed by the majority of those referring the cases (Ferran et al., 1996); other researchers have reported an even larger proportion of individuals with pseudodementia, with 32–41% of dementia cases referred for psychiatric services eventually receiving a diagnosis of DEP with reversible cognitive changes (Maynard, 2003; Rabins, 1981). Likewise the growing prevalence of AD has been well established, with some regions of the United States expected to experience double-digit percentage increases in AD cases between the years 2000 to 2025 (Alzheimer's Association, 2009). Currently, AD is estimated to account for at least 60% of all dementia cases in the elderly and to affect 5.3 million Americans.

Thus far, attempts to identify features that might distinguish DEP from early AD in a quick, accurate, and affordable manner have inordinately focused on cognitive skills and often failed to determine reliable clinical differences (Nathan, Wilkinson, Stammers, & Low, 2001; Roca et al., 2008; Strang et al., 2002; Wright & Persad, 2007). In contrast, only a limited set of studies have included language measures; these initial investigations have yielded significant differences between DEP and early AD groups on both basic and high-level language production and comprehension tasks, with relatively intact proficiency among individuals with DEP and deficits among those with AD (Boone et al., 1995; Crowe & Hoogenraad, 2000; Emery, 1999; Murray, 2002; Stevens, Harvey, Kelly, Nicholl, & Pitt, 1996). Several limitations within these language studies, however, indicate that further research is warranted. First, when language skills in DEP and AD have been compared, a restricted set of tasks has been utilised. Many researchers have used only confrontation naming and verbal fluency (e.g., Boone et al., 1995; Crowe & Hoogenraad, 2000), and only one study thus far has included high-level language tasks such as ambiguous sentence interpretation (Murray, 2002). Second, some contradictory outcomes have been reported. For example, Emery (1999) found that differences between AD and DEP groups were most apparent on basic (e.g., phrase completion naming task) rather than more complex language tasks (e.g., complex syntax comprehension), whereas Murray (2002) reported the opposite pattern. Third, no prior comparisons have included discourse measures, even though discourse analysis has proven useful in identifying AD in the very earliest stages of the disease (Forbes-McKay & Venneri, 2005), distinguishing individuals with genetic risk of AD from their healthy ageing peers (Taler & Phillips, 2008), and discriminating individuals with early AD from those with early vascular dementia (Gustaw & Domagala, 2002) or mild cognitive impairment (Bschor, Kuhl, & Reisches, 2001). Furthermore, Snowden and colleagues (1996) found that low idea density in written narratives completed early in life correlated with poor cognitive function and development of AD in later life.

Accordingly, this study examined whether DEP is associated with a distinct pattern of discourse changes, and consequently whether inclusion of language sampling is warranted when attempting to discriminate DEP from early AD in elderly populations. Elderly individuals with DEP, early AD, or no psychiatric or neurological diagnoses completed a spoken narrative task in addition to formal tests of general cognition and language. The specific aims were (a) to compare the spoken narrative abilities of participants with DEP to those of participants with early AD and those of healthy ageing participants on quantitative, syntactic, and informativeness measures of verbal output, and (b) to determine if the spoken narrative abilities of the participants were related to any demographic variables and/or cognitive or language test performances.

## METHOD

### Participants

As shown in Table 1, participants included 18 with depression (DEP), 17 with AD, and 14 healthy adults (CON). Participants with DEP had been diagnosed by either a psychiatrist or general physician with major depression/unipolar or dysthymia according to DSM-IV criteria (Frances, Ross, & First, 1995); based on information from their initial interview for this study and review of their medical records, all participants with DEP had experienced recurrent episodes of depression and reported memory, concentration, and other cognitive problems. Each participant in the AD

TABLE 1
Group characteristics

| Group | Age (years) | Ed. (years) | Est. IQ[1] | Gender (M:F) | Geriatric dep. scale[2] | Hamilton dep. scale[3] | Dementia rating score[4] |
|---|---|---|---|---|---|---|---|
| *AD (n = 17)* | | | | | | | |
| M | 75.94 | 13.06 | 113.24 | 10:7 | 4.82 | 4.59 | 115.82 |
| SD | 6.64 | 2.41 | 8.14 | | 3.26 | 3.37 | 9.79 |
| Range | 60–86 | 9–16 | 99–124 | | 0–11 | 0–12 | 103–130 |
| *DEP (n = 18)* | | | | | | | |
| M | 73.78 | 14.89 | 116.24 | 4:14 | 14.94 | 25.89 | 135.72 |
| SD | 8.78 | 3.22 | 7.36 | | 3.49 | 7.53 | 4.38 |
| Range | 61–90 | 10–20 | 102–125 | | 11–21 | 16–36 | 129–143 |
| *Control (n = 14)* | | | | | | | |
| M | 73.50 | 14.36 | 116.61 | 6:8 | 2.64 | 2.21 | 139.43 |
| SD | 6.61 | 2.62 | 6.46 | | 2.92 | 2.22 | 3.16 |
| Range | 61–83 | 12–18 | 105–125 | | 0–10 | 0–6 | 132–143 |

[1]Estimated from a regression equation based on demographic variables such as occupation and years of education (Barona et al., 1984).

[2]Based on the participant's responses on the Geriatric Depression Scale (Yesavage et al., 1983), which consists of a set of yes–no questions, and on which scores above 11 are indicative of depression.

[3]Based on a trained rater's completion of the Hamilton Depression Rating Scale (Hamilton,1960) on which scores above 14 are indicative of depression.

[4]Based on the *Dementia Rating Scale* (Mattis, 1988). According to Shay et al. (1991), DRS scores can be categorised as normal (between 131 and 144, with 144 being the maximum score), mild dementia severity (between 130 and 103), or moderate dementia severity (less than 102).

group had been diagnosed by a psychiatrist and met NINCDS-ADRDA criteria for probable AD (McKhann et al., 1984). According to their caregivers and medical records, none of the participants with AD had a history of or currently presented with obvious clinical signs of depression. The medical histories of participants with DEP or AD indicated that other dementia aetiologies (e.g., tumour, vascular dementia) had been ruled out via null findings on laboratory and clinical tests. Inclusionary criteria for all participants included age 60 or older, English as a primary language, and no history of alcohol or substance dependency, head trauma, stroke, or language or learning disabilities. Additionally, all participants were required to pass the speech and visual discrimination subtests of the *Arizona Battery for Communication Disorders of Dementia* (ABCD; Bayles & Tomoeda, 1991) to ensure adequate aided or unaided hearing and vision to complete study tasks. Participants with AD also had to present with only a mild degree of cognitive impairment on the *Dementia Rating Scale* (DRS; Mattis, 1988), and those in the CON group had to show no evidence of current or past psychiatric or neurological disorder.

There were no significant differences ($p > .05$) among the three participant groups in terms of age, $F(2, 46) = 0.522$, years of education, $F(2, 46) = 1.965$, or estimated IQ (Barona, Reynolds, & Chastain, 1984), $F(2, 46) = 1.124$. The groups differed, however, in terms of gender representation, with more women than men in the DEP and CON groups but more men than women in the AD group. A significant group difference was observed on the DRS, $F(2, 46) = 60.630$, $p < .001$, with post hoc Tukey pairwise comparisons ($p < .016$, adjusted for three pair-wise comparisons) indicating greater levels of cognitive impairment among participants in the AD group versus those in the DEP and CON groups, and poorer performance by DEP versus CON participants.

Given the concerns raised regarding the validity of self-rating scales alone in dementia (e.g., Shankar & Orrell, 2000), all participants were evaluated for depression using both the *Hamilton* (Hamilton, 1960) and the *Geriatric Depression Scale* (GDS; Yesavage et al., 1983) (see Table 1). According to the cut-off scores of both depression measures, only participants in the DEP group presented with depression. Within the DEP group, 13 participants were taking an antidepressant; the remaining 6 DEP participants reported that they no longer took antidepressants because of the negative effects they had experienced when taking these drugs in the past.

## Procedures

As part of a larger research project, all participants completed a battery of attention, language, and memory tasks with task administration split across two to three 1- to 2-hour sessions to avoid subject fatigue. Task order was randomised across participants to circumvent order effects. For the current study, tests of interest included the *Test of Language Competence - Expanded* (TLC-E; Wiig & Secord, 1989) to evaluate high-level language comprehension and expression abilities, and the ABCD to assess basic cognitive abilities including language, memory, and visuospatial skills. In subsequent analyses, only the Linguistic Expression subtest and Total scores of the ABCD and the Recreating Sentence subtest of the TLC-E were used because of their direct relation to language production skills. In addition to these structured tests, participants were asked to tell a story about what was happening in Norman Rockwell's painting "The Soldier" (1945). There was no time limit for completing the spoken narrative task, and the examiner gave no feedback concerning story accuracy or appropriateness but did utilise periodic back channels (e.g., "uhhuh", "I see").

Spoken narrative samples were audiotaped, transcribed, timed, and then coded via the CHAT (Codes for the Human Analysis of Transcripts) system for automatic analyses by various CLAN (Computerised Language Analysis) programs (MacWhinney, 2000). Each sample was analysed in terms of a number of quantitative, syntactic, and informativeness variables. Quantity of output variables included the total number of utterances and words and speaking rate. To determine these variables, each narrative sample was first segmented into utterances following the guidelines of Glosser and colleagues (Glosser, Wiener, & Kaplan, 1988) and Saffran and colleagues (Saffran, Berndt, & Schwartz, 1989); that is, syntactic and prosodic boundary features were first used to identify utterances, and if these features were ambiguous, pausal patterns and semantic features were additionally considered. When calculating word totals, the rules developed by Nicholas and Brookshire (1993) were used to make decisions regarding which words to include in the word counts.

To guide the analysis of syntactic variables, which included mean length of utterance (MLU), the proportion of grammatical utterances, and the proportion of complex sentences to grammatical sentences, the procedures of Thompson and colleagues (1995) and Saffran et al. (1989) were followed. All nonword and word fillers, false starts, and word repetitions were excluded from morpheme counts when determining MLU. To determine if an utterance was grammatically complete, it had to have at least one independent clause and no syntactic errors. To be considered a grammatically complex sentence, the grammatically complete utterance had to contain at least one embedded clause or have a non-canonical form.

Three measures were used to evaluate the informativeness of the narrative samples. First, the percentage of correct information units (%CIUs) was calculated for each sample. CIUs, defined as "words that are intelligible in context, accurate in relation to the picture(s) or topic, and relevant to and informative about the content of the picture(s) or the topic" (Nicholas & Brookshire, 1993, p. 348), were identified following the criteria of Nicholas and Brookshire; %CIUs were computed by dividing the total number of CIUs in a sample by the total word count for that sample. The second measure of informativeness was the number of performance deviations per minute (PDM). According to Brookshire and Nicholas (1995), performance deviations encompass non-informative output, including words that are excluded from CIU counts. The rule-based system of Brookshire and Nicholas was followed to identify performance deviations, including word and non-word fillers, part word productions, unintelligible output, unnecessary repetitions, irrelevant words (e.g., "I like Norman Rockwell"), revisions or false starts, vague or nonspecific vocabulary (e.g., "thing"), use of "and", and inaccurate output including paraphasias (e.g., "girl" for "woman"). The last informativeness measure was the proportion of uninformative utterances (Murray, 2000). Utterances were coded as uninformative if they were incomplete or abandoned (e.g., "The soldier was . . ."), extraneous or off-topic (e.g., "My cousins lived in a tenement"), or repetitions of previously stated content. To calculate the proportion of uninformative utterances, the total number of uninformative utterances in a sample was divided by the total number of utterances in that sample.

## Inter- and intra-rater agreement

The narrative samples of two participants from each group (i.e., a total of six transcripts) were randomly chosen for re-transcription by a second listener naïve to the group membership of these participants. Point-to-point transcription agreement for utterance boundaries and words was 97% (range = 90–100%) and 93% (range = 87–100%), respectively. The majority of transcription disagreements concerned the presence or type of word and non-word fillers; all disagreements were resolved through discussion prior to further analysis of the samples.

A second set of six transcripts (i.e., the samples of two participants from each group) was randomly chosen for re-scoring by a second rater naïve to the group membership of these participants. Point-to-point inter-rater agreement was 100% for utterance counts, 99% for total word counts (range = 96–100%), 96% for grammatical sentences (range = 86–100%), 92% for grammatically complex sentences (range = 84–100%), 92% for CIUs (range = 81–100%), 98% for performance deviations (range = 96–100%), and 100% for informative utterances.

To examine intra-rater agreement, a third set of six transcripts (i.e., two participants from each group) was randomly selected for re-scoring by the original rater, at least 3 weeks following the initial coding of the transcripts. Point-to-point intra-rater agreement was 100% for utterance counts, 100% for total word counts, 100% for grammatical sentences, 100% for grammatically complex sentences, 94% for CIUs (range = 80–100%), 99% for performance deviations (range = 98–100%), and 100% for informative utterances.

## Statistical analyses

Prior to completing statistical analyses, *Fmax* (the ratio of the largest to the smallest variance) was calculated for each variable to evaluate whether the ANOVA assumption of variance homogeneity had been met (Keppel, 1991). Two language sample variables, %CIUs and the proportion of uninformative utterances, exceeded the *Fmax* criterion of 3; following arcsine transformation, however, *Fmax* for each of these variables fell below the criterion. All language sample and test data were then submitted to a series of one-way ANOVAs with group as the between-participants factor (i.e., DEP, AD, CON). Because numerous ANOVAs were planned, a conservative alpha level of $p < .005$ was adopted to guard against Type I error. Significant group effects were further analysed via independent, separate variance *t*-tests with an adjusted alpha level of $p < .016$ (i.e., .05 ÷ 3 between-group comparisons).

To identify factors that may be associated with spoken narrative skills, Pearson product–moment correlations were carried out between certain demographic and test battery variables and the narrative measures for which significant group differences were observed. Scatter diagrams and residual means and plots were checked prior to computing correlations to assure compliance with linear model assumptions (Verran & Ferketich, 1987).

## RESULTS

Group data for the quantitative, syntactic, and informativeness variables analysed in the spoken narrative samples are displayed in Table 2. No significant group differences (i.e., $p > .005$) were identified for any of the quantitative or syntactic measures. In contrast, a significant group effect was observed for each informativeness variable: $F(2, 46) = 19.626$, $p < .001$, for %CIUs, $F(2, 46) = 9.994$, $p < .001$, for PDM, and $F(2, 46) = 26.112$, $p < .001$, for the proportion of uninformative utterances. Post-hoc testing indicated that the AD group produced smaller %CIUs, more PDM, and larger proportions of uninformative

TABLE 2
Group performances on language sample measures

|  |  | AD | DEP | CON |
|---|---|---|---|---|
| *Quantitative aspects* |  |  |  |  |
| Total Words | M | 161.53 | 244.06 | 270.14 |
|  | SD | 83.98 | 125.99 | 100.77 |
|  | Range | 83–337 | 100–638 | 121–469 |
| Total Utterances | M | 18.47 | 25.67 | 26.71 |
|  | SD | 8.70 | 12.07 | 10.43 |
|  | Range | 9–44 | 13–58 | 10–46 |
| Speaking Rate | M | 112.30 | 117.66 | 133.18 |
|  | SD | 31.23 | 24.51 | 27.88 |
|  | Range | 73–173 | 75–162 | 85–182 |
| *Syntactic aspects* |  |  |  |  |
| MLU | M | 8.89 | 9.35 | 10.26 |
|  | SD | 1.91 | 1.55 | 1.20 |
|  | Range | 7–13 | 7–12 | 9–12 |
| Prop. Grammatical | M | .84 | .88 | .84 |
| Utterances | SD | .10 | .10 | .11 |
|  | Range | .70–1.0 | .64–1.0 | .63–1.0 |
| Prop. Grammatically | M | .39 | .42 | .47 |
| Complex Sentences | SD | .14 | .15 | .10 |
|  | Range | .19–.67 | .22–.69 | .31–.60 |
| *Informativeness aspects* |  |  |  |  |
| %CIUs | M | 66.45 | 79.79 | 83.31 |
|  | SD | 10.93 | 6.49 | 5.04 |
|  | Range | 46–83 | 66–90 | 77–93 |
| Performance | M | 44.45 | 29.66 | 27.05 |
| Deviations/min | SD | 16.19 | 8.33 | 8.95 |
|  | Range | 23–90 | 17–48 | 15–40 |
| Prop. Uninformative | M | .31 | .11 | .06 |
| Utterances* | SD | .15 | .06 | .05 |
|  | Range | 0.0–.60 | 0.0–.23 | 0.0–.15 |

*Utterances rated as uninformative due to repetitive, irrelevant, and/or inaccurate content.

utterances compared to the DEP group, $t(29.1) = 4.416$, $t(23.6) = -3.366$, $t(19.9) = -4.900$, respectively, and the CON group, $t(27.7) = 5.736$, $t(26.2) = -3.693$, $t(20.3) = -6.075$, respectively. None of the between-group post-hoc comparisons for the DEP and CON groups was significant, although the difference between these groups' proportions of uninformative utterances did approach our adjusted alpha level ($p < .016$), $t(28.9) = -2.507$, $p = .018$, with the DEP group producing larger proportions of uninformative utterances.

Table 3 displays the group performances on the formal, structured tests. Significant group effects were found on the test scores of interest: Linguistic Expression, $F(2, 46) = 19.144$, $p < .001$, and Total Test scores of the ABCD, $F(2, 46) = 37.338$, $p < .001$, and the Recreating Sentences TLC-E subtest, $F(2, 46) = 38.551$, $p < .001$. Post-hoc testing revealed that the AD group obtained lower ABCD Linguistic Expression, $t(24.9) = -6.036$ and $t(28.1) = -3.659$, ABCD Total Test, $t(19.8) = -8.149$ and $t(27.1) = -5.830$, and TLC-E Recreating Sentences scores, $t(19.6) = -6.622$ and $t(20.2) = -6.745$, compared to the DEP and CON groups, respectively. The DEP

TABLE 3
Group performances on linguistic and cognitive tests

|  |  | AD | DEP | CON |
|---|---|---|---|---|
| *ABCD* |  |  |  |  |
| Mental Status (max. 5) | *M* | 3.06 | 4.33 | 4.85 |
|  | *SD* | 1.03 | 0.90 | 0.36 |
|  | *Range* | 2.0–5 | 3.0–5 | 4.0–5 |
| Episodic Memory (max. 5) | *M* | 3.14 | 4.43 | 4.66 |
|  | *SD* | 0.34 | 0.43 | 0.32 |
|  | *Range* | 2.6–3.8 | 3.6–5 | 4.2–5 |
| Linguistic Expression (max. 5) | *M* | 3.69 | 4.36 | 4.75 |
|  | *SD* | 0.63 | 0.43 | 0.33 |
|  | *Range* | 2.5–5 | 3.3–5 | 4.3–5 |
| Linguistic Compreh. (max. 5) | *M* | 3.98 | 4.556 | 4.80 |
|  | *SD* | 0.81 | 0.56 | 0.19 |
|  | *Range* | 2.2–5 | 3.0–5 | 4.4–5 |
| Visuospatial (max. 5) | *M* | 4.03 | 4.73 | 4.89 |
|  | *SD* | 1.05 | 0.32 | 0.21 |
|  | *Range* | 1.5–5 | 4.0–5 | 4.5–5 |
| Total Score (max. 25) | *M* | 17.94 | 22.68 | 23.89 |
|  | *SD* | 2.84 | 1.84 | 0.90 |
|  | *Range* | 12–22 | 19–24 | 22–25 |
| *TLC-E* |  |  |  |  |
| Ambiguous Sentences (max. 39) | *M* | 14.35 | 30.33 | 32.29 |
|  | *SD* | 6.88 | 7.70 | 4.20 |
|  | *Range* | 3–27 | 16–39 | 25–39 |
| Listening Comp.: | *M* | 22.71 | 30.00 | 31.29 |
| Making Inferences (max. 36) | *SD* | 5.79 | 4.19 | 3.99 |
|  | *Range* | 14–34 | 17–36 | 25–39 |
| Oral Expression: | *M* | 45.94 | 68.67 | 69.93 |
| Recreating Sentences (max. 78) | *SD* | 14.87 | 8.59 | 5.31 |
|  | *Range* | 22–70 | 45–78 | 57–78 |

group also performed more poorly, $t(30) = -2.910$, on the ABCD Linguistic Expression scale compared to the CON group, but other DEP/CON group comparisons were not significant (i.e., $p > .016$).

For participants with AD there were modest associations between measures of narrative informativeness and ABCD test performances. That is, PDM was significantly correlated with ABCD Linguistic Expression, $r = -.503$, $p = .040$, and Total Test scores, $r = -.578$, $p = .015$, and both %CIUs and the proportion of uninformative utterances were significantly related to the ABCD Total Test score, $r = .489$, $p = .047$ and $r = -.489$, $p = .047$, respectively. For the DEP group, significant correlations were observed between %CIUs and education, $r = .497$, $p = .036$, and between GDS and PDM, $r = .493$, $p = .038$. Education was the only variable significantly correlated with informativeness (i.e., the proportion of uninformative utterances) in the control group, $r = -.547$, $p = .043$. It should be noted that for all three participants groups, the three informativeness measures were significantly (i.e., $p < .05$) correlated with each other.

## DISCUSSION

This study explored whether inclusion of language sampling and analyses might assist with resolving the diagnostic quandary of discriminating DEP and early stage

AD in elderly individuals. Specifically, the spoken narratives of individuals with DEP, AD, or no psychiatric or neurological diagnosis (CON) were compared in terms of quantitative, syntactic, and informativeness language measures. The language analysis results indicated that measures of informativeness were most useful at distinguishing the AD and DEP groups. That is, participants with AD produced smaller %CIUs, higher rates of performance deviations, and larger proportions of uninformative utterances compared to either the DEP and CON groups; furthermore, differences between the DEP and CON groups on these informativeness measures were not significant. The other discourse measures appear to hold little diagnostic potential, at least when comparing narrative samples, as nominal syntactic or quantitative differences were observed among any of the groups.

These findings accord well with prior comparisons of spoken discourse in early AD versus normal ageing (Bschor et al., 2001; Forbes-McKay & Venneri, 2005) or versus vascular dementia (Gustaw & Domagala, 2002). Although some of these studies utilised different discourse tasks (e.g., conversation), they all documented that individuals with AD, even those in the very earliest stages of the disease, provided the least informative or efficient verbal output. Likewise, several researchers have previously reported relative preservation of language form in AD (Kemper, LaBarge, Ferraro, Cheung, & Storandt, 1993; Kempler, Curtiss, & Kackson, 1987). The current results also extend the DEP literature by examining discourse and identifying a spoken narrative pattern similar to that observed in healthy ageing, in terms of quantitative, syntactic, and informativeness measures. This finding of preserved spoken narrative skills accords well with prior evaluations of verbal output in elderly individuals with DEP, albeit previous researchers solely utilised single-word and isolated sentence production tasks (Crowe & Hoogenraad, 2000; Emery, 1999; Murray, 2002; Stevens et al., 1996). Meilijson and colleagues (Mailijson, Kasher, & Elizur, 2004) did include a psychiatric control group of individuals with mixed depression-anxiety in their study of conversational pragmatic skills in schizophrenia and reported higher degrees of pragmatic inappropriateness in their schizophrenic versus depression-anxiety group; although these findings suggest perseveration of pragmatic skills in the depression-anxiety group, these researchers provided no further information pertaining to this group's verbal output or ratings.

There has been little exploration of associations between discourse characteristics and cognitive and linguistic test performance in early AD, and given the dearth of DEP discourse data, no examination of such associations in elderly with DEP. In the current AD group, significant, albeit moderate correlations were observed between informativeness discourse measures and ABCD test scores. This outcome is consistent with previous findings and the proposition that language deficits in early AD reflect deterioration in the functioning of both linguistic and cognitive abilities (Emery, 1999; Taler & Phillips, 2008). For the DEP group, discourse informativeness was correlated with their depression ratings and like the control group, with education level. Similarly, associations between depression level and degree of cognitive impairment have been reported in the DEP literature (Wright & Persad, 2007). A relation between informativeness and education level suggests that premorbid or general cognitive factors, like in healthy ageing populations (Taler & Phillips, 2008), also contribute to discourse skills in elderly individuals with DEP.

Clinically, the current data suggest that including discourse sampling and analyses, with a focus on informativeness, into comprehensive assessment protocols may lead to more accurate discrimination of DEP and early AD in the elderly. Furthermore, it is likely that only one informativeness measure needs to be analysed given that significant group effects were found for each informativeness measure and that significant correlations were found among the three informativeness measures for each participant group. However, before definitive clinical recommendations can be offered, several lines of research should be pursued to validate and extend the current findings. First, further research is needed to assure that the present findings do not underestimate the effects of DEP on discourse. For instance, there was a non-significant (i.e., $p = .018$) trend for participants with DEP to produce larger proportions of uninformative utterances compared to CON participants, and there was a modest positive correlation between depression measures and performance deviations per minute. Therefore it is plausible that both antidepressant use and relatively mild levels of depression among our DEP participants moderated the effects of depression on their narrative samples, and consequently that discourse changes might be more conspicuous in elderly individuals who have more severe levels of depression or do not take medication for their depression. Second, it should be determined whether the same discourse patterns across groups are observed when different discourse genres are utilised. For example, given that processing speed appears particularly vulnerable in elderly individuals with DEP (e.g., Murray, 2002; Nathan et al., 2001), language samples elicited during conversation or service encounters, which have inherent time demands, might yield more perceptible language changes in this clinical group. Likewise, more complex discourse tasks (e.g., unshared vs shared context conditions; picture sequences vs single picture) have greater discourse organisation and informativeness demands (Olness, 2006), and have been found to elicit poorer discourse performances from individuals in the early stages of AD (Ehrlich, Obler, & Clark, 1997; Forbes-MacKay & Venneri, 2005; March, Wales, & Pattison, 2006); thus these tasks might accentuate differences among AD, DEP, and CON groups. Finally, as elderly individuals with DEP and concomitant cognitive deficits appear to be at greater risk for developing irreversible dementia compared to their non-depressed peers and to elderly individuals with DEP but no concomitant cognitive changes (Alexopoulos, 2003; Dobie, 2002; Saez-Fonseca et al., 2007), future studies, ideally longitudinal in design (Crowe & Hoogenraad, 2000; Wright & Persad, 2007), are needed to explore whether and which discourse measures might help identify when DEP is most likely to lead to dementia.

Manuscript received 4 June 2009
Manuscript accepted 19 October 2009
First published online 29 January 2010

## REFERENCES

Alexopoulos, G. S. (2003). Clinical and biological interactions in affective and cognitive geriatric syndromes. *American Journal of Psychiatry*, *160*(5), 811–814.

Alzheimer's Association. (2009). *2009 Alzheimer's disease facts and figures*. Chicago, IL: Alzheimer's Association.

Barona, A., Reynolds, C., & Chastain, R. (1984). A demographically based index of pre-morbid intelligence for the WAIS-R. *Journal of Clinical and Consulting Psychology*, *52*, 885–887.

Bayles, K. A., & Tomoeda, C. K. (1991). *Arizona Battery for Communication Disorders of Dementia*. Tucson, AZ: Canyonlands Publishing.

Boone, K. B., Lesser, I. M., Miller, B. L., Wohl, M., Berman, N., Lee, A., et al. (1995). Cognitive functioning in older depressed outpatients: Relationship of presence and severity of depression to neuropsychological tests scores. *Neuropsychology*, *9*, 390–398.

Brookshire, R. H., & Nicholas, L. E. (1995). Performance deviations in the connected speech of adults with no brain damage and adults with aphasia. *American Journal of Speech-Language Pathology, 4,* 118–123.

Bschor, T., Kuhl, K. P., & Reischies, F. M. (2001). Spontaneous speech of patients with dementia of the Alzheimer type and mild cognitive impairment. *International Psychogeriatrics, 13,* 289–298.

Caltagirone, C., Perri, R., Carlesimo, G., & Fadda, L. (2001). Early detection and diagnosis of dementia. *Archives of Gerontology and Geriatrics, Suppl. 7,* 67–75.

Conwell, Y., Lynes, J., Duberstein, P., Cox, C., Seidlitz, L., DiGiorgio, A., et al. (2000). Completed suicide among older patients in primary care practices: A controlled study. *Journal of the American Geriatrics Society, 48,* 23–29.

Crowe, S. F., & Hoogenraad, K. (2000). Differentiation of dementia of the Alzheimer's type from depression with cognitive impairment on the basis of a cortical versus subcortical pattern of cognitive deficit. *Archives of Clinical Neuropsychology, 15*(1), 9–19.

Dobie, D. J. (2002). Depression, dementia, and pseudodementia. *Seminars in Clinical Neuropsychiatry, 7,* 170–186.

Ehrlich, J. S., Obler, L. K., & Clark, L. (1997). Ideational and semantic contributions to narrative production in adults with dementia of the Alzheimer's types. *Journal of Communication Disorders, 30,* 79–99.

Emery, V. O. (1999). On the relationship between memory and language in the dementia spectrum of depression, Alzheimer syndrome, and normal ageing. In H. E. Hamilton (Ed.), *Language and communication in old age: Multidisciplinary perspectives* (pp. 25–62). New York: Taylor & Francis.

Ferran, J., Wilson, K., Doran, M., Ghadiali, E., Johnson, F., Cooper, P., et al. (1996). The early onset dementias: A study of clinical characteristics and service use. *International Journal of Geriatric Psychiatry, 11,* 863–869.

Forbes-McKay, K., & Venneri, A. (2005). Detecting subtle spontaneous language decline in early Alzheimer's disease with a picture description task. *Neurological Science, 26,* 243–254.

Frances, A., Ross, R., & First, H. A. (1995). *DSM-IV guidebook.* Washington, DC: American Psychiatric Association.

Glosser, G., Wiener, M., & Kaplan, E. (1988). Variations in aphasic language behaviors. *Journal of Speech and Hearing Research, 53,* 115–124.

Gustaw, K., & Domagala, A. (2002). Early linguistic differential diagnosis of multi-infarct dementia and Alzheimer's disease. *Journal of Neurological Sciences, 203–204,* 302.

Hamilton, M. (1960). A rating scale for depression. *Journal of Neurology, Neurosurgery, and Psychiatry, 23,* 56–62.

Kemper, S., LaBarge, E., Ferraro, R. F., Cheung, H., & Storandt, M. (1993). On the preservation of syntax in Alzheimer's disease. *Archives of Neurology, 50,* 81–86.

Kempler, D., Curtiss, S., & Jackson, C. (1987). Syntactic preservation in Alzheimer's disease. *Journal of Speech and Hearing Research, 30,* 343–350.

Keppel, G. (1991). *Design and analysis: A researcher's handbook.* Englewood Cliffs, NJ: Prentice Hall.

Lantz, M. S., & Buchalter, E. N. (2001). Pseudodementia: Cognitive decline caused by untreated depression may be reversed with treatment. *Geriatrics, 56*(10), 42–43.

MacWhinney, B. (2000). *The CHILDES Project: Tools for analysing talk, third edition.* Mahwah, NJ: Lawrence Erlbaum Associates Inc.

March, E. G., Wales, R., & Pattison, P. (2006). The uses of nouns and deixis in discourse production in Alzheimer's disease. *Journal of Neurolinguistics, 19,* 311–340.

Mattis, S. (1988). *Dementia Rating Scale.* Odessa, FL: Psychological Assessment Resources.

Maynard, C. K. (2003). Differentiate depression from dementia. *The Nurse Practitioner, 28*(3), 18–27.

McKhann, G., Drachman, D., Folstein, M., Katzman, R., Price, D., & Stadlan, E. M. (1984). Clinical diagnosis of Alzheimer's disease: Report of the NINCDS-ADRDA Work Group under the auspices of Department of Health and Human Services Task Force on Alzheimer's Disease. *Neurology, 34,* 939–944.

Meilijson, S. R., Kasher, A., & Elizur, A. (2004). Language performance in chronic schizophrenia: A pragmatic approach. *Journal of Speech, Language, and Hearing Research, 47,* 695–713.

Murray, L. L. (2000). Spoken language production in Huntington's and Parkinson's diseases. *Journal of Speech, Language, and Hearing Research, 43,* 1350–1366.

Murray, L. L. (2002). Cognitive distinctions between depression and early Alzheimer's disease in the elderly. *Aphasiology, 16,* 573–586.

Nathan, J., Wilkinson, D., Stammers, S., & Low, J. L. (2001). The role of tests of frontal executive function in the detection of mild dementia. *International Journal of Geriatric Psychiatry, 16,* 18–26.

Nicholas, L. D., & Brookshire, R. H. (1993). A system for quantifying the informativeness and efficiency of the connected speech of adults with aphasia. *Journal of Speech and Hearing Research, 36,* 338–350.

Olness, G. (2006). Genre, verb, and coherence in picture-elicited discourse of adults with aphasia. *Aphasiology*, *20*(2–4), 175–187.

Rabins, P. V. (1981). The prevalence of reversible dementia in a psychiatric hospital. *Hospital and Community Psychiatry*, *32*, 490–492.

Roca, M., Torralva, T., Lopez, P., Marengo, J., Cetkovich, M., & Manes, F. (2008). Differentiating early dementia from major depression with the Spanish version of the Addenbrooke's Cognitive Examination. *Revue Neurologica*, *46*(6), 340–343.

Saez-Fonseca, J. A., Lee, L., & Walker, Z. (2007). Long-term outcome of depressive pseudodementia in the elderly. *Journal of Affective Disorders*, *101*, 123–129.

Saffran, E. M., Berndt, R. S., & Schwartz, M. F. (1989). The quantitative analysis of agrammatic production: Procedure and data. *Brain and Language*, *37*, 440–479.

Shankar, K. K., Orrell, M. W. (2000). Detecting and managing depression and anxiety in people with dementia. *Current Opinion in Psychiatry*, *13*, 55–59.

Shay, K. A., Duke, L. W., Conboy, T., Harrell, L. E., Callaway, R., & Folks, D. G. (1991). The clinical validity of the Mattis Dementia Rating Scale in staging Alzheimer's disease. *Journal of Geriatric Psychiatry and Neurology*, *4*, 18–25.

Snowden, D. A., Kemper, S. J., Mortimer, J. A., Greiner, L. H., Wekstein, D. R., & Markesbery, W. R. (1996). Linguistic ability in early life and cognitive function and Alzheimer's disease in late life: Findings from the Nun study. *Journal of the American Medical Association*, *275*, 528–532.

Stevens, S. J., Harvey, R. J., Kelly, C. A., Nicholl, C. G., & Pitt, B. M. N. (1996). Characteristics of language performance in four groups of patients attending a memory clinic. *International Journal of Geriatric Psychiatry*, *11*, 973–982.

Strang, J. M., Donnelly, K. Z., Grohman, K., & Kleiner, J. (2002). Verbal learning and visuomotor attention in Alzheimer's disease and geriatric depression. *Brain and Cognition*, *49*(2), 216–220.

Taler, V., & Phillips, N. (2008). Language performance in Alzheimer's disease and mild cognitive impairment: A comparative review. *Journal of Clinical and Experimental Neuropsychology*, *30*(5), 501–556.

Thompson, C. K., Shapiro, L. P., Tait, M. E., Jacobs, B. J., Schneider, S. L., & Ballard, K. J. (1995). A system for the linguistic analysis of agrammatic language production. *Brain and Language*, *51*, 124–129.

Verran, J. A., & Ferketich, S. L. (1987). Testing linear model assumptions: Residual analysis. *Nursing Research*, *36*, 127–130.

Wiig, E. H., & Secord, W. (1989). *Test of Language Competence – expanded edition*. New York: The Psychological Corporation.

Wright, S., & Persad, C. (2007). Distinguishing between depression and dementia in older persons: Neuropsychological and neuropathological correlates. *Journal of Geriatric Psychiatry and Neurology*, *20*, 189–198.

Yesavage, J. A., Brink, T. L., Rose, T. L., Lum, O., Huang, V., Adey, M., et al. (1983). Development and validation of a geriatric depression screening scale: A preliminary report. *Journal of Psychiatric Research*, *17*, 37–49.

APHASIOLOGY, 2010, 24 (6–8), 940–956

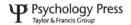

# The reliability of the Communication Disability Profile: A patient-reported outcome measure for aphasia

Wei Leng Chue and Miranda L. Rose

*LaTrobe University, Melbourne, Australia*

Kate Swinburn

*Connect – The Communication Disability Network, London, UK*

*Background*: The use of patient-reported outcome (PRO) measures is important for understanding the impact of aphasia from the perspective of the person with aphasia. However, communication difficulties may make it challenging for people with aphasia to self-report. The Communication Disability Profile (CDP) (Swinburn & Byng, 2006) is a newly published outcome measure that includes aphasia-friendly design features (e.g., pictures, simple wording, key words in bold, picture-rating scales) to support people with aphasia in self-reporting the impact of aphasia on their lives.

*Aim*: This pilot study aimed to investigate the test–retest reliability and internal consistency of the Activities, Participation, and Emotions sections of the CDP.

*Methods & Procedures*: A total of 16 participants with chronic aphasia of different severities and types were administered the CDP twice with a test–retest interval of approximately 2 weeks. Test–retest reliability was assessed using the Intraclass Correlation Coefficient (ICC) and "Minimal differences (MD) considered to be real". Internal consistency was assessed using Cronbach's alpha ($\alpha$) and corrected item–total correlations. Correlation coefficients, visual inspection, feedback, and observations were used to identify factors that may have affected the reliability or usability of the CDP.

*Outcomes & Results*: The Activities section of the CDP demonstrated high test–retest reliability with an ICC of 0.96 and a small MD value. The Participation section also demonstrated acceptable test–retest reliability (ICC = 0.89). In addition, the Activities and Participation sections demonstrated adequate internal consistency with Cronbach's alpha of more than 0.7 and corrected item–total correlations of more than 0.3. The Emotions section of the CDP did not demonstrate an acceptable level of test–retest reliability (ICC = 0.62) or internal consistency ($\alpha < 0.7$). Additionally there were no significant relationships between the severity of aphasia or comprehension abilities and the reliability of the CDP. However, increased examiner support may be required for the use of the Emotions section and when using the CDP with people with more severe aphasia.

*Conclusions*: The findings of this study provided preliminary psychometric evidence to support the use of the Activities and Participation sections of the CDP as a PRO measure by people with aphasia.

*Keywords:* Aphasia; Outcome measure; Patient reported; Reliability.

Address correspondence to: Dr Miranda L. Rose, School of Human Communication Sciences, La Trobe University, Bundoora, Australia, 3083. E-mail: M.Rose@latrobe.edu.au

http://www.psypress.com/aphasiology  DOI: 10.1080/02687030903490541

Traditionally, impairment-based interventions have been used by speech pathologists to target areas of aphasic language deficit (Duchan, 2001). However, many people with aphasia, especially those with more severe aphasia, benefit only minimally from these therapies (Parr, 2007). Many people with aphasia do not return to their pre-morbid levels of communicative functioning and continue to live for many years with marked communication difficulties. Of concern is that people with aphasia have expressed that they often do not understand the reasons for particular activities being done in therapy, and that goals of therapy were not synonymous with their own goals (Parr, 2007; Parr, Byng, Gilpin, & Ireland, 1997). Therefore there is a need for speech pathologists to consider the implications of aphasia on communication in everyday life and gear intervention towards achieving goals that clients consider to be important and relevant. The Communication Disability Profile (CDP) (Swinburn & Byng, 2006) was designed with these goals in mind.

Currently, speech pathologists who work in the field of aphasia commonly use clinician-rated measures of language impairment or functional communication. These include the Communicative Activities of Daily Living-2 (CADL-2) (Holland, Frattali, & Fromm, 1998), American Speech Language Hearing Association Assessment of Functional Communication Skills for Adults (FACS) (Frattali, Thompson, Holland, Wohl, & Ferketic, 1995), and the Therapy Outcome Measure (TOM) (John & Enderby, 2000). While clinician-rated outcome measures provide an objective and professional view of an individual's health, subjective perceptions of patients should also be considered. Increasingly, patient-reported outcome (PRO) instruments are being used to evaluate treatment (Food and Drug Administration [FDA], 2006). Although the use of PRO instruments in aphasia is new, they can be useful for a variety of reasons (Ross, 2006). First, some outcomes of intervention are known only to the patient (FDA, 2006). For instance, speech pathology intervention may have contributed to improved satisfaction or reduced loneliness, but observable or physical assessments of these concepts are not possible (Ross, 2006). In addition, PRO instruments can be used to find out the priorities and expectations of patients from treatment as their views may be different from the clinician's views (FDA, 2006). For example, the therapy goal of "socialising with new people" may be a priority goal for patients who were pre-morbidly outgoing and gregarious, but not for other patients who are more reserved.

Despite advantages of PRO measures, communication difficulties may make it challenging for people with aphasia to self-report on the impact of aphasia and their quality of life. It is suggested that the accessibility of these PRO measures can be improved with aphasia-friendly adaptations (Hirsch & Holland, 2000). For instance, the use of a multimodal approach that incorporates speech, writing, gesture, and drawing into the instructions, stimulus items, and response choices may help to reduce comprehension and response difficulties (Hirsch & Holland, 2000). Other aphasia-friendly adaptations include the use of short and simple questions, visual scales, and large print, and the provision of a closed set of response choices instead of requiring open-ended answers (Hirsch & Holland, 2000). In addition, the aphasia group at Queensland University (2001) suggested that the use of white space, pictures, and allowing additional time to read questions may help people with aphasia to better understand written materials.

Two recently published PRO measures possibly suitable for people with aphasia are the Stroke and Aphasia Quality of Life Scale-39 (SAQOL-39) (Hilari, 2003) and the Burden of Stroke Scale (BOSS) (Doyle et al., 2007). Aphasia-friendly features such as enlarged font size, key words in bold, and simple scales for rating are incorporated in the SAQOL-39 and the BOSS. However, both of these outcome measures are designed to measure the broad impact of stroke and provide limited information about the specific impact of aphasia as only a subset of items are related to communication. Questions on communication in different modalities (e.g., reading and writing) and contexts (e.g., understanding/talking to a stranger or in groups) are also not explored by these outcome measures. In addition, the SAQOL-39 and BOSS may still be unsuitable for people with more severe aphasia. Doyle, Matthews, Mikolic, Hula, and McNeil (2006) acknowledged that the BOSS may be inaccessible to people with more severe aphasia, as the BOSS psychometric studies have mainly included people with mild to moderate aphasia with relatively preserved comprehension. People with significant comprehension difficulties (< 7 of 15 on receptive domains of the Frenchay Aphasia Screening Test) were also excluded from the psychometric study of the SAQOL because they were unable to adequately self-report (Hilari, 2003). People with more severe comprehension, reading, and expression difficulties may need additional pictorial support to facilitate comprehension and response to items. An outcome measure that has included pictorial support is the Communication Outcome after Stroke (COAST) scale (Long, Hesketh, Paszek, Booth, & Bowen, 2008). The COAST demonstrated good reliability and practicality in the assessment of self-perceived communication effectiveness for people with aphasia and/or dysarthria. However, the 20-item COAST may be limited in providing comprehensive information on the modalities of reading and writing, as well as the emotional states that may be experienced by someone with communication difficulties.

## THE COMMUNICATION DISABILITY PROFILE

The Communication Disability Profile (CDP) (Swinburn & Byng, 2006) is an aphasia-focused, aphasia-friendly PRO measure. The CDP aims: to facilitate individuals with a wide range of aphasia severities and types in expressing the impact of aphasia on their lives; to quantify aspects of living with aphasia; to support joint-planning and therapy goal setting; and to explore and validate the individual's identity as someone living with aphasia. Through collaboration with people with aphasia as expert advisors, the CDP was developed and modified to incorporate pictures, change wording, and include items that contribute to understanding the impact of aphasia on everyday life.

The CDP consists of four sections: Activities, Participation, External influences, and Emotions. The Activities section explores perceived difficulties in performing everyday activities such as talking, understanding, expression, reading, and writing. The Participation section relates to the individuals' perceptions of tasks they *have to do*, *want to do*, and *how things are at home*. External influences is a picture-supported qualitative section that explores factors that facilitate or hinder participation. The Emotions section explores emotional states such as anger, frustration, determination, concepts of self-image, and levels of life satisfaction. Quantifiable data are only available for the Activities, Participation, and Emotions sections. For each item, participants provide a self-rating of a minimum score of 0, and a maximum score of 4 on a 5-point pictorial rating scale. Scale A is used to rate Activities and Participation while Scale B is used to rate Emotions. Scale C, a simple 2-point scale, can be used if participants experience difficulties with Scales A and B. Please refer to Appendix A for examples of items and scales of the CDP. The Activities section comprises 20 items, inclusive of four optional items that would be administered if non-verbal communication (e.g., using gestures or pictures) is a major mode of communication for the participant. Thus the maximum Activities score that can be achieved is either 64 or 80. The Participation section comprises 13 items that contribute to a maximum score of 52, while the Emotions section comprises 14 items that contribute to a maximum score of 56. These total scores are then converted into percentage scores, with higher scores representing more negative impacts of aphasia. The CDP was designed to be a comprehensive measure. However, clinicians may choose not to use the test in its entirety and to use elements of the CDP in a flexible way; for example, using the pictures for discussion without attempting a rating on the scale. The text or script of the CDP has also been designed to ensure that it is as accessible as possible to people with aphasia.

Preliminary analysis of the test–retest reliability of the Activities section with a sample of eight participants revealed a high correlation ($r = .92$, $p < .005$) (Best, Greenwood, Grassly, & Hickin, 2008). However, the use of the Pearson correlation coefficient as a measure of reliability may be limited as it measures the correlation or association between two sets of data but does not measure the agreement between the data (Portney & Watkins, 2000). The use of Intraclass Correlation Coefficient, a statistical index that measures both correlation and agreement is more ideal (Portney & Watkins, 2000). Furthermore, investigation of the test–retest reliability of the other sections, and with a larger sample is needed. It is also important to consider the internal consistency of an outcome measure. Items in a multi-item scale should be consistent in the sense that they should be interrelated and they should measure different aspects of the same underlying construct (Fayers & Machin, 2007; Portney & Watkins, 2000).

## AIM OF THE STUDY

The current study aimed to determine the test–retest reliability and internal consistency of the Activities, Participation, and Emotions sections of the CDP, and explore factors that may influence the reliability and usability of the CDP.

## METHOD

### Design and participants

Ethics approval was obtained from the Human Ethics Committee at La Trobe University before the study began. Participants were recruited from the Australian Aphasia Association and the Stroke Association of Victoria. The inclusion criteria were as follows: presence of aphasia for at least 1 year post-onset, no pre-aphasic history of severe cognitive decline or mental health problems as reported by participants and significant others, English as the main spoken language, corrected hearing and vision acuity adequate for paper and pencil assessment tasks as reported by participants and significant others, and judgement by examiners, and no current intervention for aphasia. The study included 16 participants with mild, moderate, severe, and very severe, fluent, or non-fluent chronic aphasia. Table 1 summarises the aphasia characteristics and background information of the participants. Please refer to Appendix B for more detailed information. The Western Aphasia Battery (WAB) (Kertesz, 1982, 2007) was used to determine the presence, type, and severity of the aphasia. The Aphasia Quotient (AQ) calculated using the WAB specified the aphasia severity of

TABLE 1
Characteristics and background information
of participants

| Participants | |
| --- | --- |
| Gender (frequency) | |
| Female | 6 |
| Male | 10 |
| Age (years) | |
| Mean (*SD*) | 66.25 (11.61) |
| Range | 51–87 |
| Years post onset (years) | |
| Mean (*SD*) | 4.22 (2.17) |
| Range | 1–8 |
| Aphasia Profile (WAB) | |
| Mild Anomic | 7 |
| Moderate Broca's | 3 |
| Severe Broca's | 1 |
| Severe Wernicke's | 2 |
| Very severe Broca's | 1 |
| Very severe Wernicke's | 1 |
| Very severe Global | 1 |

the participant: mild (AQ > 76), moderate (AQ = 51–75), severe (AQ = 26–50), very severe (AQ = < 26) (Kertesz, 2007). Parts A and B of the Reading section were also administered to obtain an understanding of the participants' reading ability.

## Procedure

The study was conducted over four or five sessions (dependent on the length of time for WAB administration) with a maximum of 2 hours per session, including rest breaks to avoid fatigue. All sessions were conducted by the first author at the participant's home, with the exception of participant 7 who preferred the sessions to be conducted at the La Trobe University Communication Clinic. The first session was a recruitment session where information about the study was explained verbally and provided in writing. Eligible participants were provided with an aphasia-friendly informed consent form to consider. The WAB was then completed over one or two sessions to determine the aphasia profile of the participant.

The CDP was then administered twice on two separate days, with the exception of Participant 15 where the CDP was administered over four sessions due to participant fatigue. The mean test–retest interval was 15 days and ranged from 14 to 21 days. Sections were administered in the order Activities, Participation, and Emotions. In line with instructions in the manual, the researcher used supported communication to facilitate the use of the CDP. The researcher read the question while gesturing and pointing to the written question and pictures. If necessary, other pictures on the page were covered to help the participant concentrate on rating a particular question. Repetition and rephrasing of questions, writing of key words, and facial expressions were used to facilitate administration. The researcher also clarified the participant's response (e.g., "So you felt a little bit frustrated this week?").

While the CDP aims to highlight aspects of participation and emotions that are affected by aphasia, the effects of aphasia and other factors (family support, physical limitations etc.) may not be easily differentiated (Swinburn & Byng, 2006). For this study, the researcher obtained an *overall* rating on aspects of participation and emotions. After that, if appropriate, reasons for the lack of participation or negative emotions were explored qualitatively. For example, if a participant with some physical limitations reported difficulty for the item on "shopping", the researcher asked "Is it because of aphasia?" while pointing to the picture that depicts aphasia. This was to clarify if the reported difficulty was due to aphasia or physical limitations. The follow-up question was asked at the researcher's discretion. For example, if the participant indicated that he had not felt lonely that week, in response to the question "Have you felt lonely?", the follow-up question was not asked. In summary, the rating per se is a rating of the overall participation level and emotions of the participant. The answer to the latter question then provides information about whether the reported difficulty was specifically attributed to aphasia or to other factors (e.g., physical limitations).

## Data analysis

All data were screened using descriptive statistics to check for assumptions of normality, homoscedasticity, and outliers. Reliability of the CDP was determined by the Intraclass Correlation Coefficient (ICC) Model (2, 1) (a two-way random effect model with absolute agreement), with values greater than 0.81 considered as good reliability. This value represents "almost perfect" reliability with reference to the arbitrary benchmark proposed by Landis and Koch (1977). A disadvantage of the ICC is that it is "unitless" (Weir, 2005). The use of an additional index such as the "Minimal Difference (MD) considered to be real" can be useful in providing a more complete estimate of reliability, as it is calculated in the "units of measure" used in the test. The MD for this study was calculated at 95% confidence level (see Figure 1). When trying to determine if a real change beyond measurement error has occurred in an individual patient, the change has to be greater than the value of the MD (Weir, 2005). Hence, a larger MD reflects a larger measurement error, and poorer reliability of the outcome measure. Although there are no clear criteria for an overall acceptable value of MD, the commonly accepted criteria are values less than 10% of the total range of measurement (Chen et al., 2007; Smidt et al., 2002). Internal consistency was assessed for both trials. Cronbach's alpha was used to report the extent to which items in a scale are correlated. Corrected item–total correlations were computed to assess whether items in a scale measured a single construct. In addition, statistical analyses of correlation were used to check for statistically significant relationships between the absolute difference of the trials and possible factors (e.g., aphasia severity as indicated by the Aphasia Quotient, comprehension abilities as indicated by comprehension sub-scores on the WAB) that may have affected reliability.

---

$$MD = 1.96 \times \sqrt{2} \times SEM$$
where Standard Error of Measurement (SEM) was estimated using the square-root of the mean square error term from the two-way repeated ANOVA (Weir, 2005).

---

**Figure 1.** Calculation of MD.

# RESULTS

## Descriptive data and visual analysis

All 16 participants completed the CDP for both trials. The mean duration for one trial of the CDP was 1 hour, and ranged from 30 minutes to 2 hours. Two participants did not provide a rating for the item "Do you deal with business or paperwork?". They indicated that this question was not applicable, as they did not deal with paperwork pre-morbidly. Thus their Participation score was obtained by dividing the raw score by 48 instead of 52. Activities, Participation, and Emotions scores and the mean difference between scores at Trial 1 (T1) and Trial 2 (T2) for all sections were normally distributed, supporting the use of the ICC and MD. The Activities and Participation sections exhibited homoscedasticity, while the Emotions section exhibited heteroscedasticity. Hence, a log transformation of the Emotions scores was performed before the computation of ICC and MD (Weir, 2005).

Table 2 summarises the mean scores for T1 and T2 and the standard deviations (*SD*), the mean and absolute difference between scores at T1 and T2, and the 95% confidence intervals (CI) for the differences. The mean section scores for T1 and T2 were similar. Additionally, the 95% CI for the difference in scores include zero, indicating that there was no significant bias towards participants scoring higher or lower at T2. The mean difference between T1 and T2 was also examined for outliers. Three outliers (participants 11, 12, and 15) were identified for the Activities section and were excluded from analyses of the Activities section. No outliers were identified for the Participation and Emotions section. The absolute difference is the numerical difference between trials without regard to its sign, and indicates the magnitude of difference between trials. Activities, Participation, and Emotions scores for individual participants and the presence of significant events or observations during the test–retest interval are presented in Table 3.

As shown in Table 3, the difference between Activities and Participation scores for T1 and T2 was small for most participants. The Emotions section demonstrated a different trend, with larger variability in the magnitude of differences between trials ranging from 0 to 28.57.

## Test–retest reliability

A high ICC of 0.96 and 95% CI (0.87 to 0.99) was found for the Activities section (see Table 4), representing "almost perfect" reliability (Landis & Koch, 1977). A high ICC of 0.89 and 95% CI (0.76 to 0.96) was obtained for the Participation section, indicating that the true reliability of the Participation section was at least "substantial".

TABLE 2
Mean scores, mean difference, and absolute difference in scores over the two trials

| Section | Mean of scores at T1 (SD) | Mean of scores at T2 (SD) | Mean difference between T1 and T2 | 95% CI of mean difference | Mean absolute difference between T1 and T2 | 95% CI of Absolute difference |
|---|---|---|---|---|---|---|
| Activities | 37.09 (17.25) | 36.17 (21.67) | 0.92 | −5.35 – 7.18 | 7.28 | 2.44 – 12.13 |
| Participation | 31.01 (16.37) | 28.96 (19.99) | 2.05 | −2.63 – 6.74 | 6.72 | 3.63 – 9.81 |
| Emotions | 26.34 (11.80) | 27.12 (13.24) | −0.78 | −8.22 – 6.65 | 10.83 | 6.36 – 15.29 |

TABLE 3
Activities, Participation, and Emotions scores of 16 participants

| Participant | A1 | A2 | P1 | P2 | E1 | E2 | Significant events/ observations between Trial 1 and Trial 2 |
|---|---|---|---|---|---|---|---|
| 1 | 20.31 | 15.63 | 9.62 | 1.92 | 3.57 | 7.14 | |
| 2 | 28.13 | 35.94 | 21.15 | 30.77 | 16.07 | 16.07 | |
| 3 | 25 | 23.44 | 26.92 | 21.15 | 25 | 12.5 | Extended family's visit |
| 4 | 52.5 | 55 | 55.77 | 59.62 | 30.36 | 51.79 | Change in family dynamics |
| 5 | 31.25 | 35.94 | 42.31 | 44.23 | 33.93 | 32.14 | |
| 6 | 64.06 | 60.94 | 51.92 | 50 | 14.29 | 37.5 | Small injury due to a fall |
| 7 | 15.63 | 17.19 | 11.54 | 11.54 | 21.43 | 17.86 | |
| 8 | 12.5 | 9.38 | 21.15 | 1.92 | 16.07 | 25 | |
| 9 | 45 | 32.5 | 28.85 | 23.08 | 26.79 | 21.43 | |
| 10 | 56.25 | 56.25 | 44.23 | 46.15 | 39.29 | 53.57 | |
| 11 | 40 | 16.25 | 34.62 | 17.31 | 28.57 | 17.86 | |
| 12 | 56.25 | 40.63 | 28.85 | 28.85 | 25 | 41.07 | Change in family environment |
| 13 | 39.06 | 42.19 | 6.25 | 16.67 | 26.79 | 23.21 | |
| 14 | 33.75 | 32.5 | 34.62 | 38.46 | 23.21 | 28.57 | |
| 15 | 60 | 91.25 | 59.62 | 65.38 | 55.36 | 26.79 | Commenced apraxia therapy between A1 and A2; significant difference in mood between E1 and E2. |
| 16 | 13.75 | 13.75 | 18.75 | 6.25 | 35.71 | 21.43 | |

A1/A2: Activities Trial 1 and Trial 2; P1/P2: Participation Trial 1 and Trial 2; E1/E2: Emotions Trial 1 and Trial 2.

TABLE 4
Results of ICC

| Section | ICC | 95% confidence interval | | F-value with True Value = 0 | Sig. |
|---|---|---|---|---|---|
| | | Lower bound | Upper bound | | |
| Activities[a] | 0.96 | 0.87 | 0.99 | 44.93 | < .01 |
| Participation | 0.89 | 0.76 | 0.96 | 16.28 | < .01 |
| Emotions | 0.62 | 0.18 | 0.85 | 4.02 | < .01 |

[a]$n = 13$; three participants were outliers and were excluded from the analysis of the Activities section.

A low ICC of 0.62 was found for the Emotions section, representing an unacceptable level of test–retest reliability. Moreover, a wide confidence interval of 0.18–0.85 was obtained.

The MD presented in Table 5 reflects the measurement error of the Activities, Participation, and Emotions sections of the CDP. For the Activities section, a person with aphasia may obtain a score difference of 9.80 on the second trial simply by chance, meeting the pre-established criteria of less than 10% of the total range of measurement. For the Participation section, however, a score difference of 17.23 difference may be expected on a second trial; this does not meet the pre-established criteria. Log-transformed Emotions scores were used to calculate the MD, which was then anti-logged to obtain values that can be interpreted in the context of the Emotions section (Bland & Altman, 1986). The results show that a person with aphasia may score 170% higher or lower on a second trial of the Emotions section. For example, if a person obtained a score of 20 for the first trial, the second trial may differ from the

TABLE 5
MD and corresponding raw scores

| Section | MD (percentage scores) | Raw score equivalents |
|---|---|---|
| Activities[a] | 9.80 | 6/64; 8/80 |
| Participation | 17.23 | 9/52 |
| Emotions | 170 | |

[a]$n$ = 13; three participants were outliers and were excluded from the analysis of the Activities section.

first trial by 170%, resulting in a score of 54. This result suggests that a large measurement error is associated with the Emotions section.

## Internal consistency

The internal consistency measures are presented in Table 6. Items in the Activities and Participation sections demonstrated acceptable internal consistency. High Cronbach's alpha values were obtained. For the corrected item–total correlations, 5 of the 20 Activities items and 5 of the 13 Participation items revealed corrected item–total correlation values that were lower than 0.3 for the first trial. However, importantly, all items displayed adequate corrected item–total correlations (> 0.30) for the second trial. The difference in results may be due to a warm-up or learning effect that will be raised in the discussion section. The Emotions section demonstrated Cronbach's alpha coefficients of 0.59 and 0.78 for T1 and T2 respectively. Indeed, higher internal consistency was observed for the second trial across all three sections. In addition, 12 of the 14 items in the Emotions section exhibited corrected item–total correlations below 0.3 (at either Trial 1 or Trial 2). Overall, the results suggest that the internal consistency of the Emotions section did not meet the acceptable level for this study.

## Outliers

Participants 11, 12, and 15 were identified as outliers who were less reliable in the rating of the Activities section across the two trials. It was noted that two of the three outliers

TABLE 6
Internal consistency of the Activities, Participation, and Emotions sections

| Section | Cronbach's alpha | | Corrected item–total correlation | |
|---|---|---|---|---|
| | T1 | T2 | T1 | T2 |
| Activities[a] | 0.85 | 0.94 | −0.05 – 0.79 (5 items < 0.3) | 0.54 – 0.88 |
| Participation[b] | 0.77 | 0.90 | 0.01 – 0.79 (5 items < 0.3) | 0.34 – 0.85 |
| Emotions | 0.59 | 0.78 | −0.10 – 0.66 (8 items < 0.3) | −0.03 – 0.71 (4 items < 0.3) |

[a]$n$ = 13; three participants were outliers and were excluded from the analysis of the Activities section.
[b]$n$ = 14; two participants did not complete all the items in the Participation sec-

TABLE 7
Correlation between severity/comprehension and the absolute difference between trials

| | Absolute difference of Activities trials | Absolute difference of Participation trials | Absolute difference of Emotions trials |
|---|---|---|---|
| Severity[a] | −0.43 (p = .10) | −0.19 (p = .49) | −0.38 (p = .14) |
| Comprehension[b] | 0.02 (p = .94) | −0.05 (p = .84) | −0.41 (p = .11) |

[a]Assessed using Pearson correlation coefficient; [b]Assessed using Spearman rank correlation coefficient.

exhibited severe aphasia. However, correlation coefficients did not indicate any significant association between the absolute difference scores and aphasia severity or auditory comprehension scores (see Table 7).

## Summary of feedback and observations

Overall, verbal feedback about the CDP was positive. Many participants (and/or their significant other) commented on the CDP's ease of usage and its relevance to everyday life with aphasia. Two participants commented that the pictures were particularly useful. Although the CDP was developed in the UK, there was minimal difficulty in terms of cultural differences when the CDP was administered to participants from the Australian population. Nevertheless, observations and participant feedback highlighted some problems in the use of the CDP. While the use of the CDP was straightforward for most participants, the examiner had to provide increased clarification and elaboration to support people with more severe aphasia in the use of the tool (e.g., writing key words, clarifying that the question was understood).

The administration and rating of the Emotions section appeared to be more complicated than the Activity and Participation sections and uses a different scale: Scale B. The Emotions section consists of questions on both negative and positive emotions. The participant is shown the picture representing the emotion and asked to rate the extent of that emotion on Scale B. For the rating of negative emotions, the picture on the left indicates a negative experience (e.g., very frustrated). However, when the scale was used to rate positive emotions, the same picture represents a positive experience (e.g., very determined).

Moreover, two questions on negative emotions and one question on positive emotions were presented on the same page. There was an increased chance of confusion as participants often associated the picture at one end of the scale with a negative experience and the picture at the other end with a positive experience. Nevertheless, increased examiner clarification and instruction assisted most participants to rate the Emotions section successfully. However, two participants with very severe Wernicke's aphasia persisted in their difficulty in using Scale B. In accordance with the instructions in the manual, one participant used Scale C (a 2-point scale) while the other participant used a consistent yes/no response to rate the Emotions section.

## DISCUSSION

Reliability is the first pre-requisite for a clinically meaningful instrument. This pilot study evaluated the test–retest reliability and internal consistency of the CDP. Two statistical analyses were used to investigate the test–retest reliability of the CDP.

While the ICC is useful in the interpretation of group-level responses, clinicians may use the MD, to evaluate whether individual changes achieved on the CDP scores represent real change (Weir, 2005).

## Activities and Participation sections

The Activities section demonstrated high test–retest reliability with an ICC of > 0.96 and an acceptable MD of 9.80. These findings support Best et al. (2008), who reported high test–retest reliability ($r$ = .92) of the Activities section. In the interpretation of clinical change in individual clients, a change of more than 9.80 for the Activities section can be considered a real change, and not a measurement error. It was decided that the Participation section has acceptable reliability as a high ICC of 0.89 was obtained. However, this conclusion needs to be taken with caution, as the MD did not meet the pre-established criteria, indicating that the Participation section may have a measurement error that is larger than acceptable. When trying to determine if a real change has occurred in the patient's perception of participation over time, the change needs to be 18 points or greater. A measured change less than the MD value may reflect measurement error.

Despite concerns that people with aphasia may not be able to use patient-reported outcome measures reliably, previous studies have found high test–retest reliability when aphasia-friendly outcome measures are used. Both the SAQOL and BOSS include aphasia-friendly features and demonstrated ICCs ranging from 0.78 to 0.99 (Doyle et al., 2007; Hilari, 2003). Hence the high ICCs demonstrated on the Activities and Participation sections of the CDP further support the notion that with adequate aphasia-friendly adaptations, people with aphasia are able to self-report their Activities and Participation status reliably despite their communication difficulties. In addition to good test–retest reliability, adequate internal consistency was also demonstrated on the Activities and Participation sections of the CDP.

## Emotions section

The Emotions section did not meet the acceptable level of test–retest reliability as demonstrated by the low ICC of 0.62 and a large MD of 170%. The low reliability may be due to a measurement error associated with the CDP itself, or may reflect the nature of the construct that was being measured (i.e., Emotions). Unlike the Activities and Participation sections, the Emotions section requires the use of a different scale (Scale B). Scale B, along with the format of questions in the Emotions section, added an increased level of complexity to the administration and self-rating of the Emotions section. The difficulty associated with the use of Scale B may have resulted in lower reliability of the Emotions section, compared to the Activities and Participation sections which used Scale A for rating.

Emotions experienced by people are inherently variable. Apart from aphasia, changes in everyday life (e.g., change in family dynamics and environments, relationships, financial matters) also contribute to emotional variability. Pallant (2005) suggests that test–retest reliability for "mood" scales is likely to be low as mood states are not likely to remain stable over a few weeks. The wide ICC confidence interval obtained for the Emotions section is consistent with Pallant's (2005) views. High test–retest reliability scores may have been demonstrated by participants whose emotions remained relatively stable over the 2-week test–retest interval. Conversely, people who experienced a change in their emotions over the test–retest interval may have achieved a higher or lower Emotions score on the second trial. Therefore the low reliability scores of the Emotions section may reflect the responsiveness of the Emotions section to detect true changes in emotions, rather than low reliability of the test itself. Thus the Emotions section could be valid, but not highly reliable.

Due to the variability of emotions, test–retest reliability may be difficult to assess. However, many current outcome measures that measure emotions demonstrate high internal consistency (Diener, Emmons, Larsen, & Griffin, 1985; Ryff, 1989; Stone, 1995; Watson & Clark, 1988). The lower internal consistency of the CDP Emotions section was inconsistent with the literature. To explain the low internal consistency of the Emotions section, we reviewed possible sub-components of the Emotions section. For example, we considered Ryff's (1989) dimensions of well-being (i.e., self-acceptance, positive relations with others, autonomy, purpose in life, environmental mastery, and personal growth). In many outcome measures that assess emotions, components of emotions are grouped into subscales, with each subscale demonstrating high internal consistency. The multi-dimensionality of the CDP Emotions section may help to explain the poor internal consistency. Furthermore, items that measure negative affect have been found to correlate with each other, but not with items that measure positive affect (Bradburn, 1969). As the Emotions section includes questions pertaining to both positive and negative affect, low internal consistency may be expected.

Moreover, the low internal consistency of the Emotions section may be reasonable, as participants with aphasia may not be expected to provide consistent ratings for each question. For example, a person with aphasia who rates him/herself as very frustrated may not feel angry at all, even though both items enquire into negative emotional states. Similarly, a person with strong family support may experience a high level of frustration but low levels of loneliness. Thus, the basis of assessing the internal consistency of the Emotions Section needs to be re-examined.

## Examination of outliers and trends

There was a trend of higher internal consistency on the second trial of the CDP. This was not consistent with the BOSS, which achieved similar internal consistency on subsequent trials (Doyle et al., 2007). Portney and Watkins (2007) suggested that the initial trial of a test is often confounded by a warm-up or learning effect with improved performance on the second trial. Although improvements in CDP scores were not globally apparent, as there was no systematic bias towards the participants scoring better on the second trial, the warm-up or learning effect may have influenced the extent to which participants rated consistently on each trial of the CDP. The trend may also be specific to the sample for this study and may not represent the internal consistency of the Emotions section that is rated by the general population of people with aphasia.

Participants 11, 12, and 15 were identified as outliers for the Activities section of the CDP. All three participants had events occur in their lives between the two CDP trials that could account for the discrepancy in their Activities sections scores. For example, participant 15 was characterised by very severe Broca's aphasia. The discrepancy in the participant's Activities scores may be attributed to the commencement of self-initiated, computer-aided apraxia therapy shortly before the second session. As the therapy was not conducted formally by a speech therapist, the participant was not excluded from the study. The participant may have experienced difficulty saying target words during apraxia therapy and become more aware of his communication impairments, contributing to higher ratings on the second trial of the Activities section. In addition, a lower Emotions score was also observed for the second trial. This corresponded to the observations regarding the huge difference in the participant's mood across the two trials of the Emotions section. Thus, severity of aphasia may not be the main factor affecting the reliability of the participant's rating. Rather, for this participant the Activities and Emotions sections of the CDP may have demonstrated responsiveness in detecting true changes in the participant's perception of his Activities and Emotional status.

## Reliability in self-ratings of people with severe aphasia

In contrast to the SAQOL-39 and the BOSS, the CDP includes pictures to further support people with aphasia in self-reporting. It is hoped that the pictures assist people with more severe aphasia to express the impact of aphasia on their lives. Despite the inclusion of participants with severe aphasia in the current study, the Activities and Participation sections of the CDP demonstrated high test–retest reliability. Moreover, there was no significant correlation between severity or comprehension abilities and the absolute difference scores between trials, indicating that severity and comprehension abilities did not impact on the overall reliability of the participants' response. Hence, these results provide preliminary support for the reliable use of the CDP by people with severe aphasia. Nevertheless, this conclusion needs to be taken with caution due to the small sample size and that three outliers (including two with very severe aphasia) were excluded from the analysis for the Activities section. In addition, the CDP may still be inaccessible to some people with extremely severe communication difficulties.

## Limitations

One of the limitations of the current study is the lack of control regarding factors that may influence the test–retest reliability of the CDP. While efforts were made to administer the two CDP trials at similar times and days of the week, this was not always achieved. The timing of the CDP administration may be important as timing can affect a person's mood (Stone, 1995; Watson & Clark, 1988) and a person's perception of the impact of aphasia on their Activities and Participation status. Similarly, there was no control over events that had occurred during the test–retest interval. Many participants experienced significant events during the test–retest interval that may have influenced the reliability of the CDP, particularly the Emotions section. Hence, the results need to be interpreted with consideration of these events. The reliability results of the Emotions section, in particular, may not reflect the true test–retest reliability of the Emotions section.

The results of this study need to be taken with caution because of the small sample size and unequal number of participants in each severity group. In addition, the Activities section results need to be considered with caution as 3 of 16 participants were excluded from the analysis of the Activities section because they were outliers. Nevertheless, this study included participants with a wide range of aphasia severity and types, approximating the aphasia characteristics of the population of people with aphasia. The sample size required to achieve sufficient power for reliability studies is dependent upon the minimum acceptable reliability and the true reliability (Fayers & Machin, 2007). For example, if 0.8 is decided as the minimum acceptable level of reliability for the Activities section, and the true reliability (as obtained in this study) was estimated as 0.9, then 46 participants are needed to obtain a power of 80% (Walter, Eliasziw, & Donner, 1998). The current pilot study should prove useful in providing estimates of the true reliability for future reliability studies on the CDP.

## CONCLUSION

This study is important, as it is the first to evaluate the reliability of the CDP in an Australian population. The Activities and Participation sections of the CDP demonstrated high reliability with a sample of people with diverse aphasia profiles, supporting the notion that people with aphasia are able to provide reliable self-ratings on outcome measures with aphasia-friendly features. This study provided preliminary psychometric evidence to support the use of the CDP as a clinically meaningful PRO measure. Future research with a larger sample size will provide more information about the psychometric properties (e.g., test–retest reliability, inter-rater reliability, validity, responsiveness etc.) of the CDP. With further research, the CDP could prove to be a useful tool that can be used successfully by people with aphasia to report the impact of aphasia and interventions on their everyday life. The aphasia-focused, patient-reported, aphasia-friendly design of the CDP could potentially contribute to our understanding of the impact of aphasia on the life of individuals, including individuals with more severe aphasia.

Finally, our experiences during this study suggest that the interviewer may need to use increased clarification and elaboration during the administration of the Emotions section, and when using the CDP with people with more severe aphasia. We support the recommendations by Best et al. (2008) and authors of the CDP (Swinburn & Byng, 2006) — the examiner should be familiar with the effects of aphasia and someone who has established rapport with the person with aphasia. Familiarity with the person with aphasia will assist the examiner in using appropriate strategies to facilitate valid use of the CDP. Training of the interviewer may also help to facilitate the administration of the CDP, in using Scales B and C.

Manuscript received 21 July 2009
Manuscript accepted 12 November 2009

## REFERENCES

Best, W., Greenwood, A., Grassly, J., & Hickin, J. (2008). Bridging the gap: Can impairment-based therapy for anomia have an impact at the psycho-social level? *International Journal of Language & Communication Disorders*, *43*(4), 390–407.

Bland, J. M., & Altman, D. G. (1986). Statistical methods for assessing agreement between two methods of clinical measurement. *Lancet, i*, 307–310.

Bradburn, N. M. (1969). *The structure of psychological well-being*. Chicago: Aldine Publishing Company.

Chen, H. M., Hsieh, C. L., Lo, S. K., Liaw, L. J., Chen, S. M., & Lin, J. H. (2007). The test-retest reliability of 2 mobility performance tests in patients with chronic stroke. *Neurorehabilitation and Neural Repair*, *21*(4), 347–352.

Diener, E., Emmons, R., Larsen, R., & Griffin, S. (1985). The Satisfaction with Life Scale. *Journal of Personality Assessment*, *49*(1), 71–75.

Doyle, P., Matthews, C., Mikolic, J., Hula, W., & McNeil, M. (2006). Do measures of language impairment predict patient-reported communication difficulty and distress as measures by the Burden of Stroke Scale (BOSS)? *Aphasiology*, *20*(2), 349–361.

Doyle, P., McNeil., M., Bost, J., Ross, K., Wambaugh, J., Hula, W., et al. (2007). The Burden of Stroke Scale (BOSS) provided valid, reliable, and responsive score estimates of functioning and well-being during the first year of recovery from stroke. *Quality of Life Research, 16*, 1389–1398.

Duchan, J. F. (2001). Impairment and social views of speech-language pathology: Clinical practices re-examined. *Advances in Speech-Language Pathology, 3*(1), 37–45.

Fayers, P. M., & Machin, D. (2007). *Quality of life: The assessment, analysis and interpretation of patient-reported outcomes* (2nd ed.). Chichester, UK: John Wiley & Sons.

Food and Drug Administration [FDA]. (2006). *Guidance for industry patient-reported outcome measures: Use in medical product development to support labeling claims.* Retrieved 26 June 2008 from: http://www.fda.gov/cder/guidance/5460dft.htm

Frattali, C. M., Thompson, C. M., Holland, A. L., Wohl, C. B., & Ferketic, M. M. (1995). *ASHA Functional Assessment of Communication Skills for Adults (FACS).* Rockville, MD: American Speech-Language-Hearing Association.

Hilari, K. (2003). *The stroke and aphasia quality of life scale – 39 item version.* London: City University.

Hirsch, F. M., & Holland, A. L. (2000). Beyond activity: Measuring participation in society and quality of life. In C. M. Frattali & L. E. Worrall (Eds.), *Neurogenic communication disorders: A functional approach* (pp. 35–54). New York: Thieme.

Holland, A. L., Frattali, C., & Fromm, D. (1998). *Communication activities of daily living* (2nd ed.). Austin, TX: Pro-Ed.

John, A., & Enderby, P. (2000). Reliability of speech and language therapists using therapy outcome measures. *International Journal of Communication Disorders, 35*(2), 287–302.

Kertesz, A. (1982). *Western Aphasia Battery.* New York: Grune & Stratton.

Kertesz, A. (2007). *The Western Aphasia Battery revised.* San Antonio, TX: PsychCorp.

Landis, J., & Kock, G. (1977). The measurement of observer agreement for categorical data. *International Biometric Society, 33*(1), 159–174.

Long, A. F., Hesketh, A., Paszek, G., Booth, M., & Bowen, A. (2008). Development of a reliable self-report outcome measure for pragmatic trials of communication therapy following stroke: The Communication Outcome after Stroke (COAST) scale. *Clinical Rehabilitation, 22*, 1083–1094.

Pallant, J. F. (2005). *SPSS survival manual: A step by step guide to data analysis using SPSS for Windows (Version 12)* (2nd ed.). Crows Nest, NSW: Allen & Unwin.

Parr, S. (2007). Living with severe aphasia: Tracking social exclusion. *Aphasiology, 21*(1), 98–123.

Parr, S., Byng, S., Gilpin, S., & Ireland, C. (1997). *Talking about aphasia: Living with loss of language after stroke.* Buckingham, UK: Open University Press.

Portney, L. G., & Watkins, M. P. (2000). *Foundations of clinical research: Applications to practice* (2nd ed.). Upper Saddle River, NJ: Prentice Hall Health.

Ross, K. B. (2006). Patient-reported outcome measures: Use in evaluation of treatment for aphasia. *Journal of Medical Speech-Language Pathology, 14*(3), ix–xi.

Ryff, C. (1989). Happiness is everything, or is it? Explorations on the meaning of psychological well-being. *Journal of Personality and Social Psychology, 57*, 1069–1081.

Smidt, N., Van der Windt, D. A., Assendelft, W., Mouritis, A., Deville, W. L., de Winter, A. F., et al. (2002). Interobserver reproducibility of the assessment of severity of complaints, grip strength, and pressure pain threshold in patients with lateral epicondylitis. *Archives of Physical Medecine & Rehabilitation, 83*, 1145–1150.

Stone, A. A. (1995). Measurement of affective response. In S. Cohen, R. C. Kessler, & L. U. Gordon (Eds.), *Measuring stress: A guide for health and social scientists* (pp. 148–174). New York: Oxford University Press.

Swinburn, K., & Byng, S. (2006). *The Communication Disability Profile.* London: Connect Press.

Walter, S. D., Eliasziw, M., & Donner, A. (1998). Sample size and optimal designs for reliability. *Statistics in medicine, 17*(10), 101–110.

Watson, D., & Clark, L. A. (1988). Development and validation of brief measures of positive and negative affect: The PANAS Scales. *Journal of Personality and Social Psychology, 54*(6), 1062–1070.

Weir, J. P. (2005). Quantifying test-retest reliability using the intraclass correlation coefficient and the SEM. *Journal of Strength and Conditioning Research, 19*(1), 231–240.

# APPENDIX A

## Examples of Communication Disability Profile (CDP) items and scales

Activities section

- During the last week, how easy is it for you to talk with a group of friends?
- During the last week, how easy is it for you to read a whole story in a newspaper?

Participation section

- How is shopping? Can you show me on the scale?
- How easy is it for you to meet friends?

Emotions section

- During the last week, have you felt frustrated?
- During the last week, have you felt determined?

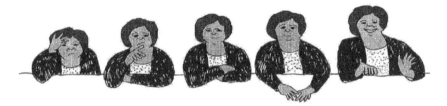

Scale A – used for the rating of the Activities and Participation sections.

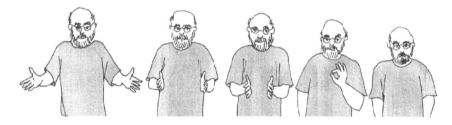

Scale B – used for the rating of the Emotions section.

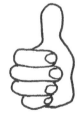 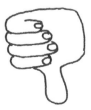

Scale C – 2-point scale.

# APPENDIX B

## Participant details

| Participant number | Gender | Age | Years post onset | Aphasia Type | Aphasia severity | AQ /100 | Reading score /60 | Spontaneous speech /20 | Comprehension /10 | Repetition /10 | Naming /10 |
|---|---|---|---|---|---|---|---|---|---|---|---|
| 1 | F | 77 | 2.17 | Anomic | Mild | 90.8 | 60 | 19 | 10 | 7.4 | 9 |
| 2 | M | 76 | 3 | Anomic | Mild | 94.2 | 60 | 19 | 10 | 8.7 | 9.4 |
| 3 | F | 55 | 3.42 | Anomic | Mild | 96 | 60 | 20 | 10 | 8.9 | 9.1 |
| 4 | M | 83 | 4 | Wernicke's | Severe | 39.4 | 29 | 10 | 5.6 | 2.3 | 1.8 |
| 5 | M | 51 | 6 | Anomic | Mild | 98 | 52 | 20 | 10 | 10 | 9 |
| 6 | F | 55 | 6 | Broca's | Moderate | 59.1 | 2 | 10 | 6.05 | 5.8 | 4.7 |
| 7 | M | 51 | 8 | Broca's | Moderate | 72.5 | 60 | 13 | 8.55 | 6.3 | 8.4 |
| 8 | M | 57 | 2 | Broca's | Moderate | 75.8 | 50 | 13 | 9.8 | 8.8 | 6.3 |
| 9 | M | 61 | 8 | Global | Very Severe | 20.2 | 14 | 4 | 5.5 | 0.6 | 0 |
| 10 | M | 66 | 6 | Anomic | Mild | 86.9 | 36 | 19 | 9.25 | 7.8 | 7.4 |
| 11 | F | 66 | 4 | Wernicke's | Very Severe | 24.2 | 29 | 7 | 5.1 | 0 | 0 |
| 12 | M | 70 | 3 | Anomic | Mild | 94.6 | 58 | 19 | 10 | 9.5 | 8.8 |
| 13 | F | 81 | 3 | Anomic | Mild | 87.4 | 51.5 | 18 | 9.9 | 7.1 | 8.7 |
| 14 | M | 62 | 1 | Wernicke's | Severe | 26.3 | 12 | 8 | 4.15 | 1 | 0 |
| 15 | M | 87 | 6 | Broca's | Very Severe | 23.4 | 4 | 3 | 5.2 | 3.2 | 0.3 |
| 16 | F | 62 | 2 | Broca's | Severe | 41.6 | 50 | 5 | 8.45 | 3.2 | 4.1 |

APHASIOLOGY, 2010, 24 (6–8), 957–968

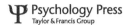

# Importance of health-related quality of life for persons with aphasia, their significant others, and SLPs: Who do we ask?

Tamara B. Cranfill

*Eastern Kentucky University, Richmond, KY, USA*

Heather Harris Wright

*Arizona State University, Tempe, AZ, USA*

*Background*: Outcomes that support improved health-related quality of life (HRQL) are increasingly identified as desirable products to aphasia intervention. Although domain importance has been examined for survivors of stroke, little research evidence exists indicating what particular HRQL domains are or are not important to persons with aphasia (PwA).

*Aims*: The study aimed to determine if persons with mild, moderate, and severe aphasia, their respective speech-language pathologists (SLPs) and respective significant others (SOs) attribute similar importance rankings to different domains and overall HRQL.

*Method & Procedures*: This study was a prospective, observational, non-randomised group design. The *Stroke and Aphasia Quality of Life Scale-39* (SAQOL-39; Hilari, Byng, Lamping, & Smith, 2003a) and the *Quality of Communication Life* scale (Paul et al., 2004) were administered to 24 PwA, their treating SLPs ($n = 7$), and SOs ($n = 24$). Importance ratings on a 5-point Likert scale were obtained for each scale item. Severity of aphasia was determined by expressive ability resulting in by chance assignment of eight participants per severity group.

*Outcomes & Results*: The SAQOL-39 physical domain was the only HRQL domain to be statistically significant with a significant group main effect, $F(2, 21) = 4.057$, $p < .05$. The SLP and SO significantly correlated with each other for importance of HRQL, but not with the PwA who had no significant correlations with the importance ratings made by the SO or the SLP on the SAQOL-39 and QCL. A total of 43% of variance in the overall importance ratings by PwA was accounted for by age, $R^2 = .434$, $F(1, 22) = 16.89$, $p < .01$.

*Conclusions*: Seeking importance ratings of HRQL domains from persons with mild, moderate, and severe aphasia may result in development of treatment goals more relevant to the PwA. Assessment of multiple HRQL domains is necessary to understanding priorities PwA place on rehabilitation outcomes across the continuum of care. Consideration for severity assignments beyond impairment-based assessments is discussed.

*Keywords:* Health-related quality of life; Aphasia; Stroke.

Address correspondence to: Tamara B. Cranfill, Eastern Kentucky University, 521 Lancaster Avenue, 245 Wallace Building, Richmond KY 40475, USA. E-mail: tamara.cranfill@eku.edu

http://www.psypress.com/aphasiology          DOI: 10.1080/02687030903452624

The term *health-related quality of life* (HRQL) is increasingly used in the medical and health science literature to refer to components of overall quality of life (QOL) that centre on or are directly affected by health, disease, disorder, and/or injury. General consensus was noted in the literature with regard to identifying the components of HRQL (Guyatt, Feeny & Patrick, 1993; Hilari, Wiggins, Roy, Byng & Smith, 2003a; Naughton & Shumaker, 2003). Health-related quality of life is defined as the impact of a health state on a person's ability to lead a fulfilling life (Hilari et al., 2003b) and examines attributes valued by individuals whose lives have been affected by illness or disease.

Many researchers agree that HRQL and associated factors are subjective and dynamic by nature (Orely & Kuyken, 1994). Because persons with aphasia (PwA) have impaired communication abilities, their participation in quality of life research is often limited. Some researchers have examined quality of life for survivors of stroke but excluded PwA from participation (e.g., Smout, Koudstaal, Ribbers, Janssen, & Passchier, 2001). Other researchers have not included speech-language pathologists (SLPs) in surveys of rehabilitation health professionals in an effort to define HRQL for survivors of stroke (e.g., McKevitt, Redfern, La-Placa, & Wolfe, 2003). Failure to include PwA, their significant others (SOs) and SLPs serving this population eliminates a substantial population of individuals impacted by stroke.

Proxy responses have been considered as an alternative to not including individuals with aphasia (Duncan et al., 2002). Duncan and colleagues (2002) determined that the best agreements were for domains that represented observable physical behaviours, and the worst agreements were on more subjective domains (e.g., memory and thinking, communication, emotion, and strength). Sneeuw, Aaronson, DeHaan, and Limburg (1997) suggested that there are significant differences in perceptions of HRQL between survivors of stroke and their proxy respondents. Proxies tended to rate the survivors of stroke as more impaired or with a lesser QOL than the survivors of stroke rated themselves.

Speech-language pathologists (SLPs) generally believe their clients experience an enhanced HRQL as a result of treatment for aphasia (Doyle, 2002, 2005; Doyle, Matthews, Mikolic, Hula, & McNeil, 2006). However, there is limited published research evidence examining the importance of HRQL domains to individuals with communication disorders, their SOs, and/or their treating SLPs. The emotional impact of aphasia (Code, Hemsley, & Herrmann, 1999) and the need to manage the psychosocial adjustment of aphasia (Müller, 1999) are identified as important aspects of aphasia management, but researchers fall short of providing a means for determining what is most important to the PwA. Understanding the importance of HRQL domains to PwA is vital to promoting their involvement in goal development and movement toward outcomes that are personally germane (King, 1996). Impairment-based assessments do not measure communication difficulty or associated psychological distress that frequently accompanies language impairment (Ross & Wertz, 2003), so they are inadequate in identifying what it means to live with aphasia. Without assessment of the individual's perspective of assigned values, interventions may be directed towards the possibility of an event, rather than the day-to-day domains important to the PwA. For example, the clinician may consider it important that the client be able to make phone calls, particularly emergency calls for assistance. Yet, unless there is an event to precipitate the need, the client may not consider this important on a day-to-day basis because the caretaker is able to provide that assistance. Identifying the importance of particular HRQL domains such as social relationships, language, mood, self-care, and family roles could reveal diagnostically distinct areas that would enable clinicians to target more specific interventions for PwA (Herrmann & Wallesch, 1990) along the continuum of care.

Health-related quality of life assessments need to reflect the importance of specific domains to the individual in relation to a given context or situation. Since aphasia is described as "a disorder of communication leading to a disorder of the person" (Sarno, 1993, p. 323), individuals with aphasia, regardless of severity, should be provided with an opportunity to supplement standardised measurement items with those regarded as personally relevant (Ross & Wertz, 2003). Indicating whether one is satisfied or dissatisfied with some aspect of one's life does not necessarily correlate to whether those aspects are important or lack importance. Individuals who recently developed paraplegia or quadriplegia following a motor vehicle accident were reported as not significantly different from recent lottery winners when asked to report their level of happiness (Ubel, Loewenstein, & Jepson, 2002). This example seems counterintuitive, but indicates the significance of the insider's perspective (Hunt, 1997) and supports the value of asking participants to rate the importance of items used to determine HRQL (King, 1996).

The primary research questions were:

1. Are there significant differences between importance ratings of four HRQL domains (physical, psychosocial, communication, and energy) and overall HRQL for participants identified with mild, moderate, and severe aphasia (determined by expressive language impairment)?
2. Are there significant differences between importance ratings of the HRQL domains and overall HRQL for different respondent types (PwA, SO, SLP)?

## METHOD

### Participants

*Person with aphasia.* A total of 24 participants with aphasia (PwA), with a mean age of 70 ($SD$ = 13.17), took part in the study. They included 10 males and 14 females from rural and urban areas. A diagnosis of aphasia was determined by performance on the *Western Aphasia Battery* (WAB; Kertesz, 1982). Overall mean score for the WAB Aphasia Quotient (AQ) was 67.4 ($SD$ = 23). All participants reported a history of English proficiency. Three participants were African-American and the remainder Caucasian. All participants met the following criteria: (1) diagnosis of aphasia; (2) history of one or more strokes, with the most recent stroke occurring at least 1 month prior to study entry; (3) current enrolment in speech-language therapy at least once per week; (4) moderate (or better) aided or unaided hearing acuity as determined by the *Hearing Handicap Inventory for the Elderly – Screening Questionnaire* (HHIE-S; Ventry & Weinstein, 1983); sensitivity when compared to an audiogram-defined hearing impairment is reported as 72–76% (Demers, 2004); (5) brain damage confined to the left hemisphere; (6) no history of other diseases that would affect communicative ability; (7) corrected visual acuity no worse than 20/100 in the better eye as determined by a pocket-size Snellen chart for illiteracy; (8) either upper extremity sufficiently preserved to indicate a clear choice; and (9) living in their own home, in a rehabilitation facility, or in an assisted living facility. Information about the PwA was obtained through medical chart review, interviews with the individual and his or her SO, and formal assessments. Table 1 provides descriptive data for PwA.

TABLE 1
Descriptive data for participants with aphasia (PwA)

| PwA | Age | Gender | Ed[1] level | Race | WAB AQ[2] | MPO[3] | SQL39[4] | QCL[5] | Amb[6] status |
|---|---|---|---|---|---|---|---|---|---|
| *Mild* | | | | | | | | | |
| 1 | 67 | M[7] | 14 | W[9] | 57.8 | 6 | 144 | 60 | Ind[11] |
| 2 | 81 | F[8] | 16 | W | 89.8 | 1 | 133 | 42 | W/C[12] |
| 3 | 86 | M | 8 | W | 91 | 1 | 133 | 72 | W/C |
| 4 | 75 | F | 12 | W | 88.3 | 2 | 154 | 75 | Cane[13] |
| 5 | 54 | F | 12 | W | 90.8 | 1 | 156 | 63 | Walker |
| 6 | 55 | M | 4 | W | 85.4 | 13 | 133 | 72 | Walker |
| 7 | 76 | F | 12 | W | 92.2 | 180 | 155 | 58 | Cane |
| 8 | 82 | M | 12 | B[10] | 88 | 2 | 129 | 73 | W/C |
| Mean | 72 | | 11.3 | | 85.4 | 25.8 | 142.1 | 64.4 | |
| (SD) | (12.2) | | (3.7) | | (11.4) | (62.5) | (11.5) | (11.1) | |
| *Moderate* | | | | | | | | | |
| 1 | 75 | M | 16 | W | 72.2 | 52 | 96 | 63 | W/C |
| 2 | 79 | F | 18 | W | 57.4 | 53 | 123 | 61 | Walker |
| 3 | 90 | M | 12 | W | 88 | 5 | 82 | 74 | W/C |
| 4 | 92 | F | 6 | W | 86.9 | 1 | 126 | 47 | W/C |
| 5 | 84 | F | 18 | W | 65.4 | 4 | 180 | 81 | W/C |
| 6 | 51 | F | 8 | B | 63.3 | 23 | 104 | 60 | Ind |
| 7 | 54 | M | 16 | W | 37.5 | 9 | 78 | 39 | Ind |
| 8 | 52 | F | 8 | B | 83.7 | 10 | 107 | 35 | Ind |
| Mean | 63.1 | | 10.9 | | 69.3 | 19.6 | 112 | 57.5 | |
| (SD) | (17.3) | | (4.5) | | (17.2) | (21.3) | (32.4) | (16.2) | |
| *Severe* | | | | | | | | | |
| 1 | 77 | F | 12 | W | 53.2 | 1 | 122 | 67 | Ind |
| 2 | 71 | F | 12 | W | 63.8 | 3 | 81 | 65 | Ind |
| 3 | 61 | M | 12 | W | 28 | 2 | 116 | 64 | W/C |
| 4 | 70 | F | 18 | W | 73.2 | 1 | 140 | 79 | W/C |
| 5 | 61 | F | 16 | W | 39.9 | 84 | 134 | 73 | Cane |
| 6 | 77 | M | 16 | W | 33.3 | 9 | 69 | 33 | Ind |
| 7 | 70 | F | 12 | W | 14.8 | 17 | 105 | 61 | Cane |
| 8 | 47 | M | 14 | W | 72.8 | 12 | 125 | 38 | Ind |
| Mean | 66.8 | | 14 | | 51.4 | 16.1 | 111.5 | 60 | |
| (SD) | (10.0) | | (2.4) | | (21.7) | (28.0) | (25.1) | (16.2) | |

[1]Education; [2]Western Aphasia Battery Aphasia Quotient; [3]months post onset of stroke; [4]Stroke and Aphasia Quality of Life Scales-39 total score; [5]Quality of Communication Life Scale total score; [6]ambulatory; [7]male; [8]female; [9]White/Caucasian; [10]Black/African-American; [11]independent; [12] wheelchair bound; [13] ambulates with cane.

Participants were excluded if: (1) they had been discharged from speech-language pathology services; (2) they lived alone without continuous family support; (3) they had history of cognitive decline or progressive disorders; (4) family or SLPs did not agree to enrol in the study; (5) their scores on *Raven's Coloured Progressive Matrices* (RCPM; Raven, Court, & Raven, 1995) placed them below the 50th percentile for their age group; (6) they scored below 14 of 20 correct (70%) on the yes/no question response section of WAB; or (7) they had a history of substance abuse within the past 12 months.

Severity was determined using a unit of information count similar to a content unit count (Yorkston & Beukelman, 1980) scored from a taped transcript of the WAB picture description task (the Picnic Scene). Units of information were judged as the amount of information conveyed and defined as a unit of expression by normal speakers (Yorkston & Beukelman, 1980). Severity rankings were conceptualised from those used by Yorkston and Beukelman (1980) for the Cookie Theft picture from the Boston Diagnostic Aphasia Examination (Goodglass & Kaplan, 1983). Participants with aphasia were categorised as presenting with severe aphasia if they produced five or fewer units of information in their description of the WAB picture. Moderate rankings were assigned to individuals producing six to eleven units of information; those producing greater than 11 units of information during WAB picture descriptions were categorised as mild. Eight participants were identified for each severity group by chance. Reliability was assessed by having two SLPs judge a series of six randomly selected speech samples previously scored by the primary investigator (PI). Judges were within ± 1 content unit of the PI score 98% of the time. Intra-rater agreement for scoring six randomly selected samples was 100%. Differences in scoring between the judges did not influence severity group assignments.

*Significant other of the participant with aphasia.* The mean age for the significant other (SO) of the PwA was 64.8 years ($SD$ = 14.1); they included 15 females and 9 males. Although a spouse or partner was preferred, adult children and parents of the PwA were allowed; they included 14 spouses, 8 adult children of the PwA, and 2 parents of the PwA. All SOs reported daily face-to-face contact with the PwA. Significant others met the following criteria: (1) reported normal aided or unaided hearing; (2) evidence of normal cognition (> 28) as measured by the *Mini-Mental State Examination* (MMSE; Folstein, Folstein, & McHugh, 1975) and by observation; (3) no history of current unmanaged psychological disorders by report and observation; (4) reported normal corrected or uncorrected visual acuity; and (5) English as the primary language. Significant others also were the primary caregiver for the PwA.

*Speech-language pathologist of the participant with aphasia.* The SLPs were licensed and ASHA certified as well as having professional experience with PwA. Multiple PwA were clients of each SLP, resulting in a total of seven SLP participants. Licensure and professional certification were determined at the time of initial contact.

## Measures

All participants (i.e., PwA, SOs, and SLPs) were administered two measures: *Stroke and Aphasia Quality of Life Scale -39* (SAQOL-39; Hilari et al., 2003a) and *Quality of Communication Life* (QCL; Paul et al., 2004) scales. The SAQOL-39 is an instrument for assessing HRQL in people who have had a stroke and who present with aphasia. The QCL is a measure of quality of communication life as a distinct, but related, aspect of general quality of life. Both measures were selected for their inclusion of individuals with varying severity levels of aphasia during development, and determination of life quality domains, since PwA have typically been excluded from validation studies for instruments to assess quality of life (Buck et al., 2004; Duncan et al., 1999; Williams, Weinberger, Harris, Clark, & Biller, 1999). A one-to-one interviewer-assisted format was employed using the recommended procedures for each instrument for all respondents. Participants were also asked to rate the importance of each individual test item using a 5-point scale (5 = very important, 4 = important, 3 = neutral/somewhat important, 2 = unimportant, 1 = very unimportant). The evaluator asked, "How important is this to you?" to elicit the responses, and then directed the participant's attention to the 5-point scale. If necessary, repetition, rephrasing, and item-specific examples were used to enhance the validity of responses and permit each participant to provide his/her own reactions. Rephrasing was necessary only for the neutral, important, and very important ratings. Verbal and nonverbal responses were accepted. The PwA responded from a personal perspective of item importance. The SLP and SO ranked items of importance based on his/her opinions of importance for the PwA.

Additional instruments were used to supplement HRQL measures. All PwA completed the *Brief Carroll Depression Scale* (B-CDS; Carroll, 1998), *Frenchay Activities Index* (FAI; Holbrook & Skilbeck, 1983), and *MOS Social Support Survey* (MOS-SS; Sherbourne & Stewart, 1991). The B-CDS is a 12-item yes/no rapid screening questionnaire with a severity score range from 0 to 12. The depression ratings provided by the B-CDS informed on possible correlations with responses on the HRQL scales, but were not used to eliminate participants from the study. The FAI is a brief measure of lifestyle consisting of 15 four-point measures and examines three major factors: domestic chores, leisure/work, and outdoor activities. The MOS-SS is a self-administered questionnaire measuring strength of perceived social support available on an ordinal 5-point scale. Five dimensions of support are measured: emotional support (four items), informational support (four items), tangible support (four items), positive social interactions (four items), and affection (three items).

## Procedure

A Latin square design was used to determine the order of presentation of HRQL assessments for each triad. Although the order of assessments was randomised, the number of assessments completed on a given day varied for the convenience of the PwA, SO, and SLP. Following informed consent, 23 PwA and SO pairs were tested on the same day. The one exception was completed on consecutive days. Responses were obtained individually without the presence of other triad members. Testing took place at the PwA's primary residence. SLPs were tested at their workplace within the same week as the PwA and SO. The average time for completion of the QCL with the PwA was 15 minutes, inclusive of importance ratings; with the SO and SLP it was 12 minutes. The SAQOL-39 averaged 23 minutes for administration, inclusive of importance ratings, for the PwA. Significant others and SLPs completed the SAQOL-39 and importance ratings in an average of 18 minutes.

## RESULTS

Reliabilities of the two HRQL scales were calculated for responses and importance ratings for each respondent group using Cronbach alpha. Reliability was acceptable for each respondent type on the SAQOL-39, range: 0.89–0.95, and QCL, range: 0.77–0.90.

### Importance of HRQL across different severities of aphasia

Several one-way analyses of variance (ANOVA) with pairwise planned comparisons using Tukey HSD were conducted to explore the impact of severity (three grouped levels: mild, moderate, severe determined by expressive ability) on importance ratings for HRQL domains (physical, communication, psychosocial, energy) and overall HRQL

(SAQOL-39 total score and QCL total score). Analysis of the four HRQL domains revealed a significant group main effect for importance of the physical domain, $F(2, 21) = 4.057$, $p < .05$. Planned comparisons revealed significant differences between the mild and moderate severity groups and the moderate and severe groups; as severity increased, importance of the physical domain also increased. No other HRQL domains yielded statistically different results. No differences among aphasia severity groups were found for importance ratings of overall HRQL.

Stepwise multiple regression was conducted to determine which independent variables—severity, age, gender, education level, time post onset of stroke, perceived support (MOS-SS), depression (B-CDS), activity level (FAI), cognition (RCPM), and WAB-AQ—were predictors for overall HRQL importance ratings by PwA. Results indicated a significant regression equation for age, $R^2 = .434$, $F(1, 22) = 16.89$, $p < .01$. This model accounted for 43% of variance in the overall importance ratings by PwA. A total of 56% of variance was accounted for with a second regression equation with scores from the RCPM and age, $R^2$ of .564, $F(1, 21) = 6.22$, $p = .021$. Age and cognition made a greater contribution to HRQL importance perceptions than other independent variables.

## Rating importance of HRQL domains among PwA, SOs, and SLPs

To explore the differences in mean importance ratings of the two scales among triad members (PwA, SO, SLP), a multivariate analysis of variance (MANOVA) of respondent type (PwA, SO, SLP) by measure (importance rating for SAQOL-39, importance rating for QCL) by severity (mild, moderate, severe expressive ability) was conducted. No significant differences were found among respondent types for importance ratings of overall HRQL on either measure. Severity assignments for the SO and SLP were based on that of the PwA. Pearson correlation coefficients further examined the association among the total importance ratings of overall HRQL on the SAQOL-39 and QCL and respondent type. As demonstrated in Table 2, ratings by the SLP and SO significantly correlated for importance of HRQL on both scales (SAQOL-39, $r = .43$, $p < .05$, and QCL, $r = .47$, $p < .05$), but not with the ratings from the PwA.

MANOVA with multiple comparisons were calculated with severity as the independent variable and respondent type (PwA, SO, SLP) and importance ratings on

TABLE 2
Correlation coefficients

| | SLP[1]-QCL | SLP-39[2] | SO[3]-QCL | SO-39 | PwA[4]-QCL | PwA-39 |
|---|---|---|---|---|---|---|
| SLP-QCL | 1.00 | .653** | .470* | .425* | .093 | −.263 |
| SLP-39 | | 1.00 | .276 | .605** | −.057 | −.168 |
| SO-QCL | | | 1.00 | .540** | .392 | .003 |
| SO-39 | | | | 1.00 | .206 | .301 |
| PwA-QCL | | | | | 1.00 | .334 |
| PwA-39 | | | | | | 1.00 |

Significant Pearson correlation coefficients examining importance ratings on the Stroke and Aphasia Quality of Life Scale-39 (SAQOL-39) and Quality of Communication Life (QCL) for respondent type. [1]Speech-language pathologists; [2]SAQOL-39; [3]significant other; [4]participants with aphasia; *significant at $p < .05$; **significant at $p < .01$.

HRQL domains (physical, communication, psychosocial, energy) as dependent variables. Statistically significant differences were found for importance of the physical domain for the three respondent types within severity groups. Significant differences for the PwA were found, $F(2, 21) = 4.057$, $p < .05$, between the moderate and severe aphasia groups. Participants with moderate aphasia attributed more importance to the physical domain's influence on HRQL than participants with severe aphasia. Significant differences for the SOs were found, $F(2, 21) = 5.56$, $p < .05$, between the mild and the moderate severity groups. The SOs of the mild group attributed more importance to the physical domain's influence on HRQL than SOs from the moderate group. The SLP importance ratings for physical domain were significantly different, $F(2, 21) = 4.65$, $p < .05$, between the mild and moderate severity groups and between the moderate and the severe groups. As aphasia severity increased, the SLP attributed more importance to the physical domain's influence on HRQL to the PwA. The physical domain was perceived as significantly more important to HRQL among respondent types compared to the psychosocial, communication, and energy domains.

## DISCUSSION

The current study examined HRQL domains (physical, communication, psychosocial, energy), overall HRQL and attribution of their importance with mild, moderate, and severe aphasia groups. SLPs and significant others (SOs) of the PwA were included in the study to compare ratings among the respondent types, thus adding another element to previous proxy research. The PwA were divided into the three severity groups based on verbal expressive ability. No significant differences were found in importance ratings for HRQL domains or overall HRQL between the different respondent groups. The SOs and SLPs rated what they perceived was the HRQL for the PwA. These results were compared to the PwA rating. Importance ratings by the SOs and SLPs were more similar to each other than ratings by the PwA.

### HRQL across different severities of aphasia

Clinical judgements based on severity of aphasia alone using verbal expressive ability do not identify the areas of greatest concern for the PwA regarding their HRQL and rehabilitation, supporting, and extending previous research in this area (Ross & Wertz, 2002). In this study, severity of physical functioning was of greater concern than communication functioning for many PwA. Although the findings add to the growing body of literature in this area, it was surprising that the aphasia groups did not significantly differ on more of the HRQL measures. One possible explanation is that importance of HRQL domains is influenced by areas other than the severity of the condition. A total of 40% of PwA were 1 month post onset of stroke. The 30-day post-onset inclusion criterion, when regaining physical independence, may outweigh the importance of communicative independence, and might have been a confounding factor. Previous researchers have found that other factors beyond aphasia severity influence perceptions of HRQL, such as self-esteem (Bakheit, Barrett, & Wood, 2004) and functional communication ability (Cruice, Worrall, Hickson, & Murison, 2003). Psychosocial and emotional adjustment of PwA varies even within different levels of aphasia severity (Hemsley & Code, 1996) resulting in broad patterns of response to stroke and aphasia being described (King, 1996).

Another possibility is that PwA viewed importance of HRQL according to their belief system rather than their communication impairment. The importance of HRQL domains and overall HRQL attributed by persons rated with mild versus severe aphasia did not vary significantly. Five of the participants with mild aphasia had higher importance ratings on the communication domain than six of the individuals in the severe group. The PwA's attribution of importance on a particular area appeared just as high for minor deficits as major ones. For example, a PwA who was able to communicate with only one-word utterances indicated the same importance for talking on the phone as a participant who had only mild word-retrieval deficits during conversation. Their abilities to perform the task differed greatly, but the importance of the activity was judged the same. Further, increased expressive language impairment did not equate to increased personal concern for improvement. Physical function, not communication, was considered more influential to overall HRQL across aphasia groups. The emotional and physical demands associated with fine and gross motor disabilities may be considerable compared to communicative disabilities. Anecdotal comments from participants suggested that the energy needed to adapt to communication limitations was less than that required for physical ability. For example, giving a nod for yes/no responses or using one-word responses to identify preferences with a broad range of communication partners requires less energy than adapting to the point of independent transfer from bed to chair or to regaining the ability to write with severe hemiparesis. This perspective may be particularly true during the initial stages of recovery.

A third possible explanation may be how severity was determined. All PwA presented with sufficient auditory comprehension ability, as this was necessary for following task instructions. However, using a verbal expressive measure of content production resulted in greater variability within the mild severity group, $(SD = 6.18)$. The moderate $(SD = 1.66)$ and severe aphasia groups $(SD = 2.12)$ had finite boundaries for identification. Assignment to the mild severity group required 12 or more content units, a potentially infinite range (i.e., range = 12–33). Greater variability within the mild severity group may have made it difficult to capture differences. Different analyses of information content within verbal expression of PwA, such as Utterance with New Information (Toro, Altmann, Raymer, Leon, Blonder, & Rothi, 2008) and main event analysis (Capilouto, Wright, & Wagovich, 2006), have also been proposed as potential measures for capturing relevant communicative changes through discourse and picture descriptions. Although not used for determination of aphasia severity, results from this study suggest further exploration on the relevance of these types of measures for severity assignment in addition to impairment models to continue to address the bias towards exclusion of individuals with mild, moderate, and severe levels of aphasia in studies of HRQL among survivors of stroke.

## HRQL ratings among PwA, SOs, and SLPs

A large amount of variance in scores was found for importance ratings for the PwA and the SO groups across both HRQL measures. Responses between the PwA and SO were not statistically different. The overall importance of HRQL ratings correlated significantly with responses between the SLP and the SO, but not with the PwA. The SLP and the SO ratings on the SAQOL-39 and QCL also significantly correlated; however, neither correlated with ratings provided by the PwA. In previous studies researchers have suggested that proxy respondents rate the survivors of stroke and aphasia as more impaired or with less QOL than the PwA rates themselves (Duncan et al., 2002; Sneeuw et al., 1997), yet proxies have been suggested as reliable raters of social communication function of PwA (Donovan, Rosenbek, Ketterson, & Velozo, 2006). Another consideration is the assumption underlying HRQL measures that the questions posed are supposed to make sense to the people answering them. It appears possible that variance could have been influenced by individuals within the respondent groups who did not want to speculate on a choice or comparison. For objective criteria, experiences of the PwA must be, in the end, submitted to the judgement of the PwA.

Importance of HRQL domains can differ across the participant groups (i.e., PwA, SO, & SLP). Additional analyses results indicated that age and cognition of the PwA had a greater influence on importance of HRQL on the SAQOL-39 than severity of aphasia. Few would argue that with age, priorities change with or without a chronic illness, such as aphasia. PwA in the study ranged in age from 46 to 92 years; cognition scores on the RCPM were within normal range ($SD = 3.2$). Personal priorities are adjusted as circumstances change under normal conditions. Gradual adjustments are not possible for PwA and their SOs, since stroke is a sudden rather than insidious event. One explanation may be that personal biases on importance attributions of life quality assigned by SOs and SLPs could not be eliminated, despite emphasis placed on taking the perspective of the PwA. Response shifts (Sprangers & Schwartz, 1999) resulting in change of values or redefinition of life quality experienced by PwA require further exploration with regard to how PwA, SOs, and SLPs accommodate the change in health state. Results from this study suggest variability of response shifts exists among triad respondents.

Caution is recommended in interpreting the data and in summing ordinal data for parametric comparisons. Statistical analyses with a larger sample may have indicated significance or non-significance in domains not identified within this study.

## Conclusions and future directions

This study offered an initial effort to examine the importance of HRQL domains to persons with mild, moderate, and severe aphasia judged by expressive ability, their SOs, and SLPs. Significant differences among aphasia severity groups were not found and the HRQL ratings for the PwA group did not significantly correlate with those of their SOs and SLPs. However, the HRQL ratings between the SO and SLPs groups did correlate significantly. Although there are limitations to the study, the results do add to the growing body of literature regarding HRQL for PwA. Future studies should include a larger sample of participants, include aphasia groups that consider severity across the language spectrum, and include aphasia groups, respective SOs, and SLPs across the recovery continuum (i.e., during rehab, post rehab). Qualitative examination of the dynamics of the triad relationship, the influence of time known in the triad relationship, and the pre-morbid value systems of the triad members may inform the profession with regard to internal variables influencing outcomes.

Despite these limitations, the results are promising and have implications for assessment and intervention for aphasia, as well as directions for future research. Physical function, not communication, was considered more influential to overall HRQL for the PwA. Assessment of multiple HRQL domains is necessary in order to understand the priorities PwA set for their rehabilitation processes. Content of

HRQL assessment should include more domains than communication-focused items to prevent bias from limiting our (i.e., SLP) perspectives about how best to help the PwA achieve an improved HRQL. Further, importance ratings of HRQL domains should be included as an essential component of overall HRQL assessment for accurate identification of treatment goals relevant to the PwA. Including assessment of the importance of HRQL domains in addition to performance of HRQL domains can provide the SLPs and SOs with a broader and more accurate understanding of the judgements PwA make about themselves and their HRQL along the continuum of care.

Intervention resources may be more appropriately designed and applied when treatment frequency, intensity, and goals are based primarily on assessment of what functional abilities are most significant to the PwA rather than severity of impairment. Asking the PwA what is and is not personally important empowers and encourages active participation in care. Such participation may provide opportunities for expression of hopes and fears not obtained with impairment-based assessments or proxy responses. Factors more important to the PwA than to others should serve as a partial guide to the role the PwA wants to play in the plan of care. Finally, further understanding of how others (i.e., SOs, SLPs, social networks) influence the perspectives of the PwA with regard to recovery would inform the profession and clinical practice.

Manuscript received 21 July 2009
Manuscript accepted 29 October 2009
First published online 7 May 2010

## REFERENCES

Bakheit, A., Barrett, L., & Wood, J. (2004). The relationship between severity of post-stroke aphasia and stated self-esteem. *Aphasiology, 18*, 759–764.

Buck, D., Jacoby, A., Massey, A., Steen, N., Sharma, A., & Ford, G. (2004). Development and validation of the NEWSQOL, The Newcastle Stroke Specific Quality of Life Scale. *Cerebrovascular Diseases, 17*, 143–152.

Capilouto, G., Wright, H. H., & Wagovich, S. (2006). Reliability of main event measurement in the discourse of individuals with aphasia. *Aphasiology, 20*, 205–216.

Carroll, B. (1998). *Carroll Depression Scales technical manual*. North Tonawanda, NY: Multi-Health Systems.

Code, C., Hemsley, G., & Herrmann, M. (1999). The emotional impact of stroke. *Seminars in Speech and Language, 20*, 19–31.

Cruice, M., Worrall, L., Hickson, L., & Murison, R. (2003). Finding a focus for quality of life with aphasia: Social and emotional health, and psychological well-being. *Aphasiology, 17*, 333–353.

Demers, K. (2004). Try this: Best nursing practices to older adults: Hearing screening (*Dermatology Nursing*, 6 August 2004). Retrieved 13 July 2006 from: http://www.medscape.com

Donovan, N., Rosenbek, J., Ketterson, T., & Velozo, C. (2006). Adding meaning to measurement: Initial Rasch analyses of the ASHA FACS Social Communication Subtest. *Aphasiology, 20*, 362–373.

Doyle, P. (2002). Measuring health outcomes in stroke survivors. *Archives of Physical Medicine and Rehabilitation, 83*, S39–43.

Doyle, P. (2005). Advancing the development and understanding of patient-based outcomes in persons with aphasia. *Perspectives on Neurophysiology and Neurogenic Speech and Language Disorders, ASHA Division 2, 15*(4), 7–9.

Doyle, P., Matthews, C., Mikolic, J., Hula, W., & McNeil, M. (2006). Do measures of language impairment predict patient-reported communication difficulty and distress as measured by the burden of strokescale (BOSS)? *Aphasiology, 20*, 349–361.

Duncan, P., Lai, S., Tyler, D., Perera, S., Reker, D., & Studenski, S. (2002). Evaluation of proxy responses to the Stroke Impact Scale. *Stroke, 33*, 2593–2599.

Duncan, P., Lai, S., Wallace, D., Embretson, S., Johnson, D., & Studenski, S. (1999). Stroke impact scale version 2.0: Evaluation of reliability, validity, and sensitivity to change. *Stroke, 30*, 2131–2140.

Folstein, M. F., Folstein, S., & McHugh, P. (1975). Mini-mental state: A practical method for grading the state of patients for the clinician. *Journal of Psychiatric Research, 12*, 189–198.

Goodglass, H., & Kaplan, E. (1983). *Boston Diagnostic Aphasia Evaluation*. Baltimore, MD: Williams & Wilkins.

Guyatt, G., Feeny, D., & Patrick, D. (1993). Measuring health-related quality of life. *Annals of Internal Medicine, 118*, 622–629.

Hemsley, G., & Code, C. (1996). Interactions between recovery in aphasia, emotional and psychosocial factors in subjects with aphasia, their significant others and speech pathologists. *Disability and Rehabilitation, 18*, 567–584.

Herrmann, M., & Wallesch, C. (1990). Expectations of psychosocial adjustment in aphasia: A MAUT study with the Code-Muller scale of psychosocial adjustment. *Aphasiology, 4*, 527–538.

Hilari, K., Byng, S., Lamping, D., & Smith, S. (2003a). Stroke and Aphasia Quality of Life Scale – 39 (SAQOL-39). Evaluation of acceptability, reliability, and validity. *Stroke, 34*, 1944–1950.

Hilari, K., Wiggins, R., Roy, P., Byng, S., & Smith, S. (2003b). Predictors of health-related quality of life (HRQL) in people with chronic aphasia. *Aphasiology, 17*(4), 365–381.

Holbrook, M., & Skilbeck, C. (1983). An activities index for use with stroke patients. *Age and Ageing, 12*, 166–170.

Hunt, S. M. (1997). The problem of quality of life. *Quality of Life Research, 6*, 205–212.

Kertesz, A. (1982). *Western Aphasia Battery*. New York: Grune & Stratton.

King, R. (1996). Quality of life after stroke. *Stroke, 27*, 1467–1472.

McKevitt, C., Redfern, J., La-Placa, V., & Wolfe, C. (2003). Defining and using quality of life: A survey of health care professionals. *Clinical Rehabilitation, 17*, 865–870.

Müller, D. (1999). Managing psychosocial adjustment to aphasia. *Seminars in Speech and Language, 20*, 85–92.

Naughton, M., & Shumaker, S. (2003). The case for domains of function in quality of life assessment. *Quality of Life Research, 12*, 73–80.

Orely, J., & Kuyken, W. (1994). *Quality of life assessment: International perspectives*. Berlin: Springer-Verlag.

Paul, D., Frattali, C., Holland, A., Thompson, C., Caperton, C., & Slater, S. (2004). *Quality of Communication Life Scale*. Rockville, MD: ASHA.

Raven, J., Court, J., & Raven, J. (1995). *Coloured Progressive Matrices*. Oxford, UK: Oxford Psychological Press.

Ross, K., & Wertz, R. (2002). Relationships between language-based disability and quality of life in chronically aphasic adults. *Aphasiology, 16*, 791–800.

Ross, K., & Wertz, R. (2003). Quality of life with and without aphasia. *Aphasiology, 17*, 355–364.

Sarno, M. (1993). Aphasia rehabilitation: Psychosocial and ethical considerations. *Aphasiology, 7*, 321–334.

Sherbourne, C., & Stewart, A. (1991). The MOS social support survey. *Social Science Medicine, 32*, 705–714.

Smout, S., Koudstaal, P., Ribbers, G., Janssen, W., & Passchier, J. (2001). Struck by stroke: A pilot study exploring quality of life and coping patterns in younger patients and spouses. *International Journal of Rehabilitation Research, 24*, 261–268.

Sneeuw, K., Aaronson, N., DeHaan, R., & Limburg, M. (1997). Assessing quality of life after stroke. *Stroke, 28*, 1541–1549.

Sprangers, M., & Schwartz, C. (1999). Integrating response shift into health-related quality of life research: A theoretical model. *Social Science & Medicine, 48*, 1507–1515.

Toro, C., Altman, L., Raymer, A., Blonder, L., & Rothi, L. (2008). Changes in aphasia discourse after contrasting treatments for anomia. *Aphasiology, 22*, 881–892.

Ubel, P., Loewenstein, G., & Jepson, C. (2002). Whose quality of life? A commentary exploring discrepancies between health state evaluations of patients and the general public. *Quality of Life Research, 12*, 599–607.

Ventry, I., & Weinstein, B. (1983). Identification of elderly people with hearing problems. *ASHA, 25*, 37–42.

Williams, L., Weinberger, M., Harris, L., Clark, D., & Biller, J. (1999). Development of a stroke-specific quality of life scale. *Stroke, 30*, 1362–1369.

Yorkston, K., & Beukelman, D. (1980). An analysis of connected speech samples of aphasic and normal speakers. *Journal of Speech and Hearing Disorders, 45*, 27–36.